Biomedical Research: Costs and Benefits

Biomedical Research: Costs and Benefits

by
Selma J. Mushkin

with the assistance of
J. Steven Landefeld

Ballinger Publishing Company, Cambridge, Massachusetts
A Subsidiary of Harper & Row, Publishers, Inc.

"This Work has been funded at least in part with Federal funds from the Department of Health, Education, and Welfare under contract number N01-OD-5-2121. The contents of this publication do not necessarily reflect the views or policies of the Department of Health, Education, and Welfare."

 This book is printed on recycled paper.

International Standard Book Number: ISBN 0-88410-549-0

Library of Congress Catalog Card Number: 79-19889

Printed in the United States of America

Library of Congress Cataloging in Publication Data

Mushkin, Selma J   1913-
  Biomedical research.

  Includes bibliographies.
  1. Medical research—United States—Cost effectiveness. 2. Diseases—Economic aspects—United States. 3. Mortality—United States. 4. Medical care, Cost of—United States. I. Title.
R854.U5M87   338.4'3   79-19889
ISBN 0-88410-549-0

This volume is dedicated
to
Herbert Ballantyne Woolley
1917-1978

Contents

List of Figures   xiii

List of Tables   xv

Acknowledgments   xxiii

Introduction
Biomedical Research: What Is It Worth?   1

Chapter One
Cost-Benefit Analysis and Biomedical Research   13

Costs of Illness   15
Defining Cost-Benefit Analysis   17
Common Units and Cost-Benefit Analysis   19
Earlier Studies   21
Pharmaceutical Industry: Rates of Return   25
Cost-Benefits in Perspective   26
New Directions   28
References   30

Chapter Two
Biomedical Research Trends   35

The Content of Biomedical Research   35
The Size of Biomedical Research   37

Issues in Biomedical Research Policies   42
Health Research and R&D Policy in General   44
The Basis for Research Outlay Estimates   54
Measuring Research Effort   60
References   76

Chapter Three
Deaths As an Assessment Indicator   79

Trends in Mortality   79
Methodology of Counts of Death   96
A Delphi Exercise for Year 2000   103
Identifying Preventable Causes of Death   110
References   113

Chapter Four
Biomedical Research and Improved Mortality
Rates   117

Earlier Studies and Their Findings   118
Case Studies   124
Developing a Model for Estimation   127
The Estimating Equation   137
Findings   138
References   156

Chapter Five
Biomedical Research and Savings in Cost
of Death   159

Pricing a Human Life   159
Savings in the Cost of Premature Death   167
Asset Value of Lifesaving   180
Contributions of Biomedical Research to Economic Gains   183
References   188

Chapter Six
Biomedical Research Priorities and Mortality   191

Present Targeting of Research Funds   191
Research Missions of the Institutes   193

Limitations of Mortality As an Allocator   195
Classification of Health Research Expenditures,
   by Disease   197
References   204

**Chapter Seven
Sickness As a Criterion of Research Program
Need and Outcome**   205

Sources of Sickness Data   208
Comparisons, by Disease   214
Indicators of Improved Health   215
Determinants of Sickness Levels   221
Trends in Sickness Data   223
The Objective Sickness Rate   228
Conclusion   233
References   235

**Chapter Eight
Biomedical Research and Disability**   239

A Model for Analysis   240
A Model Modified for the Objective Condition   248
Findings on Biomedical Research and the Objective
   Condition   250
Reduction in Objective Sickness Attributed to
   Biomedical Research   251
Work Loss and Biomedical Research   253
Postscript on Earlier Studies   257
Contribution of Biomedical Research   263
References   265

**Chapter Nine
Biomedical Research and the Economic Cost of
Sickness**   267

Estimates of Economic Cost   269
Sickness Cost and Biomedical Research   282
Simulated Cost, by Disease   285
Summary   290
References   291

Chapter Ten
The Cost of Debility   293

Types of Debility   295
Temporary Acute Sickness   295
Physical or Mental Impairment Following a Major
    Illness   302
Static or Stabilized Disability Impairments   305
Impact of Debility on Other Costs of Production   308
Summary of Debility Costs   311
References   313

Chapter Eleven
Trends in Health Expenditures   315

Growth in Health Expenditures   318
Advances in Knowledge and the Expenditure Growth   325
Patterns of Health Care   333
Expenditures, by Disease Category   337
References   342

Chapter Twelve
Health Expenditures and Biomedical Research   345

Residual Factor Analysis   345
Analysis of 1930-75 Changes   346
Biomedical Research and Health Expenditures, 1900-30   353
A Market Model   356
References   362

Chapter Thirteen
Summing Up the Burden of Illness   363

Trends in Burden of Illness   365
Indexes of Burden of Illness   369
Biomedical Advances and Impact on Burden   375
Real Gains from Rising Outlays   376
Indirect Cost Trends and the Challenge to Medicine   377
Burden of Illness on the Economy   379
Cost Estimates Expanded   383
References   394

Chapter Fourteen
Objectives and an Accounting 395

Biomedical Research Objectives 395
The Investment in Biomedical Research 398
Multiple Objectives and Investment in the Health
    Condition 400
Accounting for Industry's Biomedical R&D 402
The Partial Accounting 406
Benefits and Cost of R&D 407
Qualifications 413
An Accounting by Disease 415
Current Year Returns on R&D 419
References 420

Chapter Fifteen
New Directions 421

Gradations of Levels of Health 422
Criteria Used to Judge Measurements of Health
    Status 423
Example of a Desirable Functional Indicator 425
Consumer Preferences 429
Surveys of Preferences 430
Present Market Values as Minimum Willingness
    to Pay 431
Demand-Revealing Processes of Willingness to Pay 435
An Experimental Resource Allocation Guide 438
References 441

Index 445
About the Author 457

List of Figures

2-1	National Biomedical Research by Source of Funds	39
2-2	National Health Research: Expenditures in Current and Constant Dollars, 1967-77	41
2-3	Trends in Numbers of Biomedical PhD's, 1900-76	65
2-4	Trends in Numbers of U.S. Patents Issued for Drugs and Medicine, 1900-76	66
2-5	Trends in Numbers of Patents for Health-related Professional and Scientific Instruments	67
2-6	Trends in Numbers of New Journal Titles Published, 1900-76	68
2-7	Trends in Total Numbers of Biomedical Journals Printed, 1900-76	69
3-1	Trend in Age-adjusted Death Rate per 100,000 Population, 1900-76	81
3-2	Life Expectancy, 1900-76	82
3-3	Age-specific Death Rates, by Age, Selected Years, 1900-75	84
3-4	Percent of All Deaths of Persons Aged 65 to 74 and 75 and Over	87
3-5	Trends in Death Rates Due to Selected Infectious Diseases	88
3-6	Trends in Heart and Cancer Deaths, 1900-76	89
3-7	Percent of All Deaths in the Disease Category of Persons Aged 65 to 74 and 75 and Over	95

3-8	Total Number of Deaths, Selected Years, 1900-2000	98
4-1	Decline in Tuberculosis Death Rate, 1945-75	120
4-2	Death Rates and Sickness Rates from Measles per 100,000 Population	122
4-3	Mortality Rate and Number of Deaths from Congenital Heart Diseases between 1950 and 1970	124
4-4	Effect of Biomedical Research on Age-adjusted Death Rates	147
5-1	Present Discounted Values for Men 30 to 34 Years Old, Selected Years, 1900-2000	168
5-2	Index of Economic Costs per Death, for Ten Causes of Death, 1900 and 1975	175
5-3	Total Economic Cost of Death by Disease Category, Ten Major Causes of Death, 1975 and 2000, at 1975 Earnings Levels, Discounted at 2.5 Percent, in Billions	177
7-1	Changes in Measures of Disability	211
7-2	Impact of Sick Leave Coverage on Frequency of Work Loss by Duration, 1922-1924	225
7-3	Eight Days Sickness, Case Rates per 1,000 Workers	226
7-4	Persons Unable to Work, Institutionalized and Noninstitutionalized, Selected Years, 1900-2000	228
7-5	Institutionalized Population, Selected Years, 1900-2000	229
7-6	Institutionalized Population per 100 Employed Persons, Selected Years, 1957-76	230
9-1	Percentage of Sickness Cost, by Disease and Injury Category	283
11-1	Direct Health Expenditures, 1930-75, and Factors Accounting for the Increase	317
11-2	Direct Costs of Illness as a Percentage of the GNP for Selected Years	322
11-3	Expenditures for Health Care Relative to the Cost of Physicians' Services, 1900-2000	335
11-4	Direct Costs of Health Care, Year 2000	341
13-1	Current Dollar Costs of Illness for Selected Years	367
13-2	Constant 1975 Dollar Costs of Illness for Selected Years	368
13-3	Economic Burden of Illness as a Percent of GNP for Selected Years	380

List of Tables

2-1	National Expenditures for Medical Research, Selected Years, 1940-77	37
2-2	Health Research Expenditures, over Selected Periods	38
2-3	R&D in the Department of Health, Education, and Welfare	40
2-4	Cumulative Health Research Expenditures: Selected Periods	42
2-5	Comparative Indexes of Size of National Health Research Effort	44
2-6	Total Direct Health Expenditures and Health Research Expenditures, Selected Years, 1900-2000	45
2-7	Comparative Ranking of Health Research Projects and Principal Causes of Death and Illness, 1946	49
2-8	Federal Government Support of Research	58
2-9	Selected Indicators of Research in the Biomedical Sciences	70
2-10	Average of Annual Growth Rates of Indicators of Biomedical Research, in Percentages, 1900-75	71
2A-1	Estimated Biomedical Research Expenditures, Fiscal Year 1900-68, Actual Expenditures, 1946-68	72
2A-2	Health Research Expenditures, Fiscal Year 1976-77	76

3-1	Percentage of All Deaths Caused by Selected Infectious and Chronic Diseases, Selected Years, 1900-75	91
3-2	Age-adjusted Death Rates per 100,000 Population, Ten Major Causes of Death, Selected Years, 1900-75	92
3-3	Change in Age-adjusted Death Rates, by Major Cause, Due to Changing Disease Definitions	102
3-4	Year 2000: Number of Deaths by Age, Sex, and Cause	104
3-5	Distribution of Deaths, by Cause, for 1900 and 1975 with the Year 2000 Projections	106
3-6	Estimated Total Years of Life Lost up to Age 75	113
4-1	Estimated Reduction in Deaths in 1970 by Causes of Death Affected by Surgical Advances	123
4-2	Examples of Significant Advances and Technological Developments, 1936-62	127
4-3	Correlation Coefficients for the Data for 1930-75	134
4-4	Correlation Coefficients for the Data for 1900-75	135
4-5	Empirical Results for 1900-75; Elasticity Coefficients Adjusted for First-Order Autocorrelation	139
4-6	Empirical Results for 1930-75 with Various Lags and Alternative Death Rates; Elasticity Coefficients Adjusted for First-Order Autocorrelation	140
4-7	Empirical Results for 1930-75 with Various Distributed Lags; Elasticity Coefficients Adjusted for First-Order Autocorrelation	141
4A-1	Significant Medical Advances and Technological Developments	150
5-1	Present Value of Future Earnings, by Age and Sex, 1975 and 1976	163
5-2	Present Value of Future Earnings, Discounted at 2.5 Percent, by Age and Sex, Selected Years, 1900-2000	164
5-3	Work Experience Rates, by Age and Sex, 1975	166
5-4	Estimated Economic Cost of Premature Death, Selected Years, 1900-2000	169
5-5	Cost of Death, in Millions, by Cause of Death, Selected Years, 1900-75	170

5-6	Estimated Economic Cost per Death, Discounted at 2.5 Percent, by Major Causes of Death, Selected Years, 1900-2000	172
5-7	Index of Economic Costs per Death by Cause of Death, Selected Years, 1900-2000, Base Year 1930	174
5-8	Increases in Life Expectancy Due to the Elimination of Particular Diseases, Gains in Years of Life, and Maximum Economic Benefits of Such Elimination	176
5-9	Gains in Work-Force Years in 1975 Due to Improvements in Mortality Rates between Benchmark Year and 1975	182
5-10	Capital Asset Value of Workers in 1975 Attributable to Improvements in Mortality Rates since 1900 and 1930	183
5A-1	Labor Force Participation Rates, by Age and Sex, Selected Years, 1900-2000	185
5A-2	Mortality Losses: Actual 1975 Losses Compared to Losses Had 1930 or 1900 Mortality Rates Prevailed in 1975	186
6-1	Appropriations, Fiscal Year 1976, and Indicators of the Impact of Diseases for Eight Research Institutes at the National Institutes of Health	194
6-2	Kendall Rank Order Correlations between Alternative Rankings of Institute Interest and 1976 Institute Funding	195
6-3	Percentage Shares of Total Allocations According to Various Indicators and Algorithms	198
6-4	Disease-by-disease Rankings of NIH Extramural Grants and Contracts as Contrasted with Rankings by Deaths, Disability, and Economic Cost	202
7-1	Health Conditions by Degree of Bother for Ten Major Classes of Chronic Illness	207
7-2	Metropolitan Life Insurance Data, 1915-17, on Persons Sick and Unable to Work, Ranked by Frequency of Causes of Illness or Injury	214
7-3	Noneffective Rates on Account of Disease Condition per 1,000 Average Strength of the Army and Navy, Selected Years, 1904-74	216
7-4	Rates per 100,000 Population for Specified Reportable Diseases, 1915-17	217
7-5	Numbers of Persons Unable to Work Due to Sickness, Selected Years, 1900-2000	227

7-6	Males—Bed Disability	234
7-7	Males—Work Loss	234
8-1	Impact of Biomedical Research on Sickness Rates (Plus or Minus), and Factors Influencing Reported Sickness	245
8-2	Regression Findings Applying Navy Data on Sickness Rates as the Dependent Variable, 1926-74	251
8-3	Regression Findings Applying Army Data on Sickness as the Dependent Variable, 1930-40, 1953-73	252
8-4	Regression Findings Applying Army Data on Sickness as the Dependent Variable and a Distributive Lag for the Variable on Biomedical Research	253
8-5	Relative Share of Decrease in Objective Sickness Attributable to Biomedical Research, Medical Care, and Income Changes	254
8-6	Determinants of Changes in Work Loss over Time, by Independent Variables	256
8-7	The Impact of Biomedical Research on Work Loss Due to Sickness, 1957-76	257
8-8	Summary of Disability Literature Surveyed	260
8-9	Shares of the Reduction in Sickness Attributable to Biomedical Research	264
9-1	Costs of Illness and Injury: A Classification	270
9-2	Consumer Expenditures as a Result of Illness	271
9-3	Full-time Earnings for Male Workers, by Age, Selected Years, 1900-2000, in Current Dollars	272
9-4	Numbers of Workers Withdrawn from the Labor Force Due to Illness, Selected Years, 1900-2000	273
9-5	Percentage of Labor Force in Selected Age Groups, Male and Female, 1900-2000	275
9-6	Total Economic Cost of Sickness, Selected Years, 1900-2000	276
9-7	Total Economic Cost of Sickness Per Capita and per Selected Years, 1900-2000	276
9-8	Ratio of Economic Cost of Sickness from Start of Period to End of Period, Selected Years, 1900-2000	278
9-9	Trend in Market Sector Work Loss, 1900-2000, Work-Loss Days per Worker	279

9-10	Estimated Objective Sickness Rates per Worker, 1900-75	280
9-11	Sickness Costs for Major Disease and Injury Categories, Selected Years, 1900-2000, at 1975 Earnings Level	281
9-12	Distribution of Sickness Costs among Disease and Injury Categories, Selected Years, 1900-2000	282
9-13	Estimated Saving in Sickness Cost, over Selected Periods, 1900-75, at Standard Earnings and Labor Market Participation Rates	284
9-14	Ratio of 1975 Simulated Costs of Morbidity to Actual 1975 Costs	286
9-15	Total Sickness Cost Saving, 1930-75, Based on Simulation, by Disease and Injury Categories	290
9-16	Two Estimates of Saving in Sickness Attributable to Biomedical Advances over Designated Periods, in Billions of 1975 Dollars	291
10-1	Number and Percentage Distribution of Incidence of Acute Conditions, by Measures of Impact of Illness, According to Condition Group: United States, July 1974-June 1975	297
10-2	Incidence of Selected Acute Conditions: Per Person and by Number of Years Elapsing between Cases	298
10-3	Alternative Measures of the Incidence of Selected Acute Conditions	300
10-4	Estimated Number of Workers with Temporary Debilitating Effects Following Major Surgery	303
10-5	Static or Stabilized Impairments, Latest Year Circa 1975, of Persons Usually Working	305
10-6	Mean Values of Components of Earnings for "Well" Persons and the Gross and Adjusted Differences between "Well" and "Sick" Persons	307
10-7	Estimated Debility Losses of the Chronically Disabled, 1975	309
10-8	Determinants of Work Injury Rates: Fiscal Years 1961-75	310
10-9	Estimated Accident Costs, in Millions, Attributable to Debility, 1975	312
10-10	Approximate Cost of Debility, by Type of Cost	312
11-1	National Health Expenditures, in Billions, Selected Years, 1900-2000	318

11-2	Use Rates for Selected Health Services by Age and Sex, 1930, 1975	320
11-3	National Health Expenditures Per Capita, Selected Years, 1900-2000	324
11-4	Real Per Capita Health Expenditures, 1975 = 100, by Disease Category, Selected Years, 1900-75	326
11-5	Mean Averages of Treatment Costs, in 1971 Prices	327
11-6	Medical Care for the Most Expensive Cause of Illness, 1930	330
11-7	Percent Allocation of Direct Health Expenditures, by Class of Expenditures, 1900, 1930, 1975	336
11-8	Direct Health Expenditures, in Millions, by Disease Category, 1900, 1930, 1975	338
11-9	Distribution of Direct Health Expenditures, by Disease Category, 1900, 1930, 1975	339
11-10	Per Capita Health Expenditures, by Disease Category, 1900, 1930, 1975	340
12-1	Factors Contributing to the Increase in Health Expenditures, Fiscal Years 1930-75	348
12-2	Regression Results Obtained by Use of Adjusted Health Expenditure Per Capita as the Dependent Variable ($n = 46$)	349
12-3	Factors Contributing to Growth of Total Health Expenditures	350
12-4	Health Expenditures by Disease Category and the Impact of the Residual	352
12-5	Factors Contributing to the Increases in Health Expenditures, 1900-30	354
12-6	Empirical Results for Expenditure Regression, 1930-75	357
12-7	Health Expenditures Regressions: Alternative Measures of Health Care Providers and Health Status	359
12-8	Empirical Results Using Real Per Capita Personal Health Care Expenditures as the Dependent Variable, 1930-75	361
13-1	Percent Distribution of Economic Burden of Illness, by Disease, Selected Years, 1900-75	369
13-2	Percent Distribution of the Cost Burden of Death and Sickness, by Disease, Selected Years, 1900-75	371
13-3	Percent Distribution of Cost of Direct Use of Health Resources	372

13-4   Average Annual Growth Rate in Burden of Illness,
         1900-75   373
13-5   Economic Burden of Illness, in Billions,
         Selected Years, 1900-2000   382
13-6   Economic Burden of Illness as a Percent of
         Adjusted Gross National Product   383
13-7   An Expanded Estimate of the Burden of Illness,
         1975   385
13A-1   Total Economic Burden of Illness, in Millions,
         Fiscal Year 1975   388
13A-2   Total Economic Burden of Illness, in Millions,
         Fiscal Year 1930   390
13A-3   Total Economic Burden of Illness, in Millions,
         1900   392
14-1   Biomedical Research Expenditures, Total in
         Current Dollars and Opportunity Cost, Selected
         Periods, in Billions   399
14-2   Social and Private Rates of Return from
         Investment in Seventeen Innovations   405
14-3   Opportunity Cost of Biomedical Research and
         Some Benefit Offsets   406
14-4   Summary of the Value of Reduction in Illness
         and Premature Death Attributable to Biomedical
         Research, 1900-75 and 1930-75   408
14-5   Benefits from Biomedical Research and Research
         Costs   412
14-6   Total Savings Attributable to Biomedical
         Research, in Billions   416
14-7   Estimated Biomedical Research Outlays, Selected
         Years, 1900-75   417
14-8   Estimated Biomedical Research Outlays as a
         Percent of Total Economic Cost Burden by
         Disease, 1930, 1963, and 1975   418
15-1   Proportion of the Population with a Disease
         of Six Months' Duration, by Functional Status
         Before and After Intervention   427
15-2   Illustrative Premiums by Functional State at
         a 1 per 1,000 Risk Level   433
15-3   Voluntary Agencies' Explicit Participation
         in Priority Setting   440

Acknowledgments

A large debt is owed to the Woodrow Wilson Center for International Scholars for permitting me to write many of the chapters of this volume while a fellow of the Center, 1978-1979. The usefulness of the volume for public discussion should be a token repayment. The basic research on which this volume draws, however, was done over a period of several years by many individual staff members of the Public Services Laboratory (PSL) of Georgetown University and by consultants to PSL. The list of those who participated in the work is lengthy.

The Public Services Laboratory has, from the inception of the study, had the supportive cooperation of the NIH staff involved. The guidance and counsel of Dr. Herbert Woolley, NIH Project Manager for the study, gave invaluable help at every stage of the research—from development of methodology to thoughtful critique of results—up until the time of his death in 1978. Dr. William Copeland, his successor as Project Manager, has been equally helpful in the final months of the project.

In general the research can be thought of in three clusters. The first cluster represents the estimates of cost of illness in 1900, 1930, and 1975 as well as adjustments for greater comparability of the cost of illness estimates for 1963. Selma Mushkin, Aviva Berk, Steve Landefeld, and Lynn Parringer carried out much of this work. It was augmented by the projections to the year 2000 of the cost of disease and illness published by the U.S. Public Health Service in a special supplement of *Public Health Reports*, September-October, 1978.

Of particular interest is the new effort at measurement of the cost of debility and the first cut at estimates of the cost of pain and of the non-health sector costs of illness. Steve Landefeld was largely responsible for the work on debility and assisted Selma Mushkin in the non-health sector cost study. Cynthia Resnick collaborated in the pain cost analysis.

A second cluster represents the research carried out on research and measurements of research activity by Institutes of the National Institute of Health. Dr. Sol Schneyer, Director of the Division of Program Analysis (NIH), Selma Mushkin, and Steve Landefeld of PSL and the members of the Ad Hoc Committee at NIH participated in this work. We are grateful to the many members of this Committee, representing the various institutes at NIH, for their assistance. Dr. Woolley was especially helpful in his guidance of the almost monthly conversations that took place. Debbie Dwork did much of the search of biomedical studies in professional journals for the period 1900-1945 as well as a review of the volume of activity in biomedical research reported by research institutes for that period.

The third cluster represents the analyses carried out on the effect of biomedical research on health expenditures, mortality, and loss of work. This research profited greatly from the studies by Milton Chen, Steve Landefeld, Charles Vehorn, and Douglas Wagner.

Cynthia Resnick carried out much of the estimating work on present value of future earnings and internal rates of return in the study. The accuracy of the hundreds of figures presented is the product of her effort. Mary Susan Vehorn was very helpful in verifying statistical data.

Consultants were used as reviewers throughout the research enterprise. Among these consultants who contributed importantly to the undertaking are Teh-wei Hu, of Pennsylvania State University, Michael Grossman of the National Bureau of Economic Research, Hector Correa of the University of Pittsburg, Ezra Glazer, and Ted Woolsey. As part of a review process the NIH assembled a group of consultants who by their discussions and comments helped classify a number of issues which confronted the research staff. This group included Robert Grose of University of Michigan, Judith Lave of Carnegie-Mellon University, and Odin Anderson of University of Chicago.

Junior staff and students who worked on the research are listed below. I hope that I have not neglected to mention some, a possibility because summer students are included in the enumeration.

Tom Hrdy	Tim Park	Robin Weiss
Ann Jung	Judy Schramm	
David Lintz	Paul Smoke	

No acknowledgment in this research would be complete without referring to the editorial assistance of Esther Gould and Violet Gunther whose professionalism is clearly reflected. Ann Guillot kept the project work on an even keel; no small task when the volume of paper is considered.

Over the years, Public Services Laboratory and its predecessor the State-Local Finance Project of George Washington University have benefited from the extraordinary quality of typing of Alva Wood.

Thanks to all of you for your help.

Selma J. Mushkin

Biomedical Research: What Is It Worth?

As a nation we spend upwards of $5 billion a year from all sources on health research. The National Institutes of Health, the principal research arm of the government, has an annual budget of just over $2 billion. Is the public getting an appropriate return from those expenditures?

OBJECTIVES

Before attempting to answer that broad question, let us consider just what it is that the public seeks from biomedical research. What are the objectives to be achieved? In general, the goal is a healthier, more vigorous, more productive population. Allied with this goal is the pride that Americans have taken historically in achievements, in advancing the levels of scientific knowledge—which might be considered a goal as well. However, the public very likely would consider the former goal to be the primary aim of investments in health research, and that goal might be specified further by the following objectives, which are all closely related.

- Reduction in mortality and morbidity
- Improvement in functional states or in quality of life of those who are hit by disease
- Greater productivity of the work force and economic growth
- Reduction in health hazards
- Greater productivity of the health care system

Returns from health research would include the measured progress made on each of these objectives. However, over the years, priority has been assigned to the reductions achieved in the economic costs of disease and injury, that is, death and disability.

NIH STUDY OF COST COMPARISONS

To determine at least those returns that are associated with priority targets, the National Institutes of Health initiated a study of long-run shifts in the economic cost of disease. Has the economic cost of disease gone down? By how much? Are the declines indicative of the effects of health research on economic cost?

In response to the NIH initiative, we quantified the economic costs of disease, using an orthodox human capital methodology. Values were attached to the lives saved between one period and the next based on potential future earnings. The year 1975 was used as the standard. The same base year was also used in calculating changes in the economic cost of work-time loss due to sickness for those in the work force, those who had to withdraw from the work force, and those in mental and other institutions. The economic cost of disease includes both the indirect costs, or the loss of earnings and work time due to premature death and sickness, and the direct costs, or the nation's resources used in supplying health care to the population.

Summary data on the total economic cost of disease in 1975 show over $323 billion (at 1975 prices). Of special interest is the changing mix of costs. In 1900, about 90 percent of the costs were those of premature death and of output loss due to sickness, and 10 percent, the direct expenditures for hospitals, physicians, drugs, and so forth. By 1975 the indirect costs were about two-thirds of the total and direct costs accounted for the remaining one-third. It is projected that by the year 2000, indirect costs and direct costs will be about equivalent, each amounting to $1 trillion at year 2000 prices.[a]

Do these estimates reflect the gains from research? Not necessarily—there are too many possible patterns of interaction between health care and the progress made toward reducing premature death and sickness to draw conclusions from the direct-indirect cost comparisons over time. In some instances, higher medical care expenditures, such as those for prenatal care, reduce the cost of premature mortality. In other cases, preventive measures like vaccines reduce mortality and lower the costs for medical services. And

[a]These cost estimates and the data and assumptions on which they are based are detailed in *Public Health Reports* 93:5, September-October 1978.

in still others, higher medical care expenditures may have little impact on mortality, as in the treatment of chronic, nonlife-threatening diseases like arthritis.

Underlying the numbers are some real phenomena that point to improvements in mortality and sickness. Death rates have gone down. The reductions in infant and child mortality have been especially dramatic. The relative numbers in the population who are institutionalized or withdrawn from the work force due to illness have also dropped recently. These reductions lend support to the idea that we are better off in terms of health status now than earlier. We are spending much more, but perhaps we are getting more in return.

However, advances in medical sciences are but one of many factors that influence mortality and morbidity. Families now have higher incomes than they did at the turn of the century and in 1930. The average wage was $1.00 to 1.50 a day in 1900. By 1930, it had risen to $5, but by 1975, average daily earnings were ten times as high, or about $50. Family members today also have more education and a far better understanding of health care. Third-party payments have improved access to health services. Physicians are receiving more training. Safety standards in industry have been tightened, producing a lower rate of industrial accidents. All of these factors play a role in improving health.

On the other hand, society has grown far more complex. Stress is characteristic, and new chemical substances, many with unknown toxic qualities, have come into use. Concern about the environment and its role in illness in the population is deepening. A whole host of complex, interrelated (and sometimes offsetting) factors comes together to produce health circumstances.

ACHIEVEMENTS OF BIOMEDICAL RESEARCH

A familiar question arises. Clearly, not all of the gains in mortality can be attributed to scientific advances. But how many can be?

In the past, three different approaches have been used to quantify the role of scientific advances in mortality reduction. The first of these assumes that all mortality gains are attributable to advances in biomedical sciences but modifies this finding by noting the existence of various other factors that bear on these gains. The study of surgical procedures made by the American College of Surgeons and the American Surgical Association is representative of this approach. The second approach essentially seeks to explain mortality rate differences among regions and geographic areas, or across time, using a series of determinants, of which technology is a factor that is represented either as a residual or as a time trend. The studies by Fuchs and by Auster have used this approach. More recently, past trends in yearly death rates for a specific disease have been compared with the timing of the introduction of a specific therapy for the disease. Using this approach, McKeown and McKinlay conclude that biomedical sciences have had little influence on the death rate decline.

The role of biomedical sciences in reducing deaths thus is challenged. The challenge is not restricted to the current period. On the contrary, much of the analysis picks up in the first part of this century, a period of rapidly declining death rates, and challenges the claim that biomedical advances had much to do with the decline.

We have looked carefully at this challenge of the role of biomedical research and concluded that the method being used is essentially deficient. For any cause of death, the presumption made by McKeown and also McKinlay is that only one biomedical advance could have accounted for the decline. Such interpretation of medical advances is wrong. For example, tuberculosis deaths dropped throughout the first years of this century, yet it was not until the early 1950s that a specific therapy became available as a cure. Thus, it is argued, biomedical advance has had little impact.

Improvements in therapies for most infectious diseases were not, as is assumed, single-shot advances. The knowledge gained during the first years of the twentieth century led to incremental changes in medical care methods and public health practices. In the case of tuberculosis, for example, isolation in sanitaria of those with the disease was the chosen method of controlling spread at the start of the century, and this produced results, as did research-based, preventive measures. Measles deaths similarly dropped during that time, but it was not until the 1960s that vaccine became available. It cannot realistically be claimed that biomedical advances are measurable only by the vaccine; many new therapies for measles were used prior to its development.

We have used essentially the second, or determinants approach, to examine the impact of biomedical advances on reductions in death rates and sickness. The model applied is somewhat different from that of others, but it takes account of the mortality impacts of such factors as income, environment, stress, health care, and biomedical sciences. The main difference between earlier studies and the present one is that, for the first time, an effort is made to measure biomedical advances. To do so, we identified intermediate products of research. These include the numbers of PhD's in the biomedical sciences, patents issued for drug inventions, patents issued for surgical instruments and prosthetic appliances, and journals reporting on the biomedical sciences. Our choices of intermediate product were mainly dependent on availability of data for the 75 years from 1900 to 1975.

Analysis of the several determinants of mortality changes, by applying the several intermediate indicators of output in the measurement of biomedical advances, produced the finding that some 20 to 30 percent of the reduction in deaths over the period 1930-75 is accounted for by biomedical advance. For the longer period, 1900-75, we find that the percentages are higher, more nearly 30 to 40 percent.

We have parcelled out the improvements in mortality among the several determinants, with the resulting estimates presented here. These results in turn are based on estimating the elasticity coefficients of the several determinants. The elasticity coefficients essentially measure the rate of change in one factor that is achieved by modification of another. For example, we compute, applying a model of the determinants, that each 1 percent increase in research activity is accompanied by a decline of -0.5 to $-.10$ percent in mortality. This compares favorably with estimates of physical returns to research investment in private industry.

TRIAL AND RETRIAL

A number of different models, not just one, were used in analyzing the relationship of research activity to death rates. Surprisingly, these different models produced fairly consistent findings about the elasticity coefficients and the derived shares of mortality reduction attributable to biomedical research.

Claims for the achievements of biomedical research can easily be exaggerated, and many believe that they have been in the past. But the analysis we carried out, with its finding of 20 to 30 percent of mortality reduction attributable to research, is, if anything, on the low side of the 0 to 100 percent range. Fuchs, who produced a percentage share in analyzing the improvements in infant mortality, estimated technology's share at 40 percent.

Turning to the other priority aim—reductions in morbidity—the task becomes more difficult. It is much harder to determine what share of savings in the economic cost of sickness is due to biomedical research than to estimate the share of savings in premature death. Available statistics on time lost from work do not record improved health over time in the labor force. There has been only a small decline in average work-loss days during the twenty-one-year period of nationally reported data (1957-77). The average for the period 1957-66 was 5.8 work-loss days a year per worker. The average for the years 1967-77 was 5.2. Other data on sickness reflect no positive change over time—reported restricted-activity days have even been on the rise recently. One can hardly show that biomedical advances have reduced the economic costs of illness using only unqualified data, especially if these data show increases, not reductions, in sickness.

SICKNESS RATES: UP OR DOWN?

It is hard to believe that we are sicker now than we were at the turn of the century. Yet comparison of census data for 1890 and 1900 with today's statistics would indicate that we are. The raw, unadjusted statistics are simply misleading. Real indicators of improved health conditions abound. The population is taller today than it used to be and study results suggest that "bigger is better." Young persons mature earlier; improved nutrition and health care have contributed to this gain. Each year, new records of physical and mental performance are achieved.

Study of the statistical data points to the strong influence of socioeconomic circumstances on reported information. Sickness, as reported historically, is highly sensitive to the economic capacity to be sick, to the family's understanding of the meaning of sickness and its sequelae (such as the unattended ear infections that become otitis media), and to knowledge about what medical care can do to provide relief from sickness. Sickness, even as reported by physicians, requires a prior decision by the patient to seek care.

One respondent to a survey noted: "I wouldn't rightly know whether I am sick or not. I can't afford to stop work." Economic circumstances of the family play an important role in determining the sicknesses reported in household surveys. Income supports, such as general income maintenance programs or sickness pay, also make a sizable difference. In one early report of a natural experiment on absences from work, work-loss days per worker rose threefold with introduction of sick leave. And in reviewing early twentieth-century materials, it is plain that there were many, many cases of walking illnesses, illness in which those afflicted went about their daily chores.

The raw data as reported clearly have to be adjusted to separate out objective sickness or pathological conditions from socioeconomic sickness. Such adjustments can be made using data from other sources. Our first adjustment, involving data on work-loss days, corrected the statistics for differences in income and the potential "demand" to stay away from work. The second adjustment applied historical Army and Navy data as an index to record the decline in sickness. Only the Army and Navy data on days sick from disease were used. These data show a drop (on the average) from about twelve days sick from disease only in 1900 to about five by 1950. For the period beyond, the data suggest a further drop of one-third or so in the next twenty years to about three days on the average. Sickness rates thus declined to about one-fourth the 1900 level by 1970.

Sickness data for the armed forces, of course, are not representative of the health condition of the population as a whole. All gains in reduced sickness of the very young are excluded, but the very young are also excluded from the data on the economic cost of work time lost, as are the aged. In addition, relative work-loss days of women are not reflected. The sickness rates in the armed forces for the age groups covered may be expected to be below that in the population generally. Men with chronic illness tend to be excluded from the count by screening prior to admission and by possible subsequent discharge because of disability. Also, reported days sick represent persons who have been screened by physicians on duty, in contrast to the self-reports in civilian health surveys. While the level of sick days in the armed forces may not be representative of the general population, it does seem reasonable to think that the relative movement in sickness rates of civilians and armed forces (for disease only) might be similar. We assumed similarity in movement. We have used both the adjusted, by income, figures for the civilian population and the data for the armed forces to arrive at an estimate of the objective sickness rates.

OBJECTIVE SICKNESS

We estimate that 39 percent of reductions in objective sickness is attributable to advances in biomedical knowledge. The 39 percent share is analogous to the share of gains in mortality of 20 to 30 percent attributable to research for the period 1930-75 and the comparable figure of 30 to 40 percent for 1900-75. It is based on a model similar to that used for mortality, with work-time loss adjusted to an objective rate as the dependent variable, and income, biomedical research, and providers as independent variables.

Biomedical research does not contribute overnight to a reduction in mortality or sickness. It takes time to achieve a change. How long a process may be a matter of judgment, but the question, however, has been researched by Battelle for the National Institutes of Health with the finding of approximately a ten-year average.

LAGS

In developing the estimates shown here, we faced the problem of lags between the biomedical science activity and the achievement of a change in health status. New therapies involve a lengthy process, from generation of an idea to formulation of a process to completion of the necessary trials prior to widespread adoption. We used a ten-year lag between biomedical research activity and changes in mortality or sickness. However, various lags were, in fact, tried out and tested prior to the adoption of the ten-year period.

The point is that it takes time to change the health condition through new research findings. But what is a reasonable achievement if we wait out advances? What is the record of the past on the value of additional biomedical research activity?

FINDINGS ARE FAVORABLE

We have estimated the total value of reduction in sickness and postponement of premature death at $481 billion over the period 1930-75. Of this total, $260 billion is attributed to reduction in sickness and the remaining $221 billion is the savings achieved in the cost of premature death. When we apply the estimates mentioned earlier (shares of savings attributable to biomedical research) to these figures—20 to 30 percent to the $221 billion and 39 percent to the $260 billion—we derive estimates of $145 to $167 billion as the gains from biomedical advances over the period 1930-75.

Similar estimates for the longer period of 1900-75 indicate that the total value of the reduction in sickness and postponement of premature death is between $936 and $1,211 billion. The saving in premature death is about two-thirds of the total, and saving in sickness, about one-third. Furthermore, when we apply the 30 to 40 percent estimates of the share of the value of death reduction attributable to biomedical research over that period (1900-75) and 39 percent for sickness, we derive estimates of $300 to $480 billion as the longer run gains from biomedical advances.

While the shares of reduced mortality and sickness may not seem large, the net benefits from biomedical research turn out to be surprisingly high. This is so because we estimate the value of each premature death averted at $76,000 and the value of a work year when sickness is averted to $12,250, while research and development outlays are small by comparison.

Net benefits, measured as benefits less the opportunity cost of research, are between $115 and $137 billion over the period 1930-75 and from $227 to $402 billion over the period 1900-75. A ratio of benefits to cost of one to one would not be disadvantageous to further investment. In contrast, the benefits of biomedical research for the period 1930-75 are minimally four to six times the opportunity cost of the research and, for the period 1900-75, ten to sixteen times the opportunity cost of the research.

To permit easier comparison with R&D gains in industry and with earlier studies, the internal rate of return for these periods was calculated essentially using two different measures of the year-to-year changes attributable to the gains and costs of biomedical research. The internal rate of return is estimated at 47 percent for the period 1930-75 and within a range of 54 to 62 percent for the period 1900-75.

Public policy on health research and development requires reassessment of decisions recently taken—reassessment that takes note of the favorable returns. The returns have been large by any investment standard: biomedical research has been worth its price. Scientists, dedicated to their scientific work, have little reason to comply, without question, to a buffeting due to budgetary constraints. Putting limitations on scientific pursuits does not accord with the historical findings presented here.

RECENT YEAR RETURNS

It is often objected, with a historical study, that the gains happened long ago. What we really are concerned about here is the current or recent return for research and development.

To achieve at least a partial answer, we looked closely at the recent experience. The opportunity cost of research and development outlays that may have had an impact on mortality and work loss in 1975 was $3.4 billion. The returns on these investments in reduced deaths and sickness, when adjusted to reflect only the shares attributable to biomedical research, amount to $570.4 million. The annual return each year on the investment would be 16.7 percent. This rate is hardly an inconsequential return, or one unfavorable by other investment standards.

SAFETY, EFFICIENCY, AND COST

These estimates of the worth of biomedical research must also be considered within the context of other public policy issues. In recent years, biomedical research has become the focus of major public debate, often confused and misfocused. Research and development activities have come under critical questioning. The controversy has encompassed a range of fairly specific but very different issues, such as how to assure safety in research, how to measure the probabilities of effectiveness of new medical therapies, and how to prevent technology from increasing the cost of health care. The three purposes of safety, effectiveness, and cost control have often been merged as if they were essentially the same thing, with the result that clarity and focus have been lost. The cumulative effect appears to be widespread doubt about the worth of biomedical research given the cost impacts.

Individuals and groups who are concerned primarily with cost have suggested that controls be placed on health-related technology and that cost, efficiency, and safety review processes be instituted on the R&D that produces such technology. Their position that some technology pushes up health care costs is apparently bolstered by the view that biomedical research may be at least potentially unsafe and in any case does not produce efficacious results. Only by separating these questions is it possible to come to grips with the underlying differences in issues and to recognize that control of technology for purposes of cost containment is likely over time to raise costs rather than lower them, to constrain inventiveness in the biomedical sciences, and to prevent second-, third-, and fourth-generation engineering of scientific advances.

The cost of specific diseases over time appears to respond in different ways to new knowledge. For example, infective and parasitic diseases in general have declined in cost with advances in medical knowledge. A scarlet fever case costs less. Measles costs less. Infection, such as erysipelas, costs less, as do the pneumonias and dysentery. Neoplasms and heart diseases have increased in cost.

So much concentration has gone into the public debates on cost-increasing technologies, such as the CAT scanner, that, by and large, cost-reducing technologies have been neglected. Although no detailed study has been made, there is some evidence that such technologies as dental equipment, laboratory testing equipment, blood sampling methods, a number of surgical procedures, and the like have helped to reduce health care costs.

RESEARCH PRODUCT DEFINITION

There is still another level of questioning that has characterized discussions of advances in medicine. For about fifteen years, from mid-1955 to late 1969, death rates in the United States did not change. They remained basically constant despite the rapid rise during this period in medical care costs and the substantial advance in health research outlays. The question was repeatedly asked, "Are we spending more and getting less?" Only recently have the questioners been quieted somewhat by the decline in the death rates for 1975 and 1976.

It would be an exaggeration, however, to view the recent decline in death rates as a major change with large population effects. Perhaps more importantly, a major issue was raised when death rates were stable. A question was asked that still needs an answer: What is the real output of biomedical advances? Almost everyone agrees that there is an output of medical care and biomedical sciences whose evidence is not captured by the death rate and sickness data that are now collected.

Much study is being given to new measurements that more accurately capture the products of a great deal of research and medical care. Indicated, perhaps, is measurement of the capacity of the patient with disease to function at various levels. Such measurements are especially important in understanding the worth of biomedical research today. We have included in this study an effort to operationally define "functional states" for purposes of assessing biomedical advances. Even though such definition is considered a supplementary analysis, it is suggestive of further steps to be taken.

Chapter One

Cost Benefit Analysis and Biomedical Research

What is gained from investments in biomedical research? What is the balance between gains and funds expended?

Who benefits and who pays? Medical advances have created a high technology and raised new and disturbing ethical issues. With health care financed largely by governmental third-party payments or through Blue Cross-Blue Shield or other private insurance carriers, has the technology push created incentives for a large commitment of resources that could be used more effectively elsewhere?

It is against the backdrop of such questions that support for biomedical research must be evaluated. Two considerations today inevitably dominate any discussion of expenditure of public funds. One is the degree of public support for programs to be funded; the other is the public demand for government accountability for expenditures of tax dollars.

Recent public opinion polls indicate public support for medical care despite the general climate of concern about government efficiency. The Harris opinion polls asked the question: What do you consider to be "the two or three biggest problems facing people like yourself which you would like the next president (Congress) to do something about?" Health care was reported as the least of these problems in each of the surveys taken from 1970 to 1976.[1] The public appears to accept current practices in health care. Indeed, the results of two national telephone surveys by the National Opinion Research Center, in 1975 and in 1977, suggest that the public not only accepts current practices but is also willing to pay more for health care through the tax system.[2]

The public consensus that the health care system is working well is based on the statistical profile of reduced deaths. According to the traditional measures of mortality, medical advance has been constant—in some disease areas, such as the infective and parasitic diseases, spectacular. Biomedical research has contributed to this advance. It accounts for 20 to 30 percent of the decline in death rates over the last forty-five years and minimally $145 billion in lives saved.

But the gains from biomedical research today can no longer be reflected in a count of lives saved. Measures must be developed to assess the value of research to the quality of life. A meaningful interpretation of the benefits of technology and the expenditure of funds in the pursuit of technological advances requires some standard measure of health status, of functionality in situations of daily living.

While the American people believe in the efficacy of the medical care system and support biomedical research as the "genie in the bottle" to produce the miracle cures of the future, there is nevertheless skepticism as to the prudent use of federal funds for relevant research. Dr. Herbert B. Woolley noted that "public questioning of the value of continuing to fund biomedical research is not anti-intellectualism, but part of a national anxiety to commit public resources toward immediate social ends rather than long-term investment in acquiring useful information."[3]

The health care system, however, is not an isolated set of policies. The public is demanding an accounting for the tax dollars spent on all government programs. Therefore, program analysis and evaluation are being applied toward answering this demand. And, as one consequence, cost-benefit analyses are being applied more and more frequently to biomedical research as well as to all components of health care. Pressure is on government officials to assemble information about the value of programs and to account for the use of tax resources. Accountings will be made to determine, for example, whether a defined health research program will reduce economic costs and improve health care. Are the gains from this type of program greater than those from optional uses of the fiscal and real resources of staff and materials? Such questions give a sense of urgency to cost-benefit analysis.

In this context, the economic costs of illness (or social burdens of disease) are advanced as a basis for measurement. Increasingly, attention is being given to the quantification of costs as a yardstick for determining priorities. From 1975 to 1977, several institutes of the National Institutes of Health financed studies of the costs of diseases, among them studies of stroke, cranial neoplasms, multiple sclerosis, spinal brain injuries, cancer, and infectious diseases.

Legislation was introduced in the Ninety-third Congress by Tim Lee Carter of Kentucky, requiring the secretary of Health, Education, and Welfare to request appropriations for health programs giving priorities to diseases that have the highest mortality rate, the highest morbidity rate, the greatest adverse effect on the health of individuals in the United States, and, "because of lost wages, productivity, and cost of medical care . . . the most significant impact on the economy."[4] In addition, a committee, chaired by Dorothy Rice, director of the National Center for Health Statistics, has been established to develop uniform guidelines for cost-benefit measurement. The term "costs of diseases" is defined as the direct and indirect costs of diseases, including the costs of preventive measures, diagnoses, treatment, cure, and convalescence, as well as costs reasonably attributable to the pain and suffering, loss of income, and reduction in future earnings resulting from such diseases.[5]

More recently, the secretary of Health, Education, and Welfare has set in motion a process for defining health research principles, aiming toward a multiyear research strategy. Social cost or utility clearly is a major factor being considered in defining the strategy for research.[6]

COSTS OF ILLNESS

Cost-benefit analysis is essentially a substitute for the informational functions of the marketplace. When consumers buy goods in the market they are signalling approval of the production. If the public wants more of these goods, then prices are bid up, making it profitable to increase production. The market thus becomes the allocator of goods and production resources. Lack of a market to determine the efficient allocation of resources to biomedical research necessitates substitute methods of measuring losses and gains. In lieu of *market decision*, there is administrative decision: the administrative decision at present relies on a type of institutional arithmetic that can relate costs to the gains received as a consequence of the costs incurred. In support of such institutional arithmetic, analytical processes encourage identification of the savings in the costs of death, disabilities, and debilities that can be achieved by biomedical research.

Consensus is widespread on the need for (*a*) governmental support of biomedical research because the benefits are indivisible, and (*b*) a federal, rather than state or local, role in carrying out such research in view of spatial externalities. The federal role in biomedical research is not at issue—the U.S. government today finances almost 75 percent of all biomedical research,[7] and it has established linkages with the sector of the academic community that has a major responsibility for the conduct of biomedical research. At issue, however, is allocation. Allocation problems arise at three levels:

- The share of total economic and health resources to go to biomedical research
- The share of the biomedical research funding to be distributed among diseases and institutes
- The share of an institute's funding to go to specific projects

In previous assessments of the overall share of economic resources for biomedical research, various indexes of biomedical research funding, such as the percentage of the gross national product to be used for biomedical research or the percentage of medical care outlays for that purpose, have been applied.[8-10] Such indexes have sometimes been criticized as crude and inadequate. However, no "natural" standard or yardstick exists for determining the right amount for biomedical research and for making other allocation decisions. An optimum allocation of resources depends upon the willingness of taxpayers to devote their funds to research rather than to other health care or nonhealth services. Public opinion polls on relative willingness to spend for biomedical research are one way to determine whether the present allocation is enough, insufficient, or too much. But even these polls are inadequate, because the willingness to finance biomedical research is not tied to actual consumer budgets. Hypothetical statements on choice fall short of an operational guide that looks to multiple individual decisions or family decisions.

The indexes in use have been specifically criticized for inadequately answering such basic questions as:

- What should be supported?
- How intensively?
- Under whose guidance?
- With what mix of research from the several health disciplines?
- With what effect on early deaths, disabilities, debilities, pain, and suffering?
- With what impact on medical care facilities and cost to the taxpayer and to society?

Few persons contest that research is risky and that demonstrated results cannot be claimed in advance. Nor do they dispute that research is a cumulative process through which bits of knowledge are built one upon another, and that important medical findings are sometimes quite accidental. Among other factors, these three characteristics—cumulative findings, uncertain results, and accidental breakthrough—make any political arithmetic imperfect and incomplete.

The allocation methods used for diseases and institutes have been recently criticized. However, formula provisions in the congressional bill mentioned earlier call for such allocations. Therefore, as discussed extensively in Chapter 6, various trials have been made of alternative allocation methods in which indexes of morbidity and mortality were applied to the diseases of special concern to individual institutes.

The allocation of funds to projects within institutes has been assigned to the peer group review processes. Peer group review, more than any other allocation method, has been the subject of numerous investigations and evaluations.[11,12] The most recent study of peer group review was that of the President's Biomedical Research Panel[8]. The panel reviewed peer group processes, identified their shortcomings, and concluded that the processes, although subject to some abuses, were superior to other methods.

Cost-benefit analysis is advanced as a guide to allocation at each of three levels:

- As a process to determine the relative efficiency of using resources for biomedical research and other areas
- As a way to define relative cost of specific diseases (or the potential benefits from new preventive measures and cures) as a standard for allocation of appropriations among institutes
- As a criterion for decisionmaking among research projects by requiring cost-impact analyses of potential new therapies and diagnostic aids.

DEFINING COST-BENEFIT ANALYSIS

Although cost-benefit analysis is becoming an increasingly popular term, its meaning is variously interpreted, partly because of lack of consensus on the scope of analysis and the individual items to be included. Generally, cost-benefit analysis connotes a procedure for assessing the costs and benefits of alternative programs. Cost-benefit is largely conceived as a policy tool for obtaining more information on which to base decisions about the use of the economy's resources;

the objective is the most efficient allocation of funds in terms of resource input and benefits accrued.

Costs, as defined, are "opportunity costs," that is, the opportunities that are forgone to produce some alternative service or good. An analogy is often made to the slicing of a pie: consumption of a slice leaves that much less for other uses. The intent is to emphasize that the economy typically is characterized by scarcity of resources relative to unlimited human wants. Whatever bit of resources is devoted to a given range of policies becomes unavailable to meet some other pressing social need. In reality, the size of the pie changes from time to time as the economy grows, and health programs can contribute to that growth.

Cost-benefit views the costs of a program, for example, one in biomedical research, as the total resources of people, facilities, and equipment devoted to the program. Benefits can be measured in a variety of ways. The traditional method seeks to quantify the savings gained in terms of (a) direct cost of services saved, such as savings in medical therapy and hospitalization, and (b) the indirect costs to society saved as a consequence of reduced disabilities and fewer deaths. Indirect benefits, in this context, include gains in the output of workers who, in the absence of a health program, would not be able to work at all, and higher output from those who continue to work but whose performance is no longer impaired by illness.

Measurement of the cost of illness and, by assumption, the potential magnitude of the gains from prevention and cure has become almost routine. Rice and Cooper have contributed importantly to measurement of the aggregate economic costs of illness for 1963 and 1972.[13,14] The National Institute of Mental Health has estimated costs of mental illness several times; the most recent estimate was $36.8 billion for 1974.[15] Presumably, if mental illness were wiped out, $36.8 billion would be the value of the gain or benefits. In this study, we made similar estimates of the economic costs of illness, both direct and indirect, for the years 1900, 1930, 1975, and 2000.[16-19]

Earnings losses are often computed to take account of the continuing impact of a health measure by discounting the flow of benefits represented by future years' earnings. Discounting is based on the fact that a dollar is worth more today than it will be in the future, even when prices remain constant. It permits the conversion of future costs to present values. Because economists differ as to the amount of the discount rate, alternative rates are frequently used.

Cost-benefit comparisons are made in terms of various ratios or net-gain figures. Among the types of comparisons quantified are:

(*a*) the present value of net benefits (which equals the present value of benefits minus the present value of continuing costs); (*b*) the internal rate of returns on costs; and (*c*) benefit-cost ratios. The rate of return in (*b*) refers simply to the calculation of the amount of compound interest that would be required to raise the cost to the value of the expected future benefits. Three decision rules are often advanced in application of the values computed, namely:

- Choose programs with the highest values of net benefits
- Choose programs with the highest rate of return
- Choose programs with the highest benefit-cost ratios above one

COMMON UNITS AND COST-BENEFIT ANALYSIS

Differences of opinion about the usefulness of benefit evaluations in monetary terms pose a technical problem. Unless there is a common unit, it is not possible to compare programs. For example, we have only a monetary way to judge the relative worth or priority to be given to a biomedical research program or an immunization program for children. Yet the process of pricing the values generated by many social programs is difficult and potentially misleading. For example, valuation by existing methodology tends to weight some lives more than others, and yet the assumptions on which these relative weights are based are not fully disclosed. The monetary values calculated are not clear to officials who have an implicit set of values about, for example, children and the aged. The Alaskan Native Federation's use of the term "special people" for children and the aged illustrates the widespread existence of implicit values at variance with the basic assumptions of standard cost-benefit methodology.[20]

Moreover, not all gains can be converted to monetary values. What is the price of family stress that originates in the affliction of a parent with cancer?[21] What is the price of the pain of a child stricken with multiple sclerosis or the suffering of the parent?

Difficulties such as these suggest that costs should be related to measures of effectiveness, not just to estimates of benefits stated in monetary terms. Most people do not distinguish between cost-benefit and cost-effectiveness analyses; however, these approaches are quite different in the way program outcomes are compared. Some economists formulate the differences between cost-benefit and cost-effectiveness analysis in these terms: cost-effectiveness analysis is applied when the price of the service is known but benefits are difficult to assess in monetary terms. Thus, the question addressed by cost-effectiveness analysis is: What is the relative effectiveness of one course of action versus another in achieving a specific program result for the same cost? Some analysts use the term when making effectiveness comparisons among activities and programs that do not entail the same cost. Cost becomes one variable to be measured along with the different measures of program effectiveness. This latter process does not lend itself to a choice among comparables; rather, it leaves the process of weighting the various variables to the officials who have to make choices among programs.

There is not full agreement about the range of program objectives in biomedical research and, accordingly, about the yardsticks or units of effectiveness that might be universally applicable. An analysis of social returns, however, requires quantification that applies criteria indicating the extent of achievement of objectives. Standards for measurement, or criteria, are important to the process of comparing. It is customary to look to one or more standards so that a particular course of action and its relative effectiveness and costs can be compared to others. For educational activities, usually batteries of achievement test scores are applied; for criminal rehabilitation, recidivism rates and employment rates frequently are the basis of comparison. In the health field standard measures have been used for decades—death rates, life expectancy, infant mortality, and restricted activity days. But, as we discuss later, there is disagreement on acceptable standards of measurement, and it is important to question the usefulness of traditional measures. Without common yardsticks, however, it is difficult to find common dimensions across health programs and modalities. Differences among patients reinforce the barriers to achieving such commonality. The kind of pathological condition or illness being treated, the process of the treatment, and the patient's characteristics are factors that clearly affect program results when biomedical advances are converted to therapies. The lack of standardized symptomatology and the variation in specific modalities for treatment contribute to the lack of comparability both in cost assessment and in benefit or effectiveness assessment.

Effectiveness criteria are applied because the monetary values of the benefits of health care are difficult to calculate, or because they fail to disclose important policy variables. Dollar counts, nevertheless, remain important to policy officials for keeping score across programs and for defining possible consequences of reshaping priorities. Despite the progress made toward effectiveness assessments, judgments about outcomes are still being made in monetary terms. If a policy official wants to judge a program's value in relation to its costs, clearly the simplest method is to use a common unit of value. This is the strength of benefit valuation.

EARLIER STUDIES

A number of cost-benefit studies were carried out, some almost two decades ago, on returns to biomedical research and advances in therapy for particular diseases. Notable among these studies is the research of Weisbrod,[22] Fein,[23] Mushkin,[24] Laitin,[25] and Klarman.[26] Each of these researchers applied a human capital valuation in measuring the economic impact of disease. Weisbrod's study illustrates measurement of the internal rate of return. Klarman's study is an example of assessment of the cost of a disease and the ratio of benefits to cost. Application of their methodology to policy options generally took place almost a decade after the initial exploratory work was done.

We will examine briefly the methodology used in the earlier cost-benefit studies. In the internal rate of return study on poliomyelitis vaccine research, Weisbrod estimated benefits as (1) the gain in market value of production attributable to the reduction in mortality and morbidity caused by the disease, and (2) the opportunity cost of resources devoted to treatment and rehabilitation of its victims. The number of cases prevented was calculated as the difference between the number of cases that occurred when there was no vaccination program and the number of cases that occurred after the program was implemented. Benefits were represented by additional earnings minus consumption. Vaccination costs, as the costs required to implement the new technology, were netted out of gross benefits. In concept, the value of reduction in pain and suffering would be counted. However, Weisbrod indicated that in practice the basis for such measurement is hard to come by. The calculation of internal rates of return to research on the development of the poliomyelitis vaccine equates the stream of research costs with the stream of net benefits.

Weisbrod calculated internal rates of return for three different examples. In the first example, savings per case of poliomyelitis were assumed to be constant over time. In the second and third examples, the savings per case were assumed to be growing as a result of a productivity/earnings growth rate of 3 percent per year. For the years after 1957, the assumption of zero cases of the disease was considered to hold if all persons under age fifty were inoculated in 1957 and if, alternatively, either all (third example) or none (second example) of the infants born after 1957 would have to be inoculated in order to sustain complete control of the disease. For each of the three examples, Weisbrod used two assumptions concerning the ratio of actual to reported research costs. The first involved a ratio of one, and the second used a ratio of five under the assumption that research costs are understated. Weisbrod calculated rates of return by using the two assumptions for two time horizons, 1930-80 and 1930-2200. Generally, the estimated internal rates of return as computed range from about 4 to 12 percent, with 11 to 12 percent as the best estimate.

Klarman's paper on syphilis control [26] is an example of a study in which cost of disease averted is essentially the measure of benefits. Using syphilis as an example of calculating the potential gains to treatment of a disease, Klarman pointed out many of the practical and conceptual issues. Savings due to the elimination of direct expenditures and the indirect costs of mortality and morbidity comprise total economic costs or benefits from disease averted. The benefits of eliminating cost of pain and suffering were not included because of difficulties in measurement; however, Klarman addressed these benefits in his analysis of the costs of cardiovascular illness.[27]

Direct costs represented by expenditures for health care may be difficult to compute, owing to lack of data and the complications from multiple diseases. The determination of indirect costs or output loss is even more complex because of issues such as taxes and transfer payments, calculation of relevant earnings, and assumptions regarding the unemployment rate. Klarman considers mean earnings per worker as an optimal measure of output per worker, but agrees that median earnings suffice because of other compensating unmeasurables. In contrast to Weisbrod, Klarman argues that consumption per worker should not be subtracted from earnings. Housewives' time is valued by Klarman, according to Weisbrod's method, at the replacement value; for example, the value of domestic help and a full employment economy is also assumed. Klarman also recommends that taxes and transfers be ignored because they do not use real resources and that the stream of both costs and benefits should be discounted. Ideally, Klarman proposes, several discount rates should be used to give a range of relevant results depending upon assumption as to the rate of discount. Discounting is of particular relevance in the case of syphilis because of the long period of latency between the early stage of infection and, in the extreme, the late form—tabes dorsalis.

In Klarman's "Socioeconomic Impact of Heart Disease," the theoretical concepts applied to heart disease are similar to those applied to syphilis.[27] He discusses several new concepts, such as the reciprocal relationship of disease and economic status and how diseases affect the organization of medical practices.

Our study is modeled largely on the earlier work by Rice and her colleagues. In her 1963 report, "Estimating the Cost of Illness," Rice presents detailed tables of direct and indirect costs due to illness, disability, and death applying a human capital model.[13] Direct costs are broken down by type of medical services used. Indirect costs—costs of premature death and disability—are broken down by diagnosis, age, sex, and labor force participation rate. In costing morbidity, costs for institutionalized and noninstitutionalized populations are shown. Many of the discretionary choices on calculation were decided as Klarman had suggested; that is, mean instead of median earnings, assumption of a full employment economy, and use of more than one discount rate. Housewives' time was valued at average earnings of a domestic worker in 1963 and in terms of market prices of services rendered in 1972.[14] Essentially, the basic assumption is that the costs of disease would be saved if effective health programs were adopted. Findings are in terms of economic cost—$58 billion in 1963, for example—rather than a net figure such as benefits minus cost.

With the application of policy analysis tools in government, more particularly in the Department of Health, Education, and Welfare, costs and benefits came to be equated and in the specific terms of a set of defined programs. Gorham,[28] Grosse,[29] and Rivlin[30] contributed to this work. Cost-benefit analyses were made of a range of specific diseases. Programs were assessed by estimating the lives that could be saved and the disabilities that could be prevented as a result of additional expenditures and the ratio of benefits to costs. Such program assessments included those on the use of seat belts to avoid motor vehicle accidents; screening for tuberculosis, syphilis, certain cancers, and heart diseases; family planning; and maternal and infant care. Separate studies were made of a number of diseases. For example, analyses were made of alternative kidney disease programs, ranging from preventive screening programs to transplantation programs. Benefit-cost ratios for a screening program for children, for instance, were found to range from almost 15 to 1 to 39 to 1; benefit-cost ratios for screening adults for nephrogenic streptococci ranged from 47 to 1 to 130 to 1.[31]

The federal immunization program against measles was the subject of a 1969 analysis that simulated the number of cases of measles that would have occurred from 1963 to 1968 if the new measles vaccine had not been used.[32] Calculations were made of school days lost and work days lost due to measles; morbidity and mortality were valued based on earnings. The total cost of immunization was estimated at $108 million and the total cost of measles or the benefit from reduction in the incidence of measles at $531 million, leaving a net economic benefit of $423 million.

Studies have taken on even more specificity since the late 1960s and early 1970s, and far greater sophistication of methodology is indicated.[33-35] Albritton's study, for example, estimates the effects of the federal decision to initiate a measles eradication project as part of community health services.[36]

Albritton uses two regressions. The first estimates the change in reported measles incidence as a result of the 1966 eradication program, and the second estimates the change in disease incidence as a result of the new measles vaccine and the federally sponsored measles eradication effort. The results of the second regression are used to separate the impact of the federal intervention from the impact of other efforts aimed at eradicating measles in the period immediately following the development of the vaccine. Albritton uses this second regression to avoid an upward bias in the estimates of the impact of the federal program. The results of the regression represent estimates of the number of reported cases averted because of the federal program. Application of cost-benefit analysis is based on the regression results by use of various inflation-adjusted cost estimates formulated by Axnick and associates in a study they did for the Center for Disease Control.[32] Albritton estimates that medical and other cost savings from federally sponsored programs were more than $1 billion during the eight years from 1966 to 1974. He estimates direct economic benefits in productivity and medical care resources saved to be approximately $10.34 per $1.00 of actual program costs.

In a number of the more recent studies the researchers applied measures of effectiveness rather than benefits in dollar terms in the analysis. Zeckhauser and Shepard apply a utility function in which the unit of output is quality-adjusted life years.[37] They give an example in which a person has the choice between living the rest of his life with a specific impairment or having an operation. The operation has a probability X of restoring full function and a probability of $1-X$ of being immediately fatal. The basic problem here is: What value of X would influence the patient's decision to have or not to have the operation?

The researchers use quality-adjusted life-year value as an expected value weighted to reflect the probabilities that the respective outcomes are achieved. They urge policy officials to choose among alternative health-promoting policies in terms of individual quality of adjusted life streams.

Mushkin and Freidin, in a study of lead poisoning, used as criteria of effectiveness the number of mentally retarded averted and the number and proportion of children with an excess burden of body lead as measured by blood tests.[38] Chen and Bush, in their study of PKU, used adjusted life years and a scale of functional states.[39]

In a 1977 report, "Cost-Benefit Analysis of Treatment and Prevention of Myocardial Infarction Programs," Cretin sets out a procedure for heightening comparability across different interventions.[40] Previously, some measures of success were in terms of incidence and some were in mortality; the common denominator chosen by Cretin is total years of life added by the program. Costs include direct program expenditures and the more indirect costs, such as a cholesterol-lowering diet. Cretin considers various discount rates, comparability of populations, recurrence rates, and prevention versus intervention.

PHARMACEUTICAL INDUSTRY: RATES OF RETURN

Studies of rates of return that seek to describe the profitability of research and development to the drug industry comprise a large and growing body of literature.[41-46] In one study, by Schwartzman,[44] the pre-tax return for 1960 was estimated at 22.6 percent. The income on which rates of return are computed is adjusted for production cost of the newly developed drugs (including the costs of financing, plant, and equipment) and provision of working capital. Expenditures or investments in research and development are counted as a stream of discounted expenditures for each of the years of development. These expenditures are offset by the stream of discount income earned from these expenditures. In calculating returns Schwartzman essentially computed an internal rate that equates investment and returns so that the sum is equal to zero. Baily calculated rates of return for six large firms and found average pre-tax private rates of return to drug research in the period 1954-61 to be 25 to 30 percent.[45]

Industry's private returns are supplemented by social returns. Analysis suggests that because of imperfections in the invention market, industry cannot fully capture or retain all the benefits generated by its research contribution. There is, for one thing, a strong asymmetry between the original invention and subsequent invention. Once the knowledge has been gained that something can be done, it is relatively easy for others to develop alternatives, and the originating firms cannot capture all the gains. Lags and frictions in the process of transmission help assure that the firm that has done the research and development can appropriate some of the benefits. Social rates of return on private research and development investments have been calculated to be twice as large as private rates of return—more than 50 percent for industry as a whole and an even higher rate for the chemical industries.

COST-BENEFITS IN PERSPECTIVE

A pattern of cost-benefit analysis emerges from the studies discussed above. Although the conceptual framework of analysis has been extended and elaborated and new efforts have been made to identify a fuller range of benefits, these recent analyses underscore the conceptual limitations of assuming that the total costs of eradicating a disease could be wiped out with appropriate preventive or curative actions. This assumption, often made in the past, equated benefits with total costs, which is not always the case. For example, although the incidence of syphilis has been greatly reduced, costs are still being incurred. In the context of mental health programs Conley stated: "The only purpose for which estimates of the cost of mental illness can be used is to describe the size and the dimensions of the problem—i.e., what type of costs are incurred, who bears the burden, and what is being done about it—and so to stress the seriousness of the problem and the importance of seeking new methods of treatment."[47] In other words, neither the cost to society of illness nor the cost of providing care can be converted directly into a meaningful guide for program decision without much qualification.

Human Capital Methods

Even the conceptual framework for the calculation of costs has come under attack. As calculated, the cost of illness to society does not represent the burdens as perceived by the ill and their families, or the amount that they would willingly pay to avoid those burdens. Mishan[48] and Schelling[49] identified three levels of benefits as perceived by the individual: (a) benefits of a reduced risk of protracted illness to the individual; (b) benefits of the reduced risk of illness to family or friends; and (c) financial gains to the individual from the reduced risk of illness to society as a whole. Dorfman[50] additionally questions the traditional concepts of cost-benefit analysis, and Acton[51] quantifies alternative concepts.

During the mid-1950s, the application of investment concepts of health program costs caused much concern.[52] Valuation of human life in crass dollar terms raised basic ethical questions. But political pressures for accountability dissipated much of this opposition; cost computations became more frequent, and the relation of those cost calculations to cost-benefit analysis was clarified.

The calculation method for human capital considers, as indicated earlier, the cost for society as a whole. Among the critical weaknesses of the traditional human capital approach is the relative understatement of the value of the old, the young, women, and persons in minority groups. The understatement results from the several components of the human capital measurement. Value is determined by possible participation in the work force. Those who have retired and will no longer earn are thus assigned no value by this type of capital accounting. Similarly, women who are housewives do not participate in the work force as defined. In recognition of this problem of assigning "no value" to housewives' activities, a somewhat arbitrary decision has been made to assess the value of housewife services. A number of methods have been used, ranging from the one-half male earnings method[53] to valuation based on the opportunity costs in the occupation appropriate to housewives according to their age and education and in line with current market conditions. More frequently, housewives are assigned a value based on wages of domestics or alternatively the market value of the services (for example, cooking, cleaning, and child care) weighted to reflect the relative hours spent doing each task.[14] For women and minority group workers, it is not attachment to the work force that creates a low human capital but rather the relative level of earnings. Those who have low earnings are assigned a low value. The value question is exacerbated in the case of children and youth by the discounting of future earnings.

As indicated earlier, the appropriate rate of discount is undecided. Some economists urge the rate at which commercial capital is borrowed, others urge use of a pure time preference rate. The choice of discount rate is not inconsequential. On the contrary, the discount rate has appreciable effect on the computed values: the higher the rate, the lower the values assigned to earnings postponed for a period of time. Therefore, when relatively high rates are applied, the value of those not already in the labor force—children and youth—drops sharply. Yet, our society places high values on children and young persons.

Complicating the estimation of the cost of lost time are other technical questions concerning human capital computation, including (a) trends in work-force participation rates at different ages and for men and women; (b) the productivity growth outlook; and (c) earnings patterns over a working lifetime.[19]

Attempts to Improve Human Capital Methods

Alternative approaches have been proposed to correct the deficiencies in human investment accounting. One approach quantifies components of the cost of illness that are not now counted. Major expenditures of families and individual patients, for example, take the form of extra household expenses in the care of the sick and extra transportation costs. Governments finance ramps for the handicapped and special educational services for blind and for homebound children. Industry is called upon to take preventive measures against occupational injury and disease. There are still other costs that are not traditionally counted, such as the cost of debility resulting from a worker who is ill but reports to work and the cost of pain and disfigurement. Social costs of illness have been identified that importantly affect family life and children; they include costs originating in family stress, tension, and disruption, loss of sexual vitality, and the like.

Other approaches seek to measure the public's willingness to pay for improved health care by applying market or nonintrusive indicators of willingness. For example, the public in its collective role has decided at large cost on a public program for kidney dialysis for patients with end-stage kidney failure. Governments, by their actions, have determined that a sizable share of all medical resources shall be devoted to the care of the aged.

Market measures of risk aversion are provided that improve the values applied for wage loss due to sickness. The extra wages workers demand for taking on hazardous occupations become the basis for the count. It is possible to identify occupations with higher than average risk by workers' age, sex, education, and social background and to compare their earnings to those of workers in lower risk occupations as an approximate measure of how workers view their risks.[54]

Willingness to pay for health policies that reduce environmental risk has been measured by differences in land prices as surrogates. These differences in prices are suggestive of differences in the value attached by consumers to varying environmental conditions and have been used in this way. A sizable body of literature is concerned with the conditions that must be met before land prices can be used for this purpose.[55]

NEW DIRECTIONS

Analysis is currently, at best, in a rudimentary stage. The major contribution thus far has been the identification of some important questions that require additional probing, questions especially about health program outputs. In the process of analysis, the need for far greater clarity comes to be better understood. What, for example, is a treatment modality intended to achieve? What is a particular preventive method designed to yield? The need for specification has become clearer and has encouraged the use of certain criteria for program effectiveness, for example, reduced hospitalization. When we look to calculations of benefit, the focus is still on aggregates rather than on specific program analysis, even though more detail has been added within those aggregates.

The broad concepts of reduced deaths and work-loss days applied in analyses of health programs have proved deficient because these variables are too gross to reflect the way people value improved health and less disability even if they cannot return to work. Research, accordingly, is being directed on functional states as a means to improve the criteria for evaluation of particular physical health programs.

Wylie and White developed the "Maryland Disability Index" for measuring the effectiveness of rehabilitation services.[56] The disability scores correspond to the usual clinical judgment on the patient's condition. Katz and associates used an "Index of Independence in Activities of Daily Living" for measuring functional status of the elderly and chronically ill.[57] Karnofsky and Burchenal proposed a comprehensive set of disability levels to which they assign arbitrary intervals from 0 to 100 for use in assessing cancer chemotherapy.[58] More recently, Williamson devised an effectiveness measure called "Preventive Impairment Unit Decades" (PIUD) that expresses the extent to which an untreated patient's impairment might be prevented by a specified course of activities.[59] Torrance and associates developed a utility measure based on the von-Neumann-Morgenstern standard gamble using a time-equivalence technique.[60] Bush and co-workers formulated measures of functional-years (well years), or value-adjusted life expectancy.[61,62] The measure is derived by weighting functional level expectancies to yield a scalar value. Similarly, Zeckhauser and Shepard adopted the concept of quality-adjusted life years as an evaluative criterion.[37]

The assessment of programs requires agreement on intended outcomes and measures of progress. However, if analysis is to be used as a way to understand the effect of alternative resource allocations, more is required than forging agreement on desired outcomes and measures of such outcomes. Knowledge of which activities are encompassed within a defined research program or a defined treatment modality is crucial. If a good outcome is achieved, assessment should include a sufficient understanding of how that result was achieved, including the combination of factors that made for success.

In summary, the absence of a market and a price system consistent among health programs, which would enable us to select among health priorities, points to substitute (that is, nonmarket) methods for determining relative costs and gains. Substitute methods include (a) analysis of the relative costs of each program and the relative effectiveness of program alternatives, and (b) analysis of cost-benefit alternatives in resource allocation. In place of market decisions, administrative decisions rely on a type of political arithmetic. No ideal alternative is evident at present. However, cost-benefit analysis and cost-effectiveness for public decisionmaking are moving in the direction of developing and pursuing a range of approaches that can relate the costs of a health program to the gains received as a consequence of the costs incurred. Encouraging indications in the research methodology of cost-benefit are providing data to be applied to the health field.

As a formal and systematic approach to be used in a wide variety of situations, the traditional cost-benefit analysis falls short of providing the information required for decisionmaking. What appears to be indicated now is a greater analytical effort, more experimentation with diverse outcome measurements, and more extensive and intensive application of measurements that demonstrate validity in application. Even when the social utility of biomedical research can be quantified with a high degree of accuracy, the information at best becomes a datum to be included along with other information in understanding the choices to be made in resource allocation to biomedical research, among biomedical research objectives, and among projects within each objective.

REFERENCES

1. National opinion survey. Louis Harris and Associates, Inc., New York, 1970-76 (series).

2. National Opinion Research Center: General social survey. University of Chicago, Chicago, 1975, 1977 (series).

3. Personal communication from H.B. Woolley, Division of Program Analysis, National Institutes of Health, April 24, 1978.

4. U.S. Congress, House of Representatives: Bill to direct the Secretary of DHEW to request appropriations for programs in respect to specific diseases or categories of diseases on the basis of the relative mortality and morbidity rates of specific diseases or categories of diseases and the relative impact on the health of persons in the United States and on the economy. H.R. 16710, 93d Congress, 2d session, Washington, D.C., Sept. 18, 1974.

5. National Center for Health Statistics: Guidelines for cost of illness studies in the Public Health Service. National Center for Health Statistics, Hyattsville, Md., 1979.

6. Frederickson, D.S.: Memorandum to participants. National Conference on Health Research Principles, National Institutes of Health, Bethesda, Md., Sept. 15, 1978 (processed).

7. U.S. Department of Health, Education, and Welfare, National Institutes of Health: Basic data relating to the National Institutes of Health 1976. Washington, D.C., February 1976.

8. President's Biomedical Research Panel: Report to the President and to Congress. DHEW Publication No. 05 76-500. Washington, D.C., April 30, 1976.

9. U.S. Department of Health, Education, and Welfare, Public Health Service: Forward plan for health, fiscal years 1978-82. DHEW Publication No. 76-50046. Washington, D.C., August 1976.

10. Institute of Medicine: Policy issues in the health sciences (staff paper). National Academy of Sciences, Washington, D.C., October 1977.

11. Carter, M.: Peer review, citations and biomedical research policy: NIH grants to medical school faculty, R-1583-HEW. The Rand Corporation, Santa Monica, Calif., December 1974.

12. Noble, J.H., Jr.: Peer review: quality control of applied social research. Science 185: 916-921, Sept. 13, 1974.

13. Rice, D.P.: Estimating the cost of illness. Health Economics Series No. 6. U.S. Department of Health, Education, and Welfare, Washington, D.C., 1966.

14. Cooper, B.S., and Rice, D.P.: The economic cost of illness revisited. Soc Sec Bull 39: 21-36, February 1976.

15. Levine, D.S., and Willner, S.: The cost of mental illness, 1974. Mental Health Statistical Note 125. U.S. Department of Health, Education, and Welfare, ADMHA, Washington, D.C., February 1976.

16. Berk, A., and Paringer, L.C.: Costs of illness and disease 1900. Public Services Laboratory, Georgetown University, Washington, D.C., August 1977, revised 1979.

17. Berk, A., and Paringer, L.C.: Costs of illness and disease, fiscal year 1930. Public Services Laboratory, Georgetown University, Washington, D.C., May 1977.

18. Paringer, L.C., and Berk, A.: Costs of illness and disease, fiscal year 1975. Public Services Laboratory, Georgetown University, Washington, D.C., January 1977.

19. Mushkin, S.J., et al.: Costs of disease and illness in the United States in the year 2000. Public Health Rep 93:493-588, September-October 1978.

20. Oral communication, Native Federation, 1976.

21. Abt, C.C.: The social cost of cancer. Soc Indicators Res 2:175-190, March 1975.

22. Weisbrod, B.A.: Costs and benefits of medical research: a case study of poliomyelitis. J Polit Econ 79:527-544, May-June 1971.

23. Fein, R.: Economics of mental illness. Basic Books, New York, 1958.

24. Mushkin, S.J.: Health as an investment. J Polit Econ 70:129-159, October 1962.

25. Laitin, H.: The economics of cancer. Doctoral dissertation, Harvard University, 1956, unpublished.

26. Klarman, H.E.: Syphilis control programs. *In* Measuring benefits of government investments, edited by R. Dorfman. Brookings Institution, Washington, D.C., 1965, pp. 367-414.

27. Klarman, H.E.: Socioeconomic impact of heart disease. *In* The heart and circulation: second national Conference on Cardiovascular Diseases, edited by E.C. Andrus and C.H. Maxwell. Federation of American Societies for Experimental Biology, Bethesda, Md., 1965, pp. 693-707.

28. Gorham, W.: Sharpening the knife that cuts the public pie. Public Adm Rev 28:236-241, May-June 1968.

29. U.S. Department of Health, Education, and Welfare, Office of the Assistant Secretary for Program Coordination: Disease control programs: selected disease control programs, Program Analysis 1966-5, Washington, D.C., September 1966; and Human investment programs: selected human investment programs, Program Analysis 1966-10, Washington, D.C., October 1966.

30. Rivlin, A.M.: Systematic thinking for social action. Brookings Institution, Washington, D.C., 1971.

31. LeSourd, D.A., Fogel, M.E., and Johnston, D.R.: Benefit-cost analysis of kidney disease programs. U.S. Department of Health, Education, and Welfare, Public Health Service, Washington, D.C., August 1968 (prepared by Research Triangle Institute).

32. Axnick, N.W., Shavell, S.M., and Witte, J.J.: Benefits due to immunization against measles. Public Health Rep 84:673-680, August 1969.

33. Conley, R.W.: The economics of mental retardation. Johns Hopkins University Press, Baltimore, Md., 1973.

34. Witte, J.J., and Axnick, N.W.: The benefits from 10 years of measles immunization in the United States. Public Health Rep 90:205-207, May-June 1975.

35. Schoenbaum, S.C., Hyde, J.N., Jr., Bartoshesky, L., and Crampton, K.: Benefit-cost analysis of rubella vaccination policy. N Engl J Med 294:306-310, Feb. 5, 1976.

36. Albritton, R.B.: Cost-benefits of measles eradication: effects of a Federal intervention. Policy Analysis 4:1-21, winter 1978.

37. Zeckhauser, R., and Shepard, D.: Where now for saving lives? Law Contemp Prob 40:5-45, autumn 1976.

38. Mushkin, S.J., and Freidin, R.: Lead poisoning in children: the problem in D.C. and preventive steps. Public Services Laboratory, Georgetown University, Washington, D.C., September 1971.

39. Bush, J.W., Chen, M.M., and Patrick, D.L.: Health status index in cost effectiveness: analysis of a PKU program. *In* Health status indexes, edited by R.L. Berg. Hospital Research and Educational Trust, Chicago, 1973, pp. 172-194.

40. Cretin, S.: Cost-benefit analysis of treatment and prevention of myocardial infarction programs. Health Serv Res 12:174-189, summer 1977.

41. Mansfield, E., Jr., et al.: Research and innovation in the modern corporation. Norton Publishers, New York, 1971.

42. Grabowski, H.: The determinants of industrial research and development: a study of the chemical, drug and petroleum industries. J Polit Econ 76:292-306, March-April 1968.

43. Schnee, J.E.: Research and technological change in the ethical pharmaceutical industry. Doctoral dissertation, University of Pennsylvania, 1970, unpublished.

44. Schwartzman, D.: The expected return from pharmaceutical research. American Enterprise Institute for Public Policy Research, Washington, D.C., 1975.

45. Baily, M.N.: Research and development costs and returns, the U.S. pharmaceutical industry. J Polit Econ 70-85, January-February 1972.

46. Block, H.: True profitability measures. Regulation, economics and pharmaceutical innovation. *In* Proceedings of the Second Seminar on Economics of Pharmaceutical Innovation, edited by J.D. Cooper. American University, Washington, D.C., 1974.

47. Conley, R.W., Conwell, M., and Arrill, M.B.: An approach to measuring the cost of mental illness. Am J Psychiatry 124:755-762, December 1967.

48. Mishan, E.J.: Evaluation of life and limb: a theoretical approach. J Polit Econ 79:687-705, July-August 1971.

49. Schelling, T.C.: The life you save may be your own. *In* Problems in public expenditure analysis, edited by S.B. Chase. Brookings Institution, Washington, D.C., 1968, pp. 127-162.

50. Dorfman, N.: The social value of saving a life. *In* Health: what is it worth?, edited by S.J. Mushkin and D.W. Dunlop. Pergamon Press, Elmsford, N.Y., 1979.

51. Acton, J.P.: Measuring the social impact of heart and circulatory disease programs, R-1697-NHLI. The Rand Corporation, Santa Monica, Calif., 1975.

52. Mushkin, S.J., and Collings, F.d'A.: Economic concepts of disease and injury; a review of concepts. Public Health Rep 74:795-809, September 1959.

53. Malzberg, B.: Mortality among patients with mental disease. State Hospitals Press, Utica, N.Y., 1934; Social and biological aspects of mental diseases. State Hospitals Press, Utica, N.Y., 1940. Mental illness and the economic value of man. Paper presented at the 40th annual meeting of the National Committee for Mental Hygiene, New York, Nov. 16, 1949.

54. Thaler, R., and Rosen, S.: The value of saving a life: evidence from the labor market. *In* Household production and consumption, edited by N. Terleckyj. National Bureau of Economic Research. Columbia University Press, New York, 1975, pp. 265-297.

55. Niskanen, W.A., and Hanke, S.H.: Land prices substantially underestimate the value of environmental quality. Rev Econ Stat 59:375-376, August 1977.

56. Wylie, C.M., and White, B.K.: A measure of disability. Arch Environ Health 8:834-839, June 1964.

57. Katz, S., et al.: Studies of illness in the aged: the index of ADL—a standardized measure of biological and psychosocial function. JAMA 185:914-919, September 1963.

58. Karnofsky, D.A., and Burchenal, J.H.: The clinical evaluation of chemotherapeutic agents in cancer. *In* Evaluation of chemotherapeutic agents, edited by R. MacLeod. Columbia University Press, New York, 1949.

59. Williamson, J.W.: Prognostic epidemiology. *In* Pediatric atrophy, edited by M. Ryan. Williams and Wilkins, Baltimore, Md., 1971.

60. Torrance, G.W., Thomas, W.H., and Sackett, D.L.: A utility maximization model for evaluation of health care programs. Health Serv Res 7:118-133, summer 1972.

61. Chen, M.M., Bush, J.W., Patrick, J.L., and Blischke, W.R.: Linear models of social preferences for constructing a health status index. Paper prepared for

meeting of Operations Research Society of America, San Diego, Calif., November 1973.

62. Fanshel, S., and Bush, J.W.: A health-status index and its application to health services outcomes. Operations Res 18:1021-1066, November-December 1970.

Chapter Two

Biomedical Research Trends

Counts on the cost or, more broadly, the burden of illness are sought as one among many criteria for assessment of biomedical research. In this chapter we review briefly the history of biomedical research expenditure growth as a backdrop for later discussion of the price exacted by illness, and the returns in lower cost resulting from advances in science and their application. And we ask: What kinds of intermediate indicators of biomedical research can serve to parcel out the share of improved health status attributable to such research?

THE CONTENT OF BIOMEDICAL RESEARCH

Research in the health sciences has not dealt with an unchanging content. Its disciplines expanded over the years from the basic sciences of biochemistry, physiology, pharmacology, and biology. Epidemiology, biostatistics, and nutrition were included early in the twentieth century. Today health sciences research encompasses biophysics, bioengineering, and the behavioral sciences, including anthropology. Medical sociology, medical economics, medical ethics, and health services and their delivery are now included.

Traditional biomedical sciences now represent only a portion of the kinds of inquiry directed toward achieving a greater measure of prevention and better diagnostic, therapeutic, and rehabilitation methods. The investigation of biomedical sciences by the President's Biomedical Research Panel, for example, was broad; it included biochemistry, molecular genetics, tissue and organ biology, and pharmacology.[1] It also included nutrition, epidemiology, biostatistics, biomedical engineering, environmental toxicology, and the behavioral sciences. The conference held at the National Institutes of Health (NIH) in 1978 on principles of health research policy went even further to encompass within health research many disciplines ranging from the harder sciences to organizational research.[2]

Recognition of a broad scope of the health sciences is not new. The 1908 National Conservation Commission dealt at some length with nutrition, genetics, and the epidemiology of disease.[3] That commission report was a forerunner of later studies in the behavioral sciences that underscored both the environmental questions for investigation and the cost of illness.

Many critical health problems at the beginning of the twentieth century were environmental, in which community characteristics and practices, such as sanitary delivery of milk and provision of safe water supplies, had much to do with the health problems of the period. Over time, as health care shifted to personal health, the impact of individual characteristics of persons and families on health has come to be an important research question. For example, reduction of smoking to reduce the prevalence or severity of diseases, such as lung cancer, heart disease, or chronic obstructive lung diseases, is a vital field of health inquiry that includes methods of public communication and behavior modification. Patients' compliance with physicians' prescriptions is another, related example. More recently, emotional reaction and balances of stress and support have been recognized as important topics of health science investigation, as has bioethics.

We define biomedical research to include the wide range of disciplines that affect the extent and cost of illness, both those that underpin the understanding of environmental health measures and those that are the basis for decisions on personal health care. (The terms biomedical research and health research are used interchangeably given the scope of the definition.)

Research in this broad conceptual framework is a complex activity, whose special characteristics cannot be neglected. Certain of these characteristic features are repeatedly noted but they are restated here because of their relevance to planning and deciding about biomedical research fund allocations.

- Research is an uncertain activity; research objectives are not automatically met.
- A number of key discoveries come about as a result of chance observations. The history of invention is replete with examples of work on one problem that leads to discoveries in another.

- Research yielding antecedent knowledge may occur well in advance of some discovery to which the initial findings become critical.
- Research activities in biomedical sciences depend on many disciplines and a combination of disciplinary findings to achieve new knowledge and new applications.
- Research activities depend on the interests and enthusiasm of the individual research scientist. Scientists select problems for a wide variety of reasons, including perception of scientific opportunity and sensitivity to priorities.

THE SIZE OF BIOMEDICAL RESEARCH

What has been the magnitude of support for biomedical research in the United States? Table 2-1 shows the national expenditures for health research for selected years over the period 1940-77. National expenditures for health research increased from a level of $45 million in 1940 to approximately $4.6 billion in 1975 and $5.5 billion in 1977. The growth rates in outlays for health research for selected periods are shown in Table 2-2. As the figures suggest, there has been a slowing down of the rate of increase, with a further dropoff projected for the period ahead.

In 1900, biomedical research outlays may have been at a $157,000 level, representing primarily the initial expenditures of major research foundations, the medical schools, and private industry (see Table 2A-1 in the appendix to this chapter). Forty years later, of the $45 million total spent for biomedical research, over half represented expenditures of industry. The government's share accounted for less than 7 percent of the total. Federal support for research increased primarily in the period following World War II. By 1963, the

Table 2-1. National Expenditures for Medical Research, Selected Years, 1940-1977

(in millions)

Source of funds	1940	1963	1975	1977
Total	$45	$1,545	$4,640	$5,526
Government	3	1,008	3,038	3,612
Federal	3	919	2,799	3,351
State and local	NA	89	239	261
Industry	25	375	1,322	1,625
Private support	17	162	280	289

Source: National Institutes of Health; *Basic data relating to the National Institutes of Health.* U.S. DHEW, Washington, D.C., 1962, 1966, 1978.

Table 2-2. Health Research Expenditures, Over Selected Periods

Year	Rate of growth	Growth rate corrected for price
1900-29	13.7%	11.0%
1930-62	15.4	12.9
1963-75	9.1	4.0
1975-77	8.7	1.1
1975-2000	6.9-7.8	3.1-4.1

government's share rose to over $1 billion, or about two-thirds of the total. The relative share of each of the contributors to biomedical research is diagrammed in Figure 2-1.

Industry's portion of biomedical research outlays has been relatively stable in recent years at almost 30 percent of the total. In 1963, when biomedical research was greatly expanded over previous years, the growth of government financing overtook industry.

NIH's part in the nation's research effort is illustrated by its growth from about 6 percent of the total in 1950 to 41 percent by 1976 and 1977. In terms of HEW budget authority, some $2.5 billion was budgeted for federally funded health research in fiscal year 1977, a figure growing to almost $3.0 billion by fiscal year 1979 and marking a change of 4.3 percent between 1978 and 1979 or less than the rate of change required to keep up with inflation (Table 2-3). The change for NIH alone is even lower, 3.5 percent.

Expenditures in current dollars fail to tell the story about real resources devoted to health research. Accordingly, the expenditure numbers have been adjusted to a real price basis using a biomedical research price index developed by Westat for NIH (The Westat index is for the years 1961-75. The indexes for years prior to 1961 are computed from a simple regression of Westat's price index on the overall GNP price deflator for 1961-75.) A comparison of expenditures for biomedical research on a current and constant price basis is shown in Figure 2-2. The year 1970 represented the first time since 1947 that real resources for biomedical research declined. In 1971, there was some catching up, but 1973 saw little growth over 1972; 1975 witnessed a further decline in real resources and there has not been a return to the peak of the late 1960s. As indicated later, a drop in biomedical periodicals and in PhD's in the biomedical sciences is a likely response to these health research expenditure trends.

Year 2000 Estimates

As part of projections to the year 2000 and consistent with an economic model developed for the period discussed more fully later,

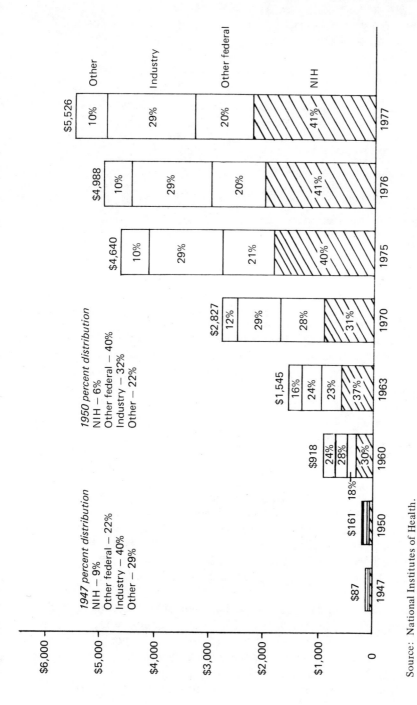

Figure 2-1. National Biomedical Research by Source of Funds, Selected Years (dollars in millions)

Source: National Institutes of Health.

1947 percent distribution
NIH — 9%
Other federal — 22%
Industry — 40%
Other — 29%

1950 percent distribution
NIH — 6%
Other federal — 40%
Industry — 32%
Other — 22%

Table 2-3. R&D in the Department of Health, Education, and Welfare (budget authority)

(in millions)

	Estimated budget			Percent change
	1977	*1978*	*1979*	*1978-1979*
Health				
National Institutes of Health	$2,240.3	$2,515.4	$2,602.6	+3.5%
Alcohol, Drug Abuse and Mental Health Administration	152.8	162.3	202.5	+24.8
Center for Disease Control	53.8	57.9	59.1	+2.1
Food and Drug Administration	41.0	47.0	47.0	—
Office of Assistant Secretary for Health	35.9	40.5	34.1	−15.8
Health Services Administration	16.2	15.8	15.8	—
Special Foreign Currency Program	1.5	11.4	11.4	—
Total	$2,541.5	$2,850.3	$2,972.5	+4.3

Source: "OMB Data for Special Analysis P."

biomedical research expenditures have been estimated to grow to $26 to $33 billion. The research and development expenditures for biomedical sciences have been estimated for the year 2000 as a way of extending outlays forward. These expenditures are estimated on the basis of the relationship between personal health care expenditures and those research outlays separately identified by the Social Security Administration in its estimates of national health expenditures.

The biomedical research included in the Social Security concept of national health expenditures is estimated at $17.2 to $21.7 billion, with the range mirroring the range of personal health expenditures as estimated for the year 2000. To these sums industrial and private nonprofit health research was added, representing that part of research costs assumed to be shifted forward into cost of production and, therefore, excluded from the research costs in the national health bill to avoid double counting. We have estimated these industrial outlays at $9 to $11 billion for 2000. In making the estimate, it was assumed that industry would continue to spend about the same share of sales for biomedical research as they did in 1976. In 1976, industry spent $1.4 billion for research, or about 10 percent of the estimated drug and eyeglass expenditures in the national health bill. We have assumed approximately this same percentage for the year 2000.

The resulting estimates may be summarized in this way:

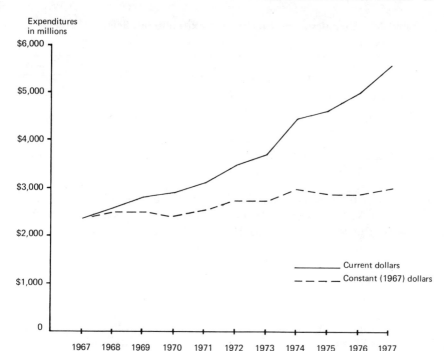

Source: National Institutes of Health.

Figure 2-2. National Health Research: Expenditures in Current and Constant Dollars, 1967-77

	(Amounts in billions)	
	1976	*2000*
Total biomedical research expenditures	$5.0	$26-33
Health research in national health bill	3.3	17-22
Industrial and private nonprofit research	1.7	9-11

These research outlays are equal to 3 percent of direct health expenditures and three-tenths to almost four-tenths of the GNP.

Total Investment in Health Research

We have attempted to estimate health research expenditures over the years for purposes of arriving at an aggregate investment for research that could be applied in analyzing investment returns.

The cumulative figures are shown in Table 2-4 for selected periods. For each of the periods, there has been a quantum jump in

Table 2-4. Cumulative Health Research Expenditures: Selected Periods
(in millions)

Selected periods	*Current dollars*	*Constant 1975 dollars*
1900-29	$ 59	$ 268
1930-62	7,580	16,926
1963-75	37,471	50,942
1900-75	45,110	68,136
1900-77	55,624	77,532
1930-77	55,565	77,264

investments for health research. The aggregate over the entire span of years 1900-75 is estimated in constant 1975 dollars at $68.1 billion, but with the years 1976 and 1977 added, the investment in health research rises to $77.5 billion in constant 1975 dollars.

ISSUES IN BIOMEDICAL RESEARCH POLICIES

Three questions are repeatedly raised in discussions of biomedical research: (1) Are we spending too much or too little of the nation's resources on biomedical research? (2) Are the funds spent where the need is greatest? (3) Are the projects selected for funding within each disease area the right ones? We examine each of these questions briefly in turn.

Are we spending too much or too little? The simple, straightforward question of too much or too little cannot be answered simply. The answer depends on the economic resources of the nation, competing claims on those resources, and relative consumer or public preferences.

In the economy, generally, competing claims are resolved by the responsiveness of production through the market system to consumer demand. The biomedical research product, however, is a public good, that is, a good enjoyed collectively; individuals cannot be excluded from the benefits of research once the research has been embodied in health practice. Benefits accrue, furthermore, not only in the country of origin but in other nations as well, depending on the rate of transmission of findings. As a result of the collective characteristics of biomedical research, the record keeping on consumer demand cannot be carried out through the marketplace. If the market could be used, those who wanted the goods would buy them at a price that is responsive to demand, and the recording of this demand would encourage new investment and new production. But biomedical research suppliers, such as NIH, have no market record of demand as a guide to their decisions to expand and invest, or to contract.

An absolute answer to the question of adequate spending for research is not technically possible. The outside limit is all the economic resources of people and materials available. Essentially, the question calls for comparison of gains from research and gains from other productive activity. Comparison, in turn, requires expression of relative preferences of individuals for this collective good, biomedical research, or an accounting of gains in relation to cost that is intended to be a proxy for the expression of individual preferences and willingness to pay. Until fairly recently, it was thought that a truthful expression of preferences could not be gained because of the prospects of a free ride—access to the gains from biomedical research without paying the price. Cost-benefit analysis offered an administrative alternative to this market-type calculus.

In the absence of comparative data on gains relative to cost of biomedical research, certain rule-of-thumb indexes are being used to judge the relative amount of resources spent for biomedical research. These indexes measure research expenditures as a percentage of gross national product, the national health bill, and total research and development outlays. Research expenditures have also been reviewed in terms of the burden or economic cost of illness.

Biomedical research, with ever-accelerating pace, claimed a larger and larger share of the nation's GNP until the late 1960s. Since then, the share has been quite stable at almost 0.3 percent of GNP (Table 2-5).

The rapid rise of health expenditures from mid-1960 to 1977 reflects itself in a somewhat smaller growth of biomedical research as a percentage of national health expenditures. Before Medicare and Medicaid, the research share was enlarged; however, since the mid-1960s, the relative share has declined (Table 2-6). The direction of the change stands out; the shift reflects a policy change with greater emphasis on more distributive equity. Use of scarce medical care resources to care for patients seemed to be preferred to use of those resources for scientific advance.

Biomedical research and development as a share of research and development rose over the decades from about 4 to 13 percent. Again, in recent years, biomedical research has grown somewhat less than all R&D.

At this time, the future of R&D expenditures is most uncertain.

Table 2-5.   Comparative Indexes of Size of National Health
Research Effort

Fiscal year	Research as percent of GNP	Research as percent of national health expenditures	Research as percent of all research and development
1946	0.04	[1]	4.44
1950	0.06	1.34	5.55
1960	0.18	3.60	6.88
1963	0.26	4.82	9.13
1970	0.29	4.13	10.96
1975	0.30	3.63	13.21
1976	0.29	3.44	12.95
1977	0.29	3.40	12.94

[1] Data for 1946 on national health expenditures were not available, so an estimate, based on 1946 personal consumption expenditures on medical care, is used here.

Sources: 1946-70: Division of Public Information, NIH: *The National Institutes of Health Almanac 1976.* U.S. DHEW, Bethesda, Md., 1976; National Institutes of Health: *Basic data relating to the National Institutes of Health.* U.S. DHEW, Washington, D.C., 1978; B.S. Cooper, N.L. Worthington, and M.F. McGee: *Compendium of national health expenditure data.* U.S. DHEW, Social Security Administration, Washington, D.C., January 1976.

1975-77: R.M. Gibson and C.R. Fisher: "National health expenditures, fiscal year 1977." *Social Security Bulletin* 41(7): July 1978.

HEALTH RESEARCH AND R&D POLICY
IN GENERAL

Until fairly recently, emphasis on the limits of scientific inquiry has combined with the unfavorable counts in the census of young persons of college age to dampen enthusiasm for federal support for research. And private industry for a variety of reasons also cut back its real effort. The economic consequences of less research and development are now being felt on the domestic job and international trade markets. A new effort is now going forward to undo past damage, to renew creative science, and to develop talent for research.

Frank Press, as director of the Office of Science and Technology and technological advisor to the president, has taken the initiative in reviews of budgetary allocations for research and development.[4] The president's first public statement on R&D policy commented on the budget review processes underway. He said that many agency heads "relegated R&D to a fairly low position of priority." But the president went on to say that he had "directed OMB to boost those R&D items much higher and they will be funded accordingly."

Science policy generally is a datum in developing principles for a five-year plan for biomedical research. The support given by the

Table 2-6. Total Direct Health Expenditures and Health Research
Expenditures, Selected Years, 1900-2000

Year	Direct health expenditures (in billions)	Health research expenditures (in millions)	Percent health research of health expenditures
1900	$ .5	$ .2	.03
1930	3.6	10.0	.3
1963	32.4	1,561.0	4.8
1975	127.7	4,640.0	3.6
2000	(1,013.6)	(26,000.0-32,000.0)	(2.6-3.3)

Sources: Health expenditures, for 1900: S.J. Mushkin and L.C. Paringer: "Direct Expenditures, 1900." Public Services Laboratory, Georgetown University, Washington, D.C., 1977; for 1930: L.C. Paringer and A. Berk: "The Cost of Illness and Disease, 1930." Public Services Laboratory, Georgetown University, Washington, D.C., 1977; for 1963: D. Rice: "Estimating the Cost of Illness." U.S. Public Health Service, Health Economics Series No. 6, 1966; for 1975: L.C. Paringer and A. Berk: "The Cost of Illness and Disease, 1975." Public Services Laboratory, Georgetown University, Washington, D.C., 1977; for year 2000: S.J. Mushkin, et al.: "Cost of Disease and Illness in the United States in the Year 2000." *Public Health Reports* 93(5):493-588, September-October 1978.

Health research expenditures, for 1900 and 1930: estimated by Public Services Laboratory; for 1963 and 1975: National Institutes of Health: *Basic Facts Relating to the National Institutes of Health.* U.S. DHEW, Bethesda, Md., March 1978; for year 2000: Public Services Laboratory estimates amended to conform with NIH definitions.

administration is reflected in federal R&D obligations. Federal R&D obligations have risen from $15.6 billion in fiscal year 1969 to $263 billion in fiscal year 1978. Most of the growth took place in the period 1976-77 when in constant dollars R&D rose 10.6 percent, only to decline to a 1.3 percent rise in constant dollars for the period 1977-78. The increase in health R&D even in current dollars was only 2.3 percent for 1977-78 compared to 7.6 percent for all R&D, including a 17 percent increase for energy development and conversion, and 8.3 percent for national defense.[5]

In June 1978 the president wrote to the chairmen and member of all the congressional committees and subcommittees responsible for appropriations for basic research. He wrote: "I want to emphasize that even relatively small reductions in key agencies—such as the National Science Foundation, or in new initiatives and growth planned for mission agencies . . . including NASA, and the Departments of Agriculture, Energy, and Defense—would defeat our objective".[6]

Some urge a quantum increase in government funding of research as well as steps to encourage and stimulate private research. Substantial increase in resources for research clearly is challenged by the stringency of the overall budget amount required to combat inflation, and priority setting in this environment of rigorous budget constraints becomes difficult. However, there is much going for science and research and development. The public remains enthusiastic about R&D despite its skepticism about many other aspects of government. The total additional outlays required for a substantial increase in funding for science would be but a small fraction of the budgets either of DOD or DHEW. In addition, the president has expressed a strong interest in advancing the nation's R&D. He has taken steps to urge Congress to maintain the real levels of spending for R&D and has led a new push for basic research initiatives, with a report from the Office of Science and Technology that the picture for research support remains encouraging. There is growing recognition of the need for a strong base of new knowledge if the nation is to grow more rapidly and to compete effectively. For a while the nation lost sight of the valuable resource that young scientists and engineers represent. As Frank Press, in his speech before the AAAS Colloquium on R&D policy, stated: "Better mechanisms must be developed for anticipating the needs of various fields and directing our talent to them".[4]

The president has launched a cabinet-level study of industrial innovation. That study, a Domestic Policy Review involving some thirty federal agencies and offices, is now well underway.[7] That review, among other things, is to consider:

- Encouraging the formation of small, high-technology firms because of their significant contribution to employment growth, as well as innovation
- Increasing efforts to develop advanced technologies that are receiving high-priority support from foreign governments because of the implication for the future competitiveness of U.S. industry

New policy initiatives for research and development have been initiated by the administration in competitive agricultural research, mineral policy, earthquake hazard reduction, and human nutrition. Energy research is a major effort that includes nuclear waste management and solar energy processes.

If there is to be a long-term health R&D policy, it will need to be developed with full awareness of the overall national policy for science, including policies on scientific manpower. Expenditures for R&D may be increased in the future. What the balance might be between biomedical research and other R&D, however, may depend on the future assessment of the relative economic role of biomedical research in our international competitive economy.[7] Biomedical research by this standard should fare well, for the United States is, after all, a major exporter of medical know-how.

Are the funds spent where the need for biomedical research is greatest? This question centers on priorities for biomedical research within the national aggregates related to measures of need. General dearth of information, combined with considerations of scientific feasibility and scientific interest, focused research, almost from the outset of federal involvement, on diseases with high death rates. Federal funds early on were allocated to research on the infectious and communicable diseases. The Hygienic Laboratory at the Public Health Service facility on Staten Island, set up in 1887 to help carry out research, gained congressional recognition in 1901 as a "laboratory for the investigation of infectious and contagious diseases and matters pertaining to public health." Through the years and even after the Hygienic Laboratory became the National Institutes of Health in 1930, the main emphasis continued to be on the communicable diseases—tuberculosis and venereal diseases, as well as yellow fever, cholera, and leprosy. In 1937, when the National Cancer Institute was created, the emphasis shifted somewhat; however, reaction to the shifting causes of death was delayed.

The three principal private research centers at the beginning of the 1900s, the Rockefeller Institute for Medical Research, the Rockefeller Foundation, and the Carnegie Institution of Washington, also concentrated their efforts on the major communicable and infectious diseases. The control of hookworm in the South, for example, was a principal charge of the Rockefeller Institute. In those early years, funds were targeted for two aspects of biomedical research: (1) the advance of rudimentary physiology, biology, and other basic biomedical sciences, and (2) control of diseases that were of major importance to national policy, such as yellow fever for defense purposes and hookworm, malaria, and tuberculosis for reasons of economic development.

The emphasis for much of the federally supported research continued to be on the infectious diseases even after the primary disease problems had changed. The Steelman Report of 1947 took exception to the then current priorities by noting:

> A comparison of the 10 principal causes of illness and death with the 10 principal diseases under investigation (in 1947) shows that something less than a high correlation exists. . . . There is virtually no research in the Federal programs on civilian accidents, cerebral hemorrhage, rheumatism and allied disease, nephritis, or influenza—all of which occupy important places in the lists of illness or death.[8]

Table 2-7 shows the comparison of research projects supported by federal research agencies and mortality and illness rates as presented in the Steelman Report. That report set a pattern of comparison of research fund allocations and disease problems that has persisted over the decades. Illness data then sparse and far from current have been greatly improved. A number of indexes of health status are now reported through the data collection activities of the National Center for Health Statistics that at least partially document need. As indicated in Chapter 1, there is some sentiment toward use of formulas for allocation that would take into account mortality, morbidity, and the cost of illness.

A number of factors are at issue in determining priorities among diseases. One such factor is the potential for a scientific advance in one (or another) of the biomedical disciplines that in concert with expanded knowledge in other disciplines can lead to progress toward understanding and cure or control of a disease. Another factor is the relative significance of the disease in terms of death and disability. Scientific capacity and interest also significantly influence the research that is undertaken. Automatic formula allocations based on standard yardsticks would be ineffective even if the data for a formula standard were adequate for the task; they are not. Persons concerned about the continuing heavy dependence on mortality data as a basis for judging, for example, are emphasizing the lack of consideration of the impaired life that is sometimes the result of postponed deaths. Others are asking for data on persons who have a disease but are able to function fully.

In Chapter 6, we examine at some length the present targeting of biomedical research funds in relation to deaths and other indexes.

Are the projects selected the right ones? Early in the agency's operations, the National Institutes of Health established a peer group review process for screening proposals submitted for research projects and for making recommendations on funding. The peer group review has served over the decades to sort out projects and to apply the scientific views of experts to project selection.

In 1976, the president's Biomedical Research Panel reviewed the processes and operation of the peer groups and found that they worked well as project selection agents.[1]

Recently, two other questions about research projects have surfaced: (*a*) the potential impact of research on medical care costs, and (*b*) the potential impact of applied research projects on health status. Because of the extent to which newer advances take the form of devices requiring major capital outlays, such as the CAT scanner or cardiac intensive care equipment, it is argued that research increases

Table 2-7. Comparative Ranking of Health Research Projects and Principal Causes of Death and Illness, 1946

Rank	Research projects	Principal causes of death[1]	Principal causes of illness
1	Cancer, other tumors	Diseases of the heart[2]	Diseases of the respiratory system
2	Venereal diseases	Cancer and other malignant tumors	Communicable diseases of childhood
3	Other infections of a bacillary or amebic origin	Intercranial lesions of vascular origin	Confinements
4	Malaria, other tropical diseases	Accidents, including motor vehicle	Accidents
5	Cardiovascular, cardiovascular-renal diseases	Nephritis	Cardiovascular, cardiovascular-renal diseases
6	General morbidity and mortality	Penumonia and influenza	Tonsillitis
7	Tuberculosis	Tuberculosis	Diseases of the digestive system
8	Other virus and rickettsial diseases	Diabetes mellitus	Other and ill-defined diseases
9	Dental, oral diseases	Premature birth	Rheumatism and allied diseases
10	Mental diseases	Senility, ill-defined, other causes	Nervous and mental diseases

[1] Press release, U.S. Public Health Service, December 27, 1946.
[2] Including diseases of coronary arteries, angina pectoris, rheumatic heart disease, and other heart diseases.
Source: Reference 8.

high-cost technology and further exacerbates the rising cost of medical care. A recently proposed review procedure essentially requires that a statement on a medical care cost impact accompany grant applications. Problems of anticipating with some certainty discovery and invention are set aside in this type of proposal, as are engineering principles about cost reduction over time when third- and fourth-generation equipment is designed and produced. Restrictive regulation can, it is urged, have adverse effects on R&D.

Measurement of health status effects of research projects is still another formulation. Dunlop, for example, has reviewed diabetes research projects for their relative impact on disability rates and deaths and concluded that research funds are not targeted in a balanced way between therapies and cures and between cures and primary prevention.[9]

In general, the debate on project support fails to differentiate the purposes of new types of assessment. Safety, efficacy (or effectiveness), and cost containment are the three overriding concerns.

Safety

Safety is used here in the special sense of control of potential hazards that might be unleased in scientific probing. Traditions of free inquiry are challenged by recombinant DNA research. Is some research to be barred or rigidly controlled because of hazards, or not? As one commentator posed the question: "Should certain lines of inquiry simply be ruled out-of-bounds as too perilous for frail mankind?"

The purpose of safety controls is to prevent illness. Scientists raised the issue of inadvertent creation of hazardous organisms in the course of research. And scientists participated in a voluntary moratorium on recombinant DNA research pending development of safety guidelines by NIH. Clarity in the formulation of safety standards would help answer the critical questions. What research is to be monitored? By whom? Who is to decide? How are decisions on enforcement to be made? With what sanctions?

Less basic safety questions are defined here under the objective of "efficacy." These include the challenges to safety arising from statistics on unnecessary patient deaths and such studies as that of Illich.[10]

Efficacy

A second objective is efficacy or effectiveness of health care and biomedical research embodied in such care. The purpose here is to (a) better inform providers of care; (b) inform consumers of care;

and (c) improve the regulation of drugs, instruments, and so forth in safety and efficacy. Problems of efficacy do not necessarily arise out of new research. On the contrary, familiar therapies often have not been assessed. Far more effective research is needed to carry out the assessments required.

Despite a decade or more of urging, the assessment of comparative therapies for their effectiveness is still most deficient. In the absence of the required research medical protocols are established, but the kind of information that could document the effectiveness of these and other alternatives is often lacking, especially information defining effectiveness in terms of the functional status of the patient. Information now available to physicians and other providers of medical care about the probabilities of outcomes in applying alternative therapies is seriously deficient. Physicians do not have the necessary facts, and patients can hardly receive answers to such questions as: What good will this medicine or procedure do? What are the chances that it will cure? What are the chances that it will control the disease? What are the adverse effects? What are the probabilities of different reactions? How does one modality compare with other possible procedures?

Part of the explanation for the lack of information on medical treatments lies in the physicians' control over medical care decisions. Yet, it is clear that the characteristics of the patient comprise one input into the effectiveness of medical care, and the patient's compliance with a medical regimen is certainly another. As long as a physician continues to decide about care as guardian for the patient, the need to know about the probabilities of consequences is muted. However, a series of factors is converging to give new emphasis to the patient's need for information in order to make decisions. Those factors include medical malpractice suits, the higher educational level of today's patients compared with that of earlier years, and the awakened sense of consumer participation.

Deficiencies in information about optional modalities are being addressed. For some time, the Office of Technology Assessment of the Congress has been identifying cases of technology requiring efficacy measurement. The recent study of electronic fetal monitoring is an outstanding example.[11] Further, a new office of technology assessment has been set up under the assistant secretary for health, DHEW, to encourage research demonstrations and evaluations respecting

- Factors that affect the use of health care technologies
- Methods of disseminating information about technologies

- The effectiveness and social, ethical, and economic impacts of particular medical technology[1][2]

Scholars at the School of Public Health at Harvard University,[1][3] among others, are engaged in the type of research that will yield assessments of therapies. University-based centers, such as the cancer centers throughout the nation and the heart centers, are intended to provide a base of data along with their examinations of consequences of alternative modalities. However, the imprecision of medical research may be suggested by Gifford and Feinstein's studies of unsupported or invalid conclusions due to statistical problems in medical manuscripts.[1][4],[1][5]

Corrective action that broadens the research to provide basic data on optional therapies to deal with diseases makes sense for both providers of care and patients. In the absence of such information, therapies are prescribed in shades of darkness. Machinery for collecting the necessary data on therapies from practitioners has been set in motion for some disease categories; more machinery of this kind is needed. Biostatistical and biometric techniques applied to the therapeutic data should help establish probabilities of cures, and of control of disease, at various functional levels. A number of questions still need to be resolved: How large an effort? Over what time period? With what incentives? Administered by whom? And with what machinery for dissemination?

Assessments of the effectiveness of known therapies need to be carefully distinguished from assessments for cost control purposes that would extend to new biomedical research proposals. Confusion in purpose seems widespread, with resulting ambiguity in the proposals for change. Indeed, there is reason to view the use of controls on research for cost containment as potentially damaging to scientific advancement if not to cost of patient care.

In place of calls for information about what course of treatment should be used, for whom, and under what circumstances, the rhetoric has shifted to technology and controls of new technology with a total confusion of technology and biomedical research. The statement is often made that new medical technology does not, as was earlier assumed, mean better patient care. Furthermore, it is alleged that new technology may indeed be harmful to patients. A study of hospital care at Yale Medical School is cited to show the extent of iatrogenic medicine.[1][6] Twenty percent of the center's patients were found to have suffered from complications, ranging from minor to fatal, from the diagnostic tests, drugs, and therapeutic measures prescribed for them.

New technology can mean any change in the process of providing care, including more (or less) repetitive testing, or introduction of different equipment, or use of different occupational groups in the provision of care. New technology may embody new biomedical research findings, but technology encompasses more than biomedical research results.

Cost Containment

Cost containment controls assume that the knowledge base on cost of illness and disease is greater than it is. As indicated in Chapter 1, the orthodox methods of measurement are being criticized on both conceptual and empirical grounds. Agreement about substitute measurements is not close at hand. Willingness-to-pay indicators are also subject to weaknesses, both conceptually and empirically. How can willingness be measured with any degree of precision when the questions asked are hypothetical? Income constraints condition decisions even about life-and-death matters. In any case, interest rates to be applied in evaluations are uncertain, and when interest rates are as high as they now are, the tendency is to limit yields to short-term payoffs with a resulting myopia in public investment.

Moreover, controls introduce a number of costs of their own, including those of administration and of compliance. Important in cost regulation is the impact of the regulation on subsequent inventive activity. Will controlling first-generation machines prevent the development of second-, third-, and fourth-generation machines?

The debate has centered on technology and cost containment with a spillover into biomedical research. Unnoticed are two important consequences that have taken place. Talented young persons equipped by training and intellectual capacity to contribute to advances in biomedical sciences are finding other employment with far less challenge as a result of curtailed outlays for R&D. Industry in the health-related fields, pharmaceutical firms for example, has done little more in the area of R&D than keep up with inflation. R&D of the ethical drug manufacturers went up 9 percent between 1976 and 1977 and also between 1975 and 1976, in contrast to a 14.1 percent rise the year before.[17]

These consequences are due to the concerns about technology and cost, coupled with the relegation of biomedical research support to "a usual item" in the budget. However, the amount of research and development funds is such a small part of the federal undertaking and of the total research and development effort that a position actually could be taken on R&D that differs from the position of the general budget without adding to inflation. Indeed, by contributing through increased productivity to the goods produced, biomedical R&D may relieve inflationary pressures.

THE BASIS FOR RESEARCH OUTLAY ESTIMATES

For the estimates presented, we have had to do much data analysis to come up with a set of figures. We tried several ways during the course of the present study to document research and development activity in the biomedical sciences for earlier years. These ways may be identified as follows:

- We reviewed the literature on expenditures for research from both public and private sources and, in particular, the Office of Management and Budget documents to try to ascertain the budgetary obligations or congressional appropriations for research. Operations of the Hygiene Laboratory, for example, can be identified historically, but the total funding includes expenditures that go beyond even the broad definition of biomedical research formulated at the outset. Estimates obtained from secondary sources do not appear to fit a pattern and in any case are fragmentary.
- The Pharmaceutical Manufacturers' Association participated with us in an inquiry to the major pharmaceutical firms to determine their 1900 and early year R&D. Firms were asked to report their R&D outlays or, if these were not available, the man-years of professional effort devoted to research. Only three firms responded and two of these indicated that they did not have the information.
- A detailed assessment for each five-year period has been made of biomedical research articles with the expectation that such an assessment would yield information on the name of the researcher, his or her affiliation, and source of financial support. This exercise yielded important insights into the volume and scientific character of research prior to World War II; it did not yield the data required to extend the biomedical R&D expenditures back in time.
- Finding the route of compilation of data closed, we estimated biomedical research expenditures in the early years using indicators of the volume of biomedical research activity as variables. More specifically, we ran a regression of biomedical research expenditures as the dependent variable and a composite index, including the stock of PhD's in the biomedical sciences, patents

issued over a seven-year period for drugs, and the periodical publications in the biomedical sciences as the independent variable.

Literature on Research Expenditures

A review of the literature failed to produce specific estimates of fiscal expenditures for biomedical research during the years 1900[18] to 1940. Neither scholarly, nor philanthropic, nor government sources state in a sequential way precise amounts spent by any one organization, let alone a conglomerate figure for national expenditure.[19-26]

Data collection on research was initiated in the mid-1950s by the National Science Foundation. Prior to that time, there were fragmentary data or only sporadic studies, such as the study for the WPA project,[27] the report of the National Resources Committee,[26] and the President's Scientific Research Board,[28] from which data were drawn as indicated earlier. Expenditure data for the years prior to the 1950s are hardly precise. The two most noted sources for this type of information, Shryock's *American Medical Research*[29] and Strickland's *Politics, Science, and Dread Disease,*[30] while mentioning an increase in money spent over time, deal with the subject only in a general way. The Resource Analysis Branch of the Office of Program Planning, National Institutes of Health, has very little solid data for the years prior to 1940. Similarly, although the Rockefeller Archive Center in North Tarrytown, New York, has both annual and cumulative bursar reports and graphs, the figures do not accurately reflect the amount of money spent on biomedical research because the Rutherford donations, government funds, and industry's research are not included.

Other likely sources also failed to yield substantive data. Private charitable expenditures for biomedical research are not well defined. This is due to a number of factors: (a) there is no one source or reference that details these expenditures; (b) for the major component of private charitable expenditures, foundations, a source giving expenditures is available, but only for 1930, 1931, 1932, and 1934; (c) although there are a number of secondary sources that mention specific amounts expended by the charitable groups, their estimates are poorly documented and often conflicting; and most importantly (d) the universe of these private groups is ill defined. As an example of the last case, some sources mention "the research institutes" as spending a given amount, yet there is no explanation of who is included in a research institute and what is the difference, if any, between a large foundation's quoted expenditures on biomedical research and the expenditures of a research group founded in its name.

Despite all these drawbacks, one fact is patently obvious: the private groups took the lead in biomedical research. Far more dedicated to the human cause than was the federal government, their expenditures exceeded that of the government until World War II.

The major foundations are reported as having donated $18.6 million, or 35.5 percent, of the 1930 total expenditures.[20] Among the foundations of primary importance were the Rockefeller Foundation, Duke Endowment, Commonwealth Fund, Milbank Memorial Fund, and Julius Rosenwald Fund. Some events in this early period are of special note:

- A research program was initiated at Hopkins in 1893 by Welch, who by 1900 reported that "pathology is everywhere recognized." Osler's text convinced John D. Rockefeller that medical science, "while as yet able to do little, had enormous possibility for human welfare."[29]
- In 1902, Rockefeller gave $1 million to a Rockefeller Board for research, including research in medicine and public health. By 1913, it had funds, as the Rockefeller Foundation, of $3 million.[29]
- According to a *Science Magazine* article of January 13, 1922, by 1921 there were 565 funds established to support scientific research with an annual yield of $17 million. Of these established funds, 135 with an annual income of $4 million were strictly for medical research.[31]

These partial reports of foundation funding for 1902 and 1921 were not used in estimating total R&D spending by year. We essentially had no appropriate way of complementing the numbers for sources other than through information voluntarily provided. The 1902 and 1921 figures cited here suggest, however, that the findings of the overall estimating equation tend to understate R&D in the first part of the century.

The Pharmaceutical Manufacturers Association has data beginning in 1950 that summarize the R&D expenditures of its members,[32] and it has also collected data since 1966, on R&D expenditures for drugs according to therapeutic purpose.[33]

Federal expenditures were reviewed in greater depth than expenditures of private sources; federal budget documents, consolidated financial reports, and annual reports of the relevant agencies were examined. The annual reports of the Veterans' Bureau, the Public

Health and Marine Hospital Service, and the Army's Surgeon General, however, do not separate R&D from other associated activities.

The review of the literature on research expenditures identified certain major changes in federal research activity:

- Early studies of the Hygienic Laboratory at the Staten Island Marine Hospital dealt with cholera, tuberculosis, typhoid fever, and diphtheria. The research mission of the Hygienic Laboratory was broadened to investigations of "infectious and contagious diseases and matters pertaining to the public health."
- During World War I, the National Hygienic Laboratory devoted a considerable effort to war-related diseases.
- In 1922, Public Health Service investigators set up a special cancer investigation laboratory at Harvard Medical School.[34]
- The expenditures by the Public Health Service on research during the 1920s are reported to have averaged slightly over $325,000 a year.[35]
- In 1930, when the Ransdell Act which created NIH was passed, the amounts for research increased.
- During the period 1930-38, federal enactments supported research on syphilis and gonorrhea and cancer.[36]
- The National Resources Committee, in its report to the Congress in 1939, presented estimates of $2.0 million for public health research for 1937 (Table 2-8) and $2.7 million for 1938.[26]
- In 1931, the Public Health Service established the Rocky Mountain Spotted Fever Laboratory in Montana.[34]
- The enactment of Title VI of the Social Security Act of 1935 authorized $2 million annually for the "investigation of disease and problems of sanitation." Actual appropriations were far below the authorization.[37]
- One of the most valuable developments to emerge from the federal medical research in the 1930s was an improved typhus vaccine that was credited with the record of "no typhus deaths during World War II."[38]
- The Public Health Service Act of 1944 empowered the surgeon general to make grants to universities, hospitals, laboratories, and other public and private institutes, as well as to individuals. This initiated the current disbursement of research funds to extramural institutions and modern research financing policies.

An early Basic Data volume from NIH presented estimates of national expenditures for medical research for a period beginning in

Table 2-8.   Federal Government Support of Research
(in thousands)

	1937
Total	$2,177
Public Health Service	2,017
Medical Department, War Department	15
Medicine and Surgery, Navy	19
St. Elizabeth's Hospital	42
Veterans' Administration	84

Source: Reference 26. Includes research on natural sciences and technology by identified health and medical agencies.

1940.[39] These 1940 figures, together with the most recent Basic Data volume estimates, are shown in Table 2-1, and for the period beginning in 1946, in Table 2A-2 in the appendix.

While piecemeal figures, public and private, were found or could be estimated for the early years of the century, the data did not seem hard enough to warrant its compilation into an aggregate.

Inquiry to Pharmaceutical Firms

With the assistance of the Pharmaceutical Manufacturers' Association, an inquiry was sent to the major pharmaceutical companies asking them to identify the amount spent on R&D or the number of biomedical scientists at work in the laboratory.

The letter to drug companies, in the form of a memorandum from the vice-president of the PMA, more specifically asked: "If you have in company historical files data on research activity in the 1900-50 period, it would be helpful. Primarily sought is quantitative data so that a time series for expenditures and/or personnel in research in the drug industry can be established."

The response was meager, perhaps because little research was being done. Although it is reported that Parke Davis and Company built a research laboratory in 1902 the production of many chemical synthetics was dominated by German-based firms. It was not until after World War I and the taking over of property (including patents) by the Alien Property Custodian that a U.S. industry was established, although consumer protection legislation of 1906, which set pharmacopoeia and national formulary standards, forced pharmaceutical manufacturers to establish laboratories for biological and chemical assay.[40] During this period in the early twentieth century there is a presumption, at least, that research and development of industry was carried out mainly in Europe.

Assessment of Biomedical Studies

Another methodology was tried, based on the idea that the best way to arrive at a meaningful ballpark figure (a more precise estimation is not attempted) is to consult the biomedical research literature itself; the figure must be based on the evidence of primary sources. The methodology assumes that there is a relationship between research done and published articles. It also assumes that examining work produced at five-year intervals will provide a fairly accurate reflection of work done during the entire period. The methodology involved four major steps.

1. The five most eminent biomedical research journals of the first half of the twentieth century were selected. Obviously, it does not necessarily follow that well-recognized scholarly journals today were so considered in the past. Thus, there are two methods by which such journals can be chosen. The first is to ask historians of science and medicine to name contemporary journals. The second is to review bibliographies of contemporary articles, noting which journals were most often cited. The methods were combined—the first indicated the right direction, the second showed the following journals to be the most eminent American sources of biomedical scholarship in the early twentieth century:

   - *The Journal of Biological Chemistry*, Volume 1: 1905
   - *The Journal of the Boston Society of Medical Sciences*, Volume 1: 1896, later renamed *The Journal of Medical Research* (1901-24), again renamed *The American Journal of Pathology* (1924-present)
   - *The Journal of Experimental Medicine*, Volume 1: 1896
   - *The Journal of Immunology*, Volume 1: 1916
   - *The Journal of Infectious Diseases*, Volume 1: 1904

2. Each journal was reviewed at five-year intervals, article by article. Where the author was based and special sources of funding, if any were noted.

3. The number and percentage of the total number of articles reviewed, written from each home base (or site of research), were derived. Thus, we know, for example, that the Rockefeller Institute for Medical Research produced ninety-five articles, or 17.6 percent of the total number of articles tallied in the sample for the year 1925.

4. The data compiled also show the number of times each granting agency was cited in the reviewed articles and the percentage of the

total number of support citations. Thus, the Chemical Foundation awarded ten separate grants, or 10.3 percent of the total number of grants awarded to the reviewed sample in 1930.

The last step was intended to lead to actual compilation of figures representing money spent on biomedical research. However, as suggested by the response of the pharmaceutical firms, direct inquiry does not appear fruitful.

Regression Analysis of Research Expenditures

Having failed to achieve a compilation from published or other sources, estimates were made of biomedical research outlays for the early years of the twentieth century.

National health research expenditures were estimated on the basis of biomedical research activity. A regression was run with biomedical research expenditures as the dependent variable against a composite variable that included the stock of PhD's in the biomedical sciences, drug patents, and journals in the biomedical sciences. Each of these variables was weighted equally in arriving at the composite. Drug patents issued over a seven-year period were included for greater comparability with the figures on the stock of PhD's in the biomedical sciences and with the number of journals published.

Table 2A-1 in the appendix shows the estimated amounts by year over the period 1900-68. The actual expenditures data and estimates are compared in columns 2 and 5. The fit of actual and estimated despite a high R^2 is not as close as might be desired. But in the absence of other data, the estimates seemed sufficient for purposes of relating research outlays and gains from biomedical research advances.

(The regression equation is Ln BioExpend = .775 + 2.51 Ln BioResearch Effort R^2 = .959 F = 20.46.)

MEASURING RESEARCH EFFORT

Assessment of returns on biomedical research requires determination of the amount of resources for research. Knowing the amount spent for research, however, tells us little about the achievements in biomedical sciences and in health care as a result of the expenditures made. The essential achievements of research are the improvements in mortality, disability, debility, and quality of life. However, many factors contribute to the reduction in mortality. To parcel out the gains made in reduction in mortality requires intermediate yardsticks measuring the quantity and quality of the research effort.

A number of different indicators are used to assess the quantity and quality of biomedical research. A familiar indicator of quality is the number of Nobel Prize winners who are employees of the National Institutes of Health or grantees whose work has been supported by the NIH. The record of quality achievements—of excellence—is attested to by the impressive numbers who have gained recognition through Nobel Prizes. Other indicators of quality are also used, such as bibliometric studies of citations of research that has been supported.[41,42] Neither of these quality measures can be applied, however, in a historical analysis of biomedical research advances. What is essentially known about Nobel Prize winners is whether in a particular year an NIH scientist or a scientist whose work was supported by NIH received an award. Certainly the achievements of these individually identified scientists do not stand as proxy for all the ongoing research in a particular year. The first American citizen to receive the Nobel Prize (first awarded in 1901) was Karl Landsteiner, in 1930, for his work at the Rockefeller Institute on the grouping of human blood. Thomas Hunt Morgan followed in 1933 for his study of the hereditary function of chromosomes. Bibliometric studies of citations of research work supported are particularly useful in appraising individual pieces of research; when applied in a comprehensive way, however, the product is simply the number of times research administered or supported by NIH has been cited. In any case, the data do not extend back for a period sufficient for purposes of the present study. Citation references tell little about how the references are used. Are there many citations because the research was outstandingly poor or off the track? Or are the citations indicative of progress? Because of this problem, we have fallen back on those indicators of the quantity of biomedical research that may yield a perspective on the role of the research in the essential achievements of reduced mortality, disability, debility, and improved quality of life.

The indicators we have selected measure aspects of a research effort but hardly all the features desirable for assessment criteria. What types of materials are available that can inform us about the research effort? Most useful would be measures that would capture the essential characteristics of biomedical research work and its variation year by year. However, we could find no single series of data that extended back in time and that fully captured breakthroughs in biomedical research. Data availability became an important criterion. Still another selection criterion was the comprehensiveness of the available data. How large a scope of the research work was encompassed by these data?

A set of indicators of the quantity of biomedical research resulted from the examination of data. The indicators are:

- Patents issued for drugs
- Patents issued for biomedical scientific instruments
- Number of new drugs approved by FDA for marketing
- Number of biomedical periodicals reporting research findings
- Number of persons who receive a PhD degree in biomedical sciences

Only two of the series, namely, biomedical research periodicals and PhD's in the biomedical sciences, are fairly comprehensive in scope. Efforts to broaden the scope of coverage of the data or to provide supplementary information failed. For example, we tried to include among the number of biomedical research scientists a count of epidemiologists, or of those with MPH degrees, but the data were not adequate for the present study which extends back to 1900.

Other indicators were explored. A simple count of the number of multidisciplinary fields of research appeared to be suggestive of the increasing complexity of biomedical sciences, but the requisite information about the numbers in multidisciplines, such as biochemistry or bioengineering, was not available. (We have separately explored data on the year in which each professional organization for a particular specialty was formed.)

The two more comprehensive measures are of very different kinds. One represents the basic resources for a research product, namely, the research force available for scientific exploration; the other, in some measure, reflects the product of scientific work as evidenced by the periodicals that have appeared to record research findings.

Neither of these two more comprehensive indicators provides guidance on the quality of the research performed. Each is purely a quantity count that tells us little about the excellence of the research done or the significance of the contribution to medicine and patient care.

Drug patents, surgical instrument patents, and new drugs approved for marketing are deficient as indicators of biomedical research. Lacking comprehensiveness, they focus instead on aspects of biomedical research output that are representative more of applied industrial research than of the broad range of scientific research, including basic research. It might be argued that these indicators show what the pharmaceutical and scientific instrument industries have achieved rather than the achievements of the bench scientist exploring a fundamental scientific question. Much biomedical research activity is directed, however, at building intellectual capital. Such capacity building is required to make advances in applied fields, such as drug therapy. Nonetheless, a complementarity between fundamental research and applied areas of research has been repeatedly emphasized. Brooks recently noted: "There is a large grey area in between 'pure' science at one end, and highly targeted applied research at the other, where the difficulty of assessment arises primarily from the inability to agree on the relative weights to be assigned to truth and utility in evaluation."[4 3] And he cites as examples of grey areas the testing of chemicals for toxicity, the carrying out of chemical analyses, and some kinds of work on systematic biology, which "are usually battlegrounds for academic scientists and scientists from industry or government." Moreover, he goes on to mention a development made possible by fundamental biochemistry and cellular biology: "Probably the most important advance in recent years in our ability to detect carcinogens in the environment has come from the development of bacterial tests for mutagenesis, typified by the Ames test."[4 3]

As a plausible hypothesis, the argument can be advanced that the degree of applied drug and surgical instrument research, as evidenced by patents or new drug approvals, mirrors the overall biomedical research effort. The use of such proxies for biomedical research is further reinforced by the relative stability, at least in recent years, in the share of research expenditures made by industry and others. Again, however, the number of patents and drug approvals tells us little about the quality of the research.

An important advantage of the patent data is the long historical period that the information covers. Patent data from the eighteenth century are available. New drug approvals as an indicator are less useful because of the far shorter period for which the statistics exist as well as the FDA's changing methods of regulation, in the past (of drugs) and the present (of appliances and drugs).

In summary, there are a limited number of indicators of biomedical advances that can be applied in assessing the relative roles of research and other factors in reducing mortality and sickness. None of the measures are fully adequate or precise. For example, research carried out in other countries is only partially represented in the data. The journal counts include foreign periodicals. Some of the patents issued in the United States are for inventions developed abroad and the same is true of new drugs when foreign firms desire to market in the United States. The number of PhD's in the biomedical sciences is a domestic, U.S., count.

The limitations, while important, appear less serious than the optional process applied in studies carried out earlier, namely, to represent "technology" as a time trend, or as a residual factor. Perhaps even more misleading are those studies that assume that all gains in mortality, morbidity, debility, or quality of life are a result of biomedical advances without taking account of other important determinants of change in health status.

Figures 2-3- 2-7 show the growth in biomedical research activity, as indicated by the several indexes. New drugs approved for marketing by the FDA were not charted because the data do not extend back in years, and because changes in regulation and practices by FDA resulted in a break in the series.

The trend data are of several kinds. The number of PhD degrees essentially measures input into the research effort. The other indexes, patents and periodicals, are essentially process or "intermediate output" measures. ("Intermediate output" as used differentiates between the health status improvements made by biomedical research and the inventions and publications that are the means to those improvements.) Some measures, the drug and medical instrument patents, relate more closely to industrial output than to output by government and university research. The number of periodicals may evidence increasing professionalization and specialization. In the biomedical sciences, as in other disciplinary fields, the pressures to publish, as a symbol of academic performance for tenure and related purposes, are great, and access to means of publication is very important. As the number of degree holders has risen, so has the number of periodicals that are available to publish the results of new contributions to scientific knowledge.

As the several series indicate (Figures 2-3- 2-6), the nation's research effort increased in the 1920s, and a quantum rise was achieved by the creation and expansion of the National Institutes of Health and the post-World War II appropriations. Growth, indeed, was a watchword during the 1950s when an amazing set of research institutions was fashioned, institutions that have gained recognition for scientific excellence both at home and abroad.

After several decades of slow upward movement, the number of PhD's in the biomedical sciences started a major upward climb in the 1950s and rose markedly almost year by year, except for the two most recent years, in which the number declined (Figure 2-3). The turning point for growth was essentially the close of World War II.

Drug patents follow a similar historical course, with relative stability in the number of patents issued until the 1930s, when there was a marked upward movement toward a new plateau, reached about 1950. Since then, the trend has been clearly upward (Figure 2-4).

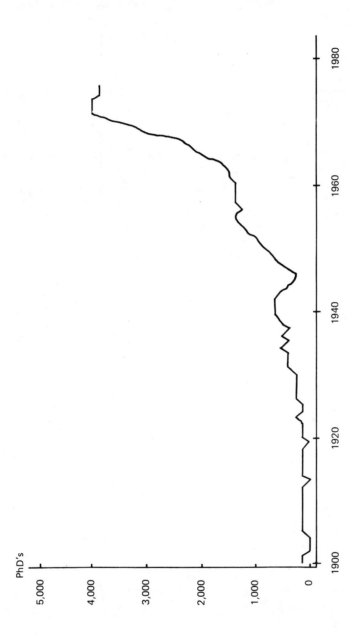

Figure 2-3. Trends in Numbers of Biomedical PhD's, 1900-76

Sources: U.S. Bureau of the Census: *Historical Statistics of the United States, Colonial Times to 1970,* Bicentennial Edition. Washington, D.C., 1975; and *Summary Reports 1975.* National Research Council, National Academy of Sciences, Washington, D.C. From 1920 on includes doctorates in basic medical sciences, medical sciences, and other biological sciences. Data before 1920 derived by assuming that a constant percentage of all doctorates were biomedical PhD's.

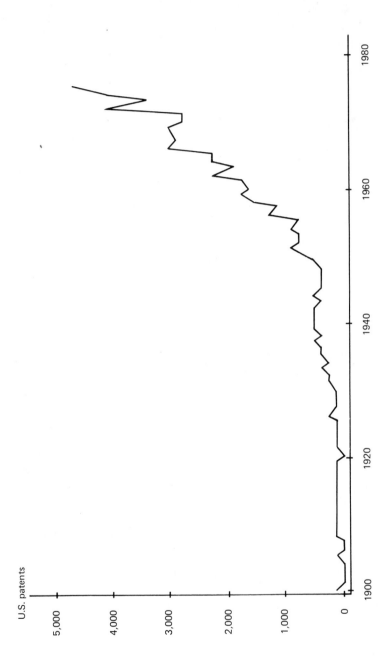

Source: U.S. Department of Commerce, Patent and Trademark Office, OTAF: Special report in response to the request of Public Services Laboratory, Georgetown University, August 1976.

Figure 2-4. Trends in Numbers of U.S. Patents Issued for Drugs and Medicine, 1900-76

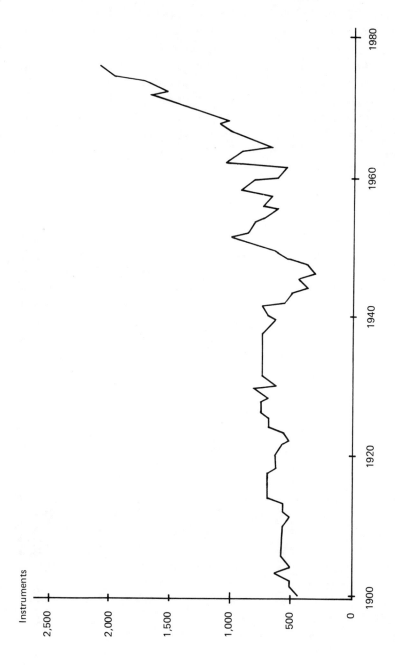

Source: U.S. Department of Commerce, Patent and Trademark Office, OTAF: Special report in response to the request of Public Services Laboratory, Georgetown University, August 1976.

Figure 2-5. Trends in Numbers of Patents for Health-related Professional and Scientific Instruments

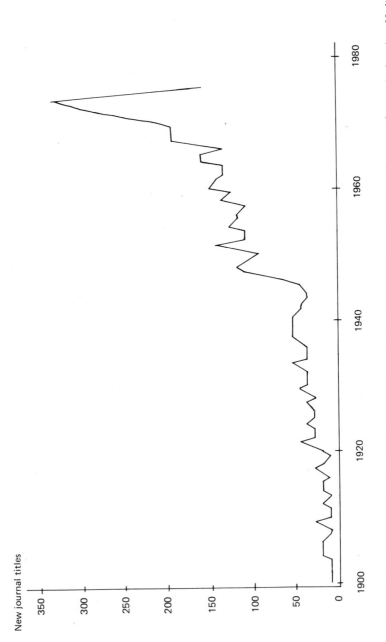

Source: M.E. Corning and M.M. Cummings: "Biomedical Communications," in J.Z. Bowers and E. Purcell (eds.), *Advances in American Medicine: Essays at the Bicentennial*, vol. 2. Josiah Macy, Jr. Foundation, New York, 1976.

Figure 2-6. Trends in Numbers of New Journal Titles Published, 1900-76

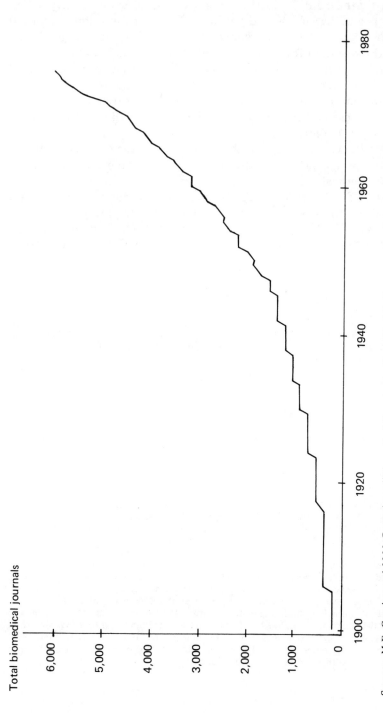

Total biomedical journals

Source: M.E. Corning and M.M. Cummings: "Biomedical Communications," in J.Z. Bowers and E. Purcell (eds.), *Advances in American Medicine: Essays at the Bicentennial*, vol. 2, Josiah Macy, Jr. Foundation, New York, 1976.

Figure 2-7. Trends in Total Numbers of Biomedical Journals Printed, 1900-76

Patents for scientific instruments show more variation. By 1976, the number of patents issued was about double the number granted per year around 1960. In contrast, the number of drug patents increased more than fourfold during this same period (Figure 2-5).

Journals in the biomedical sciences follow a trend similar to PhD degrees granted and patents issued. Although the post-World War II spurt was sharper for new journals than for the other indexes, their growth was less and their dropoff in 1975 and 1976 was greater than in other series (Figure 2-6).

While all series moved up, the growth rates vary (Tables 2-9 and 2-10). In the first decade of the century, the number of new journals in the biomedical sciences rose more rapidly than patents granted or even biomedical science degrees issued. The next decade again witnessed rapid growth in the number of new journals, and an acceleration of the rise in PhD degrees issued. The drug patent decrease in the second decade is more a result of the specific years at

Table 2-9.   Selected Indicators of Research in the Biomedical Sciences

Year	Drug patents	Instrument patents	Ph.D.'s in biomedical sciences	New biomedical journal titles	Number of biomedical journals published
1900	65	425	69	7	194
1910	82	543	80	11	319
1920	56	595	112	18	468
1930	187	630	311	30	769
1940	524	702	626	51	1,191
1950	649	800	868	95	1,859
1960	1,585	648	1,430	150	3,084
1963	1,887	907	1,611	135	3,496
1970	2,809	1,437	3,650	210	4,732
1975	4,575	2,139	3,884	157	6,064

Sources: Drug and health-related instrument patents were obtained from the Patent and Trademark Office, Department of Commerce, in an OTAF special report in response to the request of the Public Services Laboratory, Georgetown University, August 1976. The number of biomedical Ph.D.'s is the sum of Ph.D.'s awarded in basic medical sciences, medical sciences, and other biological sciences, as reported in *Historical Statistics of the United States: Colonial Times to 1970,* Bicentennial Edition. Washington, D.C., 1975, p. 387; and *Summary Reports, 1975,* of the National Research Council, National Academy of Sciences. Observations before 1920 were projected as a constant proportion of all Ph.D.'s awarded in those years. The number of new biomedical journal titles and the total number of biomedical journals published are derived from M.E. Corning and M.M. Cummings: "Biomedical Communications," in J.Z. Bowers and E. Purcell (eds.), *Advances in American Medicine: Essays at the Bicentennial,* vol. 2, Josiah Macy, Jr. Foundation, New York, 1976. Both of our journal series are lagged one year, and both are based on a series of "open SERLINE titles" as reported in Corning and Cummings.

Table 2-10. **Average of Annual Growth Rates of Indicators of Biomedical Research, in Percentages, 1900-75**

Period	Drug patents	Instrument patents	Ph.D.'s in biomedical sciences	New journals in biomedical sciences	Cumulated new journals in biomedical sciences
1900-10	2.3	2.5	1.5	4.5	5.0
1910-20	−3.8	.9	3.4	4.9	3.8
1920-30	12.1	.6	10.2	5.1	5.0
1930-40	10.3	1.1	7.0	5.3	4.4
1940-50	2.1	1.3	3.3	6.2	4.5
1950-60	8.9	−2.1	5.0	4.6	5.1
1960-63	5.8	11.2	4.0	−3.5	4.2
1963-70	5.7	6.6	11.7	6.3	4.3
1970-75	9.8	8.0	1.2	−5.8	5.0
1900-30	3.5	1.3	5.0	4.9	4.6
1930-63	7.0	1.1	5.0	4.6	4.6
1963-75	7.4	7.1	7.3	1.3	4.6
1930-75	7.1	2.7	5.6	3.7	4.6

the beginning and end dates of the decade than of the whole decade. Generally, the movement was slightly up rather than down, but in some years relatively few patents were issued. The 1920s saw a rapid growth in drug patents and in PhD's; the peak growth rates for drug patents were attained in that decade. This rapid growth occurred again between 1970 and 1975. The peak for PhD's occurred during the period 1963-70, the time when the largest numbers of college-age students were passing through the educational pipeline. The rate of growth then exceeded by 1.5 percentage points the rise in degrees awarded during the period 1920-30.

Biomedical research, as we know it today, is largely a post-World War II phenomenon. It flourished during the 1950s, 1960s, and 1970s, despite stability in federal funding for several of the early years in the 1970s. A more recently recorded drop is undoubtedly due to persons turning away from the biomedical sciences because of the lack of real substantial growth.

The outlook for biomedical research, as we indicated at the outset, is far from plain. There are diverse forces at work that could lead to another quantum jump in the magnitude of research. However, there are also forces that could constrain the aggregate to levels that provide little real advance when price impacts are taken into account.

In Chapter 6, the question of biomedical research priorities is discussed.

APPENDIX

Table 2A-1. Estimated Biomedical Research Expenditures, Fiscal Year 1900-68, Actual Expenditures, 1946-68 and Related Data Series

Year	Actual biomedical research expenditures (in millions of constant dollars)	Biomedical price index (1975=100) N	Estimated biomedical expenditures (in millions of current dollars)	(in millions of constant dollars)	Composite index of biomedical research effort
1900		11.1	0.157	1.4	0.352
1901		11.0	0.176	1.6	0.368
1902		11.4	0.206	1.8	0.391
1903		11.5	0.238	2.1	0.415
1904		11.7	0.281	2.4	0.443
1905		12.0	0.325	2.7	0.470
1906		12.3	0.375	3.1	0.497
1907		12.9	0.437	5.4	0.527
1908		12.7	0.510	4.0	0.562
1909		13.3	0.556	4.1	0.581
1910		13.6	0.628	4.6	0.610
1911		13.5	0.715	5.3	0.643
1912		14.1	0.785	5.6	0.667
1913		14.0	0.819	5.8	0.678
1914		14.3	0.878	6.1	0.697
1915		15.0	0.978	6.5	0.728
1916		17.0	1.093	6.4	0.761
1917		21.4	1.238	5.8	0.800
1918		24.3	1.381	5.7	0.835
1919		28.0	1.609	5.7	0.888
1920		32.2	2.080	6.5	0.983
1921		26.4	2.470	9.4	1.053

Year						
1922	24.2	2.810	11.6	1.108		
1923	24.8	3.350	13.5	1.189		
1924	24.8	3.826	15.4	1.253		
1925	25.1	4.354	17.3	1.319		
1926	24.7	5.088	20.6	1.404		
1927	24.7	5.964	24.1	1.495		
1928	24.1	7.018	29.1	1.595		
1929	24.5	8.381	34.2	1.712		
1930	24.0	10.018	41.7	1.838		
1931	23.7	12.453	52.5	2.004		
1932	21.4	15.221	71.1	2.171		
1933	19.1	18.112	94.8	2.327		
1934	18.0	21.112	117.3	2.473		
1935	20.1	24.450	121.6	2.622		
1936	20.3	28.131	138.6	2.772		
1937	20.4	31.429	154.1	2.897		
1938	21.3	34.482	161.9	3.006		
1939	21.1	37.392	177.2	3.104		
1940	20.5	38.742	189.0	3.149		
1941	21.1	39.889	189.1	3.185		
1942	22.9	41.422	189.0	3.234		
1943	25.6	44.415	173.5	3.325		
1944	26.8	50.248	187.5	3.492		
1945	27.4	58.031	211.8	3.698		
1946	28.1	69.06	245.8	3.963	281	79
1947	32.7	81.74	250.0	4.238	266	87
1948	37.4	99.48	266.0	4.583	332	124
1949	40.2	115.13	286.4	4.857	366	147

Table 2A-1 continued

Year	Actual biomedical research expenditures		Biomedical price index (1975=100) N	Estimated biomedical expenditures		Composite index of biomedical research effort
	(in millions of current dollars)	(in millions of constant dollars)		(in millions of current dollars)	(in millions of constant dollars)	
1950	161	406	39.7	143.79	362.2	5.306
1951	175	431	40.6	172.26	424.3	5.702
1952	197	452	43.6	208.37	477.9	6.150
1953	214	484	44.2	259.04	686.1	6.707
1954	237	528	44.9	313.30	697.8	7.234
1955	261	572	45.6	374.65	821.6	7.768
1956	312	670	46.6	471.83	1,012.5	8.514
1957	440	913	48.2	541.01	1,122.4	8.991
1958	543	1,088	49.9	639.60	1,281.8	9.610
1959	648	1,276	50.8	732.34	1,442.6	10.145
1960	932	1,792	52.0	869.59	1,672.3	10.860
1961	1,129	2,163	52.2	1,020.36	1,954.7	11.573
1962	1,372	2,569	53.4	1,107.68	2,074.3	11.958
1963	1,561	2,859	54.6	1,254.39	2,298.3	12.567
1964	1,730	3,089	56.0	1,425.58	2,545.7	13.221
1965	1,925	3,336	57.7	1,563.41	2,709.5	13.716
1966	2,147	3,590	59.8	1,888.42	3,157.9	14.786
1967	2,380	3,808	62.5	2,092.51	3,348.0	15.403
1968	2,600	3,969	65.5	2,398.58	3,662.0	16.263

Sources: Biomedical research expenditures are from *NIH Almanac, 1976*, DHEW Publication No. (NIH) 76-5, p. 125, and *Basic Data Relating to the National Institutes of Health, 1978*. The biomedical research price deflator is the index computed by S.A. Jaffe and R. Valiant: Biomedical Research and Development Price Indexes, 1961-1976. Rockville, Westat, Inc., 1977 (revised 1978). Figures before 1961 were extrapolated based on trends in the GNP price deflator and using a regression equation of the Westat index on the GNP deflator for the years 1961-75 in double logarithmic form. The regression estimate is

$$\text{Ln(Westat)} = -.30973 + 1.07291 \ \text{Ln(GNP deflator)}$$
$$(38.79)$$

$$R^2 = .992$$

Estimates of biomedical research expenditures for the 1900-45 period were computed from a regression equation of actual expenditures on a composite index of biomedical research effort over the 1946-65 period. The index of biomedical research effort is composed of an average of standardized values of the stock of Ph.D.'s in the biosciences, the number of drug patents in the succeeding seven years, and the number of biomedical journals published. The regression equation is

$$\text{Ln(Biomedical research expenditures)} = .77 + 2.51 \ \text{(LnBiomedical research effort)}$$

$$R^2 = .959$$

where the estimated equation is adjusted (20.46) for first order autocorrelation using a variant of the Cochrane-Orcutt procedure. Since data on the components of the composite index of biomedical research effort do exist back to 1900, this estimating equation can be used to project biomedical research expenditures back to 1900. Data on drug patents were obtained from a special tabulation conducted by the U.S. Patent Office. Biomedical Ph.D.'s are available back in *Historical Statistics of the United States, Colonial Times to 1970*, Volume I, p. 387, and biomedical journals are compiled from M.E. Corning and M.M. Cummings: "Biomedical Communications" in J.C. Bowers and E. Purcell (eds.), *Advances in American Medicine: Essays at the Bicentennial*, vol. 2, Josiah Macy, Jr. Foundation, New York, 1976.

Table 2A-2. Health Research Expenditures, Fiscal Year 1976-77
(dollars in millions)

Year	Expenditures (in current dollars)	Biomedical price index 1975=100	Expenditures (in constant dollars)
1946	$ 79	28.1	$ 281.1
1947	87	32.7	266.1
1948	124	37.4	331.6
1949	147	40.2	365.7
1950	161	39.7	405.5
1951	175	40.6	431.0
1952	197	43.6	451.8
1953	214	44.2	484.2
1954	237	44.9	527.8
1955	261	45.6	572.4
1956	312	46.6	669.5
1957	440	48.2	912.9
1958	543	49.9	1,088.2
1959	648	50.8	1,275.6
1960	932	52.0	1,792.3
1961	1,129	52.2	2,162.8
1962	1,372	53.4	2,569.3
1963	1,561	54.6	2,859.0
1964	1,730	56.0	3,089.3
1965	1,925	57.7	3,336.2
1966	2,147	59.8	3,590.3
1967	2,380	62.5	3,808.0
1968	2,600	65.5	3,969.5
1969	2,806	68.9	4,072.6
1970	2,856	73.3	3,896.3
1971	3,162	77.5	4,080.0
1972	3,515	81.3	4,323.5
1973	3,734	85.1	4,387.8
1974	4,415	90.3	4,889.3
1975	4,640	100.0	4,640.0
1976	4,988	107.3	4,648.6
1977	5,526	116.4	4,747.4

Sources: Research expenditures are from *NIH Almanac 1976*, DHEW Publication No. (HRA) 76-5, p. 125, and *Basic Data Relating to the National Institutes of Health, 1978*, DHEW, table 1. The biomedical research price deflator is the index computed by S.A. Jaffe and R. Valiant: Biomedical Research and Development Price Indexes, 1961-1976. Rockville, Westat, Inc., 1977 (revised 1978). Figures before 1961 were extrapolated based on trends in the GNP price deflator and using a regression equation of the Westat index on the GNP deflator for the years 1961-75 in double logarithmic form. The regression estimate is

$$\text{Ln(Westat)} = -.30973 + 1.07291 \quad \text{Ln(GNP deflator)}$$
$$(38.79)$$

$R^2 = .992.$

REFERENCES

1. U.S. Department of Health, Education, and Welfare: Report of the President's Biomedical Research Panel. Appendix A. The place of biomedical

science in medicine and the state of the science. DHEW Publication No. (OS) 76-501, Washington, D.C., April 30, 1976.

2. National Institutes of Health: National conference on health research principles. Background papers. Bethesda, Md., Oct. 3-4, 1978.

3. Report of the National Conservation Commission, Vol. III. U.S. Senate Document No. 676, 60th Congress, 2nd sess., Washington, D.C., February 1909.

4. Quoted in Press, F.: Remarks at the AAAS Colloquium on R&D Policy. Washington, D.C., June 20, 1978, p. 10.

5. National Science Foundation: Survey of science research series NSF 77-326. An analysis of federal R&D funding. Washington, D.C. (undated).

6. Shapley, W.H., and Phillips, D.I.: Research and development AAAS Report III. AAAS, Washington, D.C., 1978, p. 17.

7. Press, F.: Remarks at the manufacturing chemists association. Panel discussion on the innovation gap. New York, Nov. 21, 1978.

8. Steelman, J.R.: The nation's medical research. *In* Science and Public Policy by the President's Scientific Research Board, Washington, D.C., Oct. 18, 1947, p. 86.

9. Dunlop, D.W.: Returns to biomedical research in chronic diseases: a case study of resource allocation. *In* Health: what is it worth?, edited by S.J. Mushkin and D.W. Dunlop. Pergamon Press, Elmsford, N.Y., 1979.

10. Illich, I.: Medical nemesis. Pantheon, New York, 1976.

11. Banta, H.D., and Thacker, S.B.: The premature delivery of medical technology: a case report. National Center for Health Services Research Announcement, Hyattsville, Md., Dec. 3, 1978.

12. Sec. 309 of Public Law 95-623, Nov. 9, 1978.

13. Bunker, J., Mosteller, F., and Barnes, B.: Costs, risks, and benefits of surgery. Oxford University Press, New York, 1976.

14. Feinstein, A.R.: Clinical biostatistics. A survey of statistical procedures in 25 leading medical journals. Clinical Pharmacology and Therapeutics 15: 97, 1974.

15. Gifford, R.H., and Feinstein, A.R.: A critique of methodology in studies of anticoagulants therapy for acute myocardial infarction. New England Journal of Medicine 280:351-357, Feb. 13, 1969.

16. Schimmel, E.M.: The hazards of hospitalization. Annals Internal Medicine 60:100, January 1964.

17. Pharmaceutical Manufacturers Association: Preliminary facts and figures. Pharmaceutical Manufacturers Association, Washington, D.C., 1979.

18. McGee, W.J.: Hearings before the Committee on Interstate and Foreign Commerce of the House of Representatives. Bills to establish a Department of Commerce, Labor, Industries and Manufacture, March 31, 1902, p. 129.

19. Lester, R.M.: 40 years of Carnegie giving. Carnegie Corporation of New York, New York, 1941.

20. Karter, T.: Voluntary agency expenditures for health and welfare from philanthropic contributions, 1930-55. Soc Sec Bull, February 1958, p. 2.

21. Nicolson, D.W.: 20 years of medical research. National TB Association, New York, 1943.

22. Reports: Science 71:191, Feb. 14, 1930.

23. Medical news. Journal of the AMA 88:489, Feb. 12, 1927.

24. Horstfall, F.L., Jr.: Federal support of biomedical sciences. *In* National Academy of Sciences, Basic research and national goals. Report to the U.S. House of Representatives Committee on Science and Astronautics, 1965.

25. Hughes, R.M.: Research a natural resource. Vol. I. National Resources Commission, U.S. Government Printing Office, Washington, D.C., 1939.

26. National Resources Committee: 76th Cong., 1st sess., H.R. Doc. 122, U.S. Government Printing Office, Washington, D.C., 1939.

27. WPA: Report to the President of the United States showing the financial status of funds provided in the emergency relief appropriation acts of December 31, 1937, table VIIIB, p. 169.

28. Auerbach, Lewis E.: Scientists in the new deal: a prewar episode in the relations between science and government in the United States. Minerva 3:457-482, winter 1965.

29. Shryock, R.H.: American medical research, past and present. The Commonwealth Fund, New York, 1947, p. 90.

30. Strickland, S.: Politics, science, and dread disease. Harvard University Press, Cambridge, 1972.

31. Udden, J.A.: Research funds in the United States. Science Magazine, Jan. 13, 1922. (Based on bulletin of National Research Council of March 1921, which reports funds available for scientific research compiled by Callie Hull.)

32. Pharmaceutical Manufacturers Association: Sales and R&D expenditures, 1950-69. Pharmaceutical Manufacturers Association, Washington, D.C., 1970.

33. Pharmaceutical Manufacturers Association: Applied research and development, 1966 drugs by therapeutic purposes. Pharmaceutical Manufacturers Association, Washington, D.C., 1966.

34. Swaine, D.C.: The rise of a research empire. Science 138:1233-1237, December 1962.

35. U.S. Budget documents, 1920-30. U.S. Government Printing Office, Washington, D.C., annual.

36. Lindsay, D.R., and Allen, E.M.: Medical research: past support, future directions. Science 134:2017-2024, December 22, 1961.

37. U.S. statutes at large (1935), No. XLIX, p. 635.

38. U.S. Public Health Service: Annual report of the federal security agency. U.S. Government Printing Office, Washington, D.C., 1945, p. XV.

39. National Institutes of Health: Basic data, 1963. Office of Program Planning, OD, NIH, Bethesda, Md., 1963.

40. Young, J.H.: The medical messiahs. Princeton University Press, Princeton, 1967.

41. Price, D. de S.: General theory of bibliometric and other cumulative advantage processes. Journal American Society Information Sciences 27(5-6): 292-306, September 1976.

42. Krause, T.K., and Hillinger, C.: Citations, references, and the growth of scientific literature: a model of dynamic interaction. Journal American Society Information Sciences 22:333-336, September 1971.

43. Brooks, H.: The problem of research priorities. Daedalus 107:182, 184, spring 1978.

Chapter Three

Deaths As an Assessment Indicator

Until recently, mortality was the main index for determining need for additional health care resources (for setting priorities among health programs). Major policies were addressed to reducing mortality, and the criterion for judging the effectiveness of programs was the decrease in mortality rates.

At present, reported mortality is neither a useful measure of need for program action nor a criterion for assessing program effectiveness. Mortality rates today are relatively insensitive to the changes in medical care and advances in medical technology. The progress that has already been made in prolonging life is responsible for the insensitivity of mortality indexes.

In this chapter, we first examine trends in mortality from 1900 to the year 2000, by age and disease; second, we review briefly the methodology used, including the methods for forecasting the future; and third, we discuss optional standards for health status indicators that recognize the advances in medical knowledge in addition to other factors that contribute to declining mortality.

TRENDS IN MORTALITY

The dramatic reduction in mortality is well known. The age-adjusted death rate was 17.8 per 1,000 persons in 1900. By 1930, it had declined to 12.5 per 1,000, and by 1976 it was 6.3 per 1,000. These age-adjusted rates eliminate the impact on deaths of changes in the age distribution of the population, or, stated differently, the ages of the populations in each year are standardized.

A death rate decline of such magnitude affects the very fiber of society. The perspective of the future changes, freedom of movement is enhanced, and attitudes toward children and family are altered. The existence of large populations in crowded metropolitan areas is a result of past progress in health care, as evidenced by improvement in mortality indexes. A profound change in the human condition has been brought about by the extension of life and a reduction in uncertainty about survival from one year to the next.

The historical decline in age-adjusted death rates from 1900 to 1976 is shown in Figure 3-1. From the 1950s to 1970, little change occurred; the age-adjusted death rate declined only fractionally. Yet, this stability took place in the face of mounting outlays for health and biomedical research. Between the mid-1950s and 1970, for example, national expenditures for health services rose $51.9 billion, from $17.3 billion in 1955 to $69.2 billion in 1970, and biomedical research expenditures rose from $260 million to $2.7 billion.

In Chapter 4, we examine the relationship between biomedical research and mortality that suggests the lagged effect of such research on death rates. Other investigators have attempted to assess the contribution of medical services to changes in mortality. Auster and associates,[1] for example, found that for each 1 percent rise in health expenditures, death rates are lowered by one-tenth of 1 percent. Real health expenditures per capita from 1955 to 1965 rose 35 percent, which, according to their analysis, should have produced a 3.5 percent decline in mortality, other factors remaining unchanged. Auster and associates stated: "Our results, then, would imply that adverse environmental factors have been offsetting the advantages of increases in the quantity and quality of medical care."[1a] The study findings of Illich,[2] the McKinlays,[3] Hemminki and Paakkulainen,[4] Kass,[5] Dubos,[6] and others dispute the efficacy of medical care in postponing deaths.

As the data make clear, age-adjusted death rates have more recently shown a downturn. Death rates in 1976 were some 15 percent below those of a decade earlier. However, although the recent downward movement is favorable, it hardly matches the large declines of years ago.

Age-adjusted death rates tell the story from one perspective, life expectancy numbers tell it from another. Average life expectancy has risen between 1900 and today by more than twenty-five years. Stated differently, the average life span has risen by more than 50 percent in the first three-quarters of this century. Figure 3-2 shows the average life expectancy data over the years, recording the great

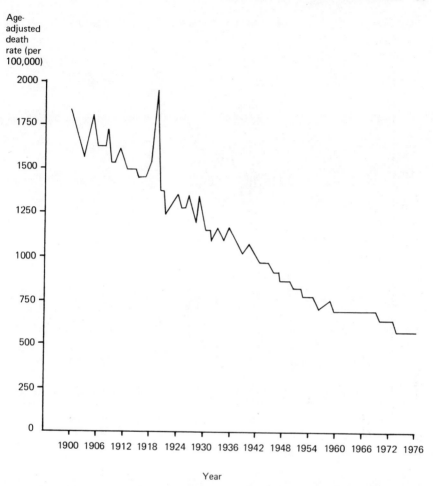

Age-adjusted death rate (per 100,000)

Year

Sources: "Death Rates by Age, Race, and Sex, United States, 1900-1953: All Causes." *Vital Statistics-Special Reports,* Vol. 43, No. 1, January 9, 1956; various annual issues of the *Vital Statistics of the United States, Volume II–Mortality–Part A.* National Center for Health Statistics, Washington, D.C.; and unpublished data from the National Center for Health Statistics, Washington, D.C.

Figure 3-1. Trend in Age-adjusted Death Rate per 100,000 Population, All Causes, 1900-76

changes that have moved life expectancy at birth from forty-seven years in 1900 to seventy-two years in 1975. About half of the twenty-five-year increase in life expectancy took place between 1900 and 1930; an additional ten years of life expectancy were added by

A. *Life Expectancy at Birth*

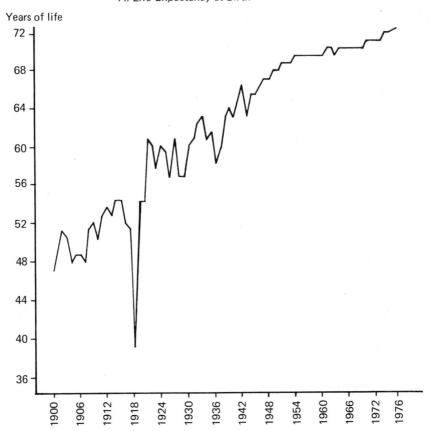

B. *Average Remaining Years of Life at Selected Ages,
Selected Years, 1900-1975*

Age	1900	1930	1963	1975
At birth	47.3	59.7	69.9	72.5
40	28.4	30.4	33.9	35.7
50	21.3	22.5	25.2	27.0
60	14.8	15.4	17.7	19.3

Sources: U.S. Bureau of the Census: *Historical Statistics of the United States, Colonial Times to 1970,* Bicentennial Edition. Washington, D.C., 1975; and U.S. Bureau of the Census: *Statistical Abstract of the United States, 1977.* Washington, D.C., 1977.

Figure 3-2. Life Expectancy, 1900-76

1963, and the remaining approximately two and one-half years, since 1963.

Figures 3-1 and 3-2 depict the marked effect of the 1918 influenza epidemic. Death rates rose sharply and life expectancy dropped.

A rise in average years of life of the magnitude this nation and others in the western world have experienced represents a change so fundamental that the full-scale societal effects are difficult to judge. However, human hopes, aspirations, and expectations have expanded. Medical science, as a contributing factor in the successes of the past, has been an integral component of those expectations. Certainly few, even Illich,[2] would dispute that better knowledge about health and hygiene has made some difference in mortality.

Profile of Age at Death

Most dramatic in the historical improvement in human life expectancy is the gain in reduced deaths among infants and young children. Over the years, the age of those who die has progressively become older.

There are various ways to show the gains in reduced mortality. Figure 3-3 shows the death rates and declines in death rates per 1,000 population in each age group for the years 1900, 1930, 1963, and 1975. The large gains are for infants under one year of age and for the one- to four-year-olds, especially from 1900 to 1930 when environmental sanitation was improved and educational levels raised. The drop in death rates in the older age groups came between 1930 and 1963—the "miracle medicine" years.

The curve representing mortality rates by age in 1900 was clearly U-shaped, with a high death rate of 185.5 per 1,000 for infants, dropping to a low at ages five to fourteen, and then rising with advancing age to 258.5 per 1,000 at ages eighty-five and over. The U-shape of the curve is moderated by the sharp drop in death rates among the young age groups in the seventy-five-year period. The reduction in infant mortality shows up dramatically. Less dramatic, but still significant, is the upward turn of death rates at later and later ages. The age at which death rates increase has advanced progressively over the years, until in 1975 there was little increase until ages thirty-five to forty-five, a sharper rise between fifty-five and sixty-five, and further acceleration of rates after age sixty-five.

Infant Mortality

Infant mortality rates are used more often than other mortality rates to judge the results of past health programs and to define new program needs. While the infant mortality rate is not a sufficiently comprehensive index, it is often the most sensitive statistical indi-

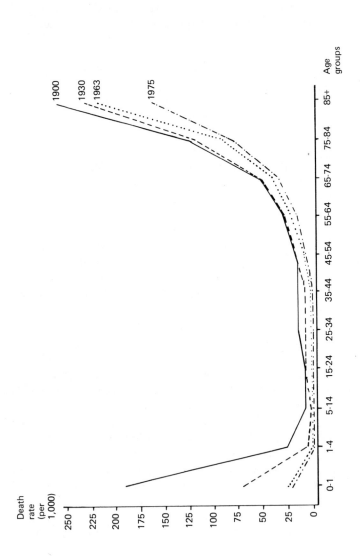

Figure 3-3. Age-specific Death Rates, by Age, Selected Years, 1900-75

Sources: F.E. Linder and R.D. Grove: *Vital Statistics Rates in the United States 1900-1940.* National Office of Vital Statistics, Washington, D.C., 1947; *Vital Statistics of the United States, 1963,* Vol. II, Mortality, Part A. National Center for Health Statistics, Washington, D.C., 1965; and "Annual Summary for the United States, 1976." *Monthly Vital Statistics Report,* Vol. 25, No. 13, December 12, 1977, National Center for Health Statistics, Hyattsville, Maryland.

cator available. Comparison of infant mortality among nations and population groups has provided standards for questioning health program deficiencies and proposing new policies. Early child and maternal health programs, before World War I and in the 1930s when a new child and maternal health program was proposed as part of the Social Security Act of 1935, looked to infant death rates as the main index of need. During the years of President Johnson's Great Society, important maternal and child health programs were identi-- fied as necessary correctives for disparities in infant mortality between states, races, and counties.

Wholey, in analyzing various infant health care programs in 1966, computed, for example, the number of infant lives that would have been saved in the United States at rates prevailing in Sweden and Great Britain.[7] Indicators of "unnecessary" infant deaths were computed from the disparities among the states and between races; excess infant death numbers were displayed with excess defined as deaths that would not have occurred if an infant mortality of 18.3 per 1,000 had prevailed instead of the actual rate.

In the mid-1960s, the death rate of infants was 24.8 per 1,000 live births. No comparison can be made with 1900 because at that time births were not recorded. However, in 1915, the first year when births were registered, of every 1,000 live-born infants, 100 died.

At the turn of the twentieth century, public health measures taken to control milk supplies, water systems, and sanitation had much to do with the reduction of diarrheal and other infectious diseases in infants. Among other things, public health workers were becoming aware of the insect as a carrier of disease, and dissemination of this information was just beginning. In 1909, Howard, in a report of the 1908 National Conservation Commission, stated that flies can be propagators of typhoid, cholera, and other infectious diseases, that rat fleas transmit the plague, and that mosquitoes carry malarial germs.[8] Another portion of this report announced that in Washington, D.C., owing to the enactment of a new law in 1895 regulating the sale of milk, the death rate from diarrhea and inflammation of the bowels among children under two years of age was reduced from 160 to 97 by 1906.[9]

In the intervening years, infant mortality from dysentery and digestive diseases was successfully controlled. By the mid-1960s, the correctives for the comparatively high U.S. infant mortality rate changed from environmental public health measures to provision of health care for poor mothers, including family planning. But this approach had a historical antecedent. A study by the Children's Bureau covering 1911 to 1915 examined the factors affecting infant mortality in eight cities.[10] The study showed a high correlation between the health of mothers and the rate of mortality of children. Among infants whose mothers died during the first year after childbirth, the death rate was four times the rate of those whose mothers survived. In addition to health of mothers, the study examined other factors, such as the differential impact on infant survival of prematurity, use of instruments at birth, artificial feedings, and mothers' ages. The study found a marked correlation between economic status and infant mortality.

Such early studies pointed to the large margin of improvement in health within the scope of existing medical knowledge. They re-emphasized the social context of medicine and the advances required in societal relationships and reduction in poverty to decrease "unnecessary" deaths. (The standards of unnecessary or premature deaths are discussed more fully later in this chapter.)

Mortality of Children

Epidemic diseases and accidents contributed importantly to the death rate of children at the beginning of the twentieth century. It was expected then that one-quarter of the children would die before reaching adulthood. In 1900, few families were free of the burdens of epidemic and often fatal diseases, such as diphtheria, whooping cough, measles, typhoid, and scarlet fever. In view of the high death rates, it is difficult to understand the slowness of the introduction of vaccines and immunization and the lags in political action to control water, food, and milk supplies. The 1900 census reported 3,500 deaths from smallpox in the United States, for example, yet in Denmark, by 1826, not a single case had appeared for a number of years.[11]

The decline of death rates in the age groups one to four and five to nine over the past decades has been far greater than declines in older age groups as the infectious and communicable diseases, particularly the childhood diseases, have been brought under control. As the data suggest, much of the improvement in child mortality was achieved between 1900 and 1930, although there were further gains between 1930 and 1963.

Today the main cause of death among children is accidents.

Concentration of Deaths by Age

The age distribution of total deaths represents still another method of showing the progress of the past and the reasons for anticipating less change in mortality for the future. Figure 3-4 shows the percentage of all deaths in each of the selected years that were accounted for by the deaths of persons sixty-five to seventy-four

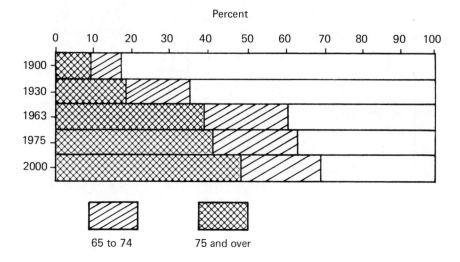

Percent

Sources: F.E. Linder and R.D. Grove, *Vital Statistics Rates in the United States 1900-1940.* National Office of Vital Statistics, Washington, D.C., 1947; *Vital Statistics of the United States, 1963,* Vol. II, Mortality, Part A. National Center for Health Statistics, Washington, D.C., 1965; unpublished data from the National Center for Health Statistics, Washington, D.C.; and S.J. Mushkin and D.P. Wagner: *Expected Mortality as a Criterion in Health Policy Evaluation.* Paper delivered at the Annual Meeting of the American Public Health Association, October 15, 1978 (processed).

Figure 3-4. Percent of All Deaths of Persons Aged 65 to 74 and 75 and over

years old and those seventy-five and older. In 1900, almost four of every ten deaths occurred in the under-five age group, and 45 percent of all deaths occurred in the under-fifteen age group. Only 17 percent of all deaths were among those sixty-five years and over. By 1930, major improvements in infant and child mortality shifted the age distribution of deaths to the older age groups. More than one-third of the deaths in 1930 were among persons sixty-five years and over. By 1975, the 1900 age profile was essentially reversed. Almost 65 percent of all deaths were among those sixty-five years and over, and 40 percent of all deaths were among those seventy-five years and over. A further postponement of death is indicated by the year 2000 estimates derived from a special study in which experts were asked their views about death rates by age and sex.[1,2]

Deaths by Cause

Progress in medicine and public health is reflected in the altered distribution of deaths by disease category. Several characteristics of the historical gains are underscored in the statistics presented in Figures 3-5 and 3-6 and Tables 3-1 and 3-2.

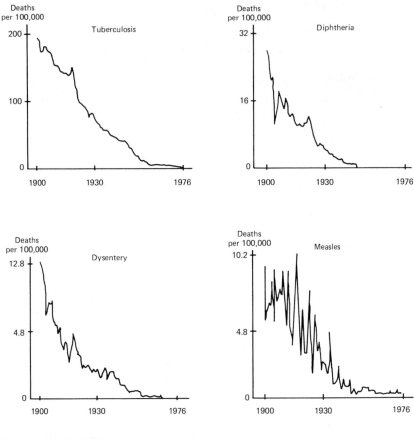

Sources: See Table 3-2.

Figure 3-5. Trends in Death Rates Due to Selected Infectious Diseases

First, the infective and parasitic diseases have been brought under control. In 1900, deaths from tuberculosis represented more than 10 percent of the total deaths; by 1975, tuberculosis deaths accounted for 0.2 of 1 percent of all deaths. Diphtheria, typhoid fever, and other infectious diseases are no longer major killers in the United States. As Table 3-1 indicates, gains in death reduction for the infective and parasitic diseases were made primarily before 1963, when major emphasis was placed on research on isolation of the bacteria causing a disease, on developing vaccines, and on public health environmental measures and related personal hygiene.

Mortality data, analyzed by Fisher for the years 1900-05,[9] indicated the prominence of diseases (as percentage of all deaths) as follows:

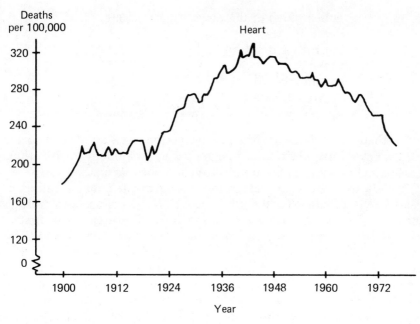

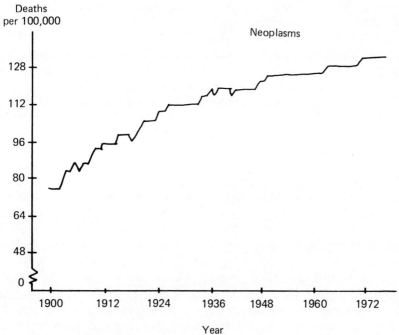

Sources: See Table 3-2.

Figure 3-6. Trends in Heart and Cancer Deaths, 1900-76

Tuberculosis of the lungs	9.9
Heart disease	8.1
Diarrhea and enteritis	7.7
Violence	7.5
Pneumonia	7.0
Bright's disease	5.6
Apoplexy	4.4

More than half of the deaths of that period were attributed to the causes listed. An additional 9 percent were attributed to ill-defined causes, including heart failure, dropsy, and convulsions.

Trends in the disease categories among the ten major causes of death help to identify the historical shift in disease patterns, as shown in Table 3-2. Major cardiovascular-renal diseases rank first in age-adjusted death rates in each of the four selected historical periods. Tuberculosis, ranking second in 1900, declined in relative importance by 1930 to fifth place but was no longer one of the ten leading killers by 1963. Influenza and pneumonia ranked third in 1900, fourth in 1930, and, despite the sharp decline in age-adjusted death rates between 1930 and 1963, influenza and pneumonia maintained fourth place in order of importance as causes of death in 1963, dropping to sixth place by 1975.

Accidents from all causes ranked eighth in 1900, advanced to fifth place in 1930 (when motor vehicle accidents were included), to fourth in 1963, and to third place by 1975. Cirrhosis of the liver and suicide appear as major causes of death only since 1963.

Figure 3-5 illustrates the historical decline in age-adjusted death rate for four selected diseases: tuberculosis, diphtheria, dysentery, and measles. The downward slopes in death rates are clearly evident. Many factors contributed to the declines, including better nutrition, housing, and working conditions, higher incomes, and improved medical knowledge, care, and public health work.

The advent of the sulfa drugs in the late 1930s and of penicillin in the 1940s led to the new "miracle" drug age and contributed to further reductions in death rates. A wide range of diseases responded to the new drugs, including syphilis, tuberculosis, nephritis, scarlet fever, and pneumonia.

The control of chronic diseases has been far less successful. Heart diseases (including renal disease) and cancer now account for more than 60 percent of total deaths. In contrast, in 1900 fewer than 4 percent of the deaths were attributed to cancer and 15 percent to heart diseases (including renal disease). Importantly, the kinds of diseases of the heart also have changed. The most prevalent heart

Table 3-1. Percentage of All Deaths Caused by Selected Infectious
and Chronic Diseases, Selected Years, 1900-75

Disease category (ICDA-8)	1900	1930	1963	1975
Selected acute diseases				
Diphtheria (032)	1.9	0.4	0.0	0.0
Typhoid (001)	1.8	0.4	0.0	0.0
Gastritis, duodenitis, enteritis, and colitis (008, 009, 535, 561, 563)	5.5	1.5	0.3	0.2[1]
Tuberculosis (010-019)	10.7	6.0	0.5	0.2
Influenza and pneumonia (470-486)	10.4	8.0	4.1	2.9
Selected chronic diseases				
Cardiovascular-renal (390-429, 440-458, 582-584)	15.0	31.4	35.2	41.9
Cancer (140-209)	3.5	8.4	15.8	19.3
Cerebrovascular (430-438)	7.1	9.0	10.9	10.3
Diabetes (250)	0.4	0.9	1.8	1.9
Cirrhosis (571)	0.4	0.4	1.2	1.7
Other diseases	43.3	33.6	30.2	21.6
Total	100.0	100.0	100.0	100.0

[1] Comparability ratio from the Seventh ICDA (Disease Nos. 543, 471, 472) to the Eighth ICDA (Disease Nos. 008, 009, 535, 561, 563) was estimated to be .643 by linear extrapolation.

Sources: Crude death rate by cause data for earlier years were adjusted to the Eighth ICDA Code by use of the comparability ratios published in "Comparability of Mortality Statistics for the Seventh and Eighth Revisions of the International Classification of Diseases, United States," Series 2, No. 66. National Center for Health Statistics, Rockville, Maryland, October 1975; "Comparability of Mortality Statistics for the Sixth and Seventh Revisions, United States, 1958." National Center for Health Statistics, *Vital Statistics-Special Reports, Selected Studies,* Vol. 51, No. 3, Washington, D.C., March 1965; "Comparability Ratios Based on Mortality Statistics for the Fifth and Sixth Revisions, United States, 1950." *Vital Statistics-Special Reports, Selected Studies,* Vol. 51, No. 3, February 1964; and "Comparison of Cause of Death Assignments by the 1929 and 1938 Revisions of the International List of Deaths in the United States, 1940." *Vital Statistics-Special Reports,* Vol. 19, No. 4, June 14, 1944. Crude death rate data for all diseases and by disease category were obtained from F.E. Linder and R.D. Grove, *Vital Statistics Rates in the United States, 1900-1940.* National Office of Vital Statistics, Washington, D.C., 1947; *Vital Statistics of the United States, 1963,* Vol. II, Mortality, Part A. National Center for Health Statistics, Washington, D.C., 1965; and "Annual Summary for the United States, 1976." *Monthly Vital Statistics Report,* Vol. 25, No. 13, December 12, 1977, National Center for Health Statistics, Hyattsville, Maryland.

diseases now are those associated with middle or old age—high blood pressure and hardening of the arteries, including coronary artery disease. Heart diseases of young persons, such as disease associated with rheumatic fever, have been checked substantially.

Table 3-2.   Age-Adjusted Death Rates per 100,000 Population, Ten Major Causes of Death,[1] Selected Years, 1900-75 (in order from cause of most deaths to cause of fewest deaths)

1900	Age-adjusted death rates per 100,000	1930	Age-adjusted death rates per 100,000
Major cardiovascular-renal disease[2]	314.5	Major cardiovascular-renal disease[2]	420.7
Tuberculosis	189.1	Cerebrovascular disease	121.4
Influenza and pneumonia	185.0	Neoplasms	111.1
Cerebrovascular disease	153.2	Influenza and pneumonia	95.5
Symptoms and ill-defined conditions	121.0	Tuberculosis	70.8
Neoplasms	75.8	Accidents (not including motor vehicles)	45.8
Gastritis, duodenitis, enteritis, colitis	74.5	Symptoms and ill-defined conditions	31.3
Accidents	61.0	Accidents—motor vehicle	27.7
Typhoid	31.2	Appendicitis and hernia	21.9
Diphtheria	27.8	Gastritis, duodenitis, enteritis, colitis	15.6

1963	Age-adjusted death rates per 100,000	1975	Age-adjusted death rates per 100,000
Major cardiovascular-renal disease[2]	317.9	Major cardiovascular-renal disease[2]	243.8
Neoplasms	127.0	Neoplasms	130.9
Cerebrovascular disease	75.9	Cerebrovascular disease	54.5
Influenza and pneumonia	28.9	Accidents (not including motor vehicle)	23.5
Accidents (not including motor vehicle)	24.6	Accidents—motor vehicle	21.3
Accidents—motor vehicle	24.1	Influenza and pneumonia	16.6
Diabetes mellitus	13.8	Cirrhosis of the liver	13.8
Cirrhosis of the liver	11.3	Suicide	12.6
Symptoms and ill-defined conditions	10.9	Symptoms and ill-defined conditions	12.3
Suicide	10.7	Diabetes mellitus	11.6

[1] Age-adjusted death rates have been adjusted for changes in disease classifications over the various editions of the International Classifications of Disease. Comparability ratios by disease category have been used to adjust age-adjusted death rates, as reported in each of the seven earlier ICDA disease codes to the Eighth ICDA Code. The raw data and comparability ratios are from various National Center for Health Statistics and Vital Statistics publications, including: F.E. Linder and R.D. Grove: *Vital Statistics Rates in the United States, 1900-1940.* U.S. Public Health Service, Washington, D.C., 1947; "Death Rates by Age, Race, and Sex, United States 1900-1953: All Causes." *Vital Statistics-Special Reports,* Vol. 43, No. 1, January 9, 1956 (No. 2-31, Vol. 43 of *Vital Statistics-Special Reports* report age-adjusted death rates by cause for 30 causes of death); R.D. Grove and A.M. Hetzel: *Vital Statistics Rates in the United States, 1940-1960.* U.S. Public Health Service, National Center for Health Statistics, Washington, D.C., 1968; *Mortality Trends for Leading Causes of Death, United States, 1950-1969.* National Center for Health Statistics, Series 20, No. 16, Rockville, Maryland, 1974; and *Comparability of Mortality Statistics for the Seventh and Eighth Revisions of the International Classification of Diseases, United States.* National Center for Health Statistics, Series 2, No. 66, Rockville, Maryland, 1975.

[2] Major cardiovascular-renal includes ICDA 390-428, 440-458, 582-584, but excludes cerebrovascular diseases (430-438). Deaths are aggregated according to this category because of the difficulties of separating renal disease from cardiovascular disease in a consistent manner for all years.

Cancer deaths are still advancing (Figure 3-6). Part of this increase undoubtedly is due to better reporting, better diagnosis, and greater emphasis on early casefinding; nevertheless, part of the rise is real and of concern. In contrast, the climb of death rates from heart diseases is reversing. Since 1940 the rate has gone down, and the rate of decline accelerated from 1972 to 1976.

The increase in chronic diseases as a cause of death originates in the very successes that were achieved in controlling the infectious and communicable diseases. Diseases that primarily affected the young have been controlled. The recent concentration of deaths in the older age groups and the projected continuation of past trends are illustrated in Figure 3-7 for four major causes of death—cancer, diseases of the heart, vascular diseases, and respiratory diseases. Almost 85 percent of all vascular deaths in 1975 were among the sixty-five years and over age group. Indeed, 60 percent of the vascular deaths were in the seventy-five years and over age group. By the year 2000, it is projected, nearly 90 percent of vascular deaths will occur among aged persons. Deaths from cancer tend to occur in a somewhat younger age group. However, in 1975, 60 percent of all those who died from cancer were sixty-five years or older.

Total Predicted Deaths, by Age and Sex
Predicted changes for the year 2000 are small compared to the dramatic gains in reduced mortality during the first half of this century.

While age-adjusted death rates, as predicted, change by only a small percentage, improvements, as well as setbacks, are predicted within the reported averages that will certainly have a marked effect on society. For one thing, infant and childhood deaths are predicted to turn down. The cancer and diabetes death rates in children are estimated to decline some 40 percent. With the infectious diseases brought under control, heart impairment attributable to sequelae of infections is expected to be checked. The expectation of survival in children reinforces the value of human life, especially when birth rates also have declined. The sense of human control over environment is reinforced, erasing any remaining shreds of fatalism.

In addition, predictions, discussed more fully later, point to some redress of the imbalance between the death rates of women and men. Today's problems of aging are often associated with the longer life expectancy of women and with the numbers of widows who are alone and lonely. In 1975, the life expectancy at birth of women was

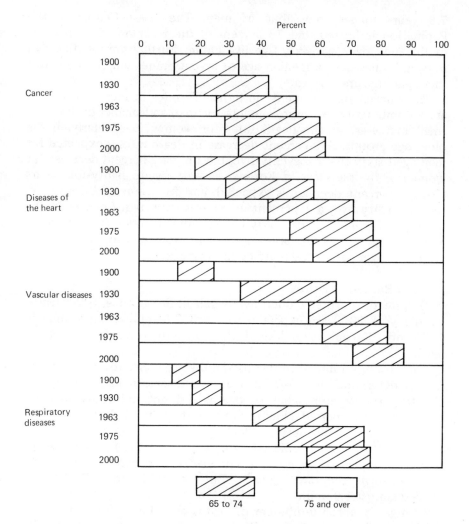

Figure 3-7. Percent of All Deaths in the Disease Category of Persons Aged 65 to 74 and 75 and over

Sources: F.E. Linder and R.D. Grove: *Vital Statistics Rates in the United States 1900-1940.* National Office of Vital Statistics, Washington, D.C., 1947; *Vital Statistics of the United States, 1963,* Vol. II, Mortality, Part A. National Center for Health Statistics, Washington, D.C., 1965; unpublished data from the National Center for Health Statistics, Washington, D.C.; Year 2000 estimates in S.J. Mushkin and D. Wagner; *Expected Mortality as a Criterion in Health Policy Evaluation.* Paper delivered at the Annual Meeting of the American Public Health Association, November 2, 1977 (processed).

7.8 years longer than that of men. The latest Census of the Population indicated that 38 percent of the women and 14 percent of the men over age sixty-five live alone. Furthermore, patients in nursing homes have a median age of seventy-nine, and 66 percent of these patients are women.

The uneven improvements in mortality rates of men and women are a combination of improvements for men and smaller declines, or small increases, in the death rates for women, particularly in the older age groups. A 9-percent decrease in death rates is expected for men aged sixty-five to seventy-five, but only a 2-percent decrease for women of the same age.[1][2] For men seventy-five to eighty-four years old, a 6-percent decrease is expected, and for women aged seventy-five to eighty-five, a 1 percent increase is expected. Changes in the lifestyle of women, particularly changes that increase stress in daily activities, as well as the larger number of women who have smoked cigarettes over past decades are cited as causes.

Total Burden of Death

Despite the further reductions overall in death rates, total deaths by the year 2000 are expected to reach 2.6 million, more than in 1975 and 1976 and 1.2 million deaths above the estimated year 1900 level.

The absolute number of deaths and the age concentration of those deaths determine the costs of death, as discussed in a subsequent chapter. The total number of deaths did not uniformly increase throughout the period (Figure 3-8). In fact, total deaths in 1930 were below the 1900 level, reflecting both birthrate reduction and the gains in mortality achieved by better sanitation, improved health practices, expansion in medical knowledge, and better living conditions through economic growth. But by 1975 and 1976, deaths totaled almost 1.9 million.

Changes in absolute number of deaths over the century reflect the total size of the population, its age and sex composition, and the characteristics of death rate trends by age and sex. Figure 3-8 mirrors the combination of those factors. A continuation of predicted death rates into the decades beyond 2000, given the World War II "baby boom" age cohort means peak deaths by the years 2010-30 and even a larger rise in the proportion of the deaths represented by those sixty-five years of age and over than shown here for year 2000.

METHODOLOGY OF COUNTS OF DEATH

The historical mortality figures presented earlier were based on two sets of adjustments of data before 1975. The first set was designed to adjust for the incomplete recording of deaths in 1900 and the second, for differences in disease classification from one code to the next. While the adjustments are far from precise, they yield a set of figures for 1900 and on deaths by cause that are more nearly comparable from year to year than are unadjusted numbers.

Compilations of U.S. mortality statistics began in 1900. At that time, however, the registration of deaths was still imperfect in many parts of the country. Hence the Census Bureau, responsible for the initial collection of mortality data, limited vital statistics tables to geographic areas in which registration was believed to be reasonably complete and accurate, namely, the Death-Registration Area (DRA). This area consisted originally of ten states and the District of Columbia, called the Death-Registration States (DRS), plus a number of cities in nonregistration states. As registration improved, more states were added to the Death-Registration Area until, in 1933, it finally included the entire continental United States.

Published death rates for the DRS in 1900 included deaths in states that accounted for only about twenty million of the country's population of 76 million, and these states were primarily in the northeast and north central regions. Limitation of recorded death data, therefore, has biased historical series that purported to represent the nation. The best possible estimate of mortality in the rest of the country would require intensive study of local data and a thorough examination, beyond the scope of this study, of cost of illness.

However, examination of statistics for eight major causes of death in 1930, when the death registration area was nearly complete, revealed that the ratio of the death rate in all registration states in 1930 to the death rate in the original states in that same year ranged from 1.49 for diarrhea and enteritis, to 0.81 for diseases of the heart.[13] The wide range indicated differences in the mortality experience of the 1900 registration states and of the country as a whole. The registration states tended to be urban, wealthier than the nonregistration states, and to have more medical and diagnostic facilities. An estimate accounting for at least some of the differences could be made from available data that would improve the historical comparisons.

The following procedure was used:

1. Start with data from the rate volume for seven cause-of-death groups for which rates by cause and age in 1900 were shown. The following seven groups accounted for 46.8 percent of all deaths in the DRS in 1900.

   Tuberculosis (all forms)

In millions

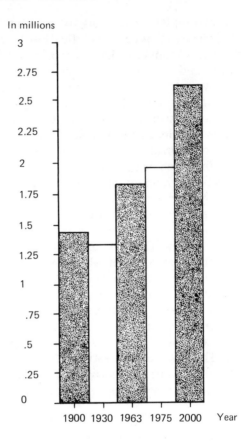

Sources: Crude death rate by cause data for earlier years were adjusted to the Eighth ICDA Code by use of the comparability ratios published in "Comparability of Mortality Statistics for the Seventh and Eighth Revisions of the International Classification of Diseases, United States," Series 2, No. 66. National Center for Health Statistics, Rockville, Maryland, October 1975; "Comparability of Mortality Statistics for the Sixth and Seventh Revisions: United States, 1958." National Center for Health Statistics, *Vital Statistics-Special Reports, Selected Studies,* Vol. 51, No. 3, Washington, D.C., March 1955; "Comparability Ratios Based on Mortality Statistics for the Fifth and Sixth Revisions: United States, 1950." *Vital Statistics-Special Reports, Selected Studies,* Vol. 51, No. 3, February 1964; and "Comparison of Cause of Death Assignments by the 1929 and 1938 Revisions of the International List of Deaths in the United States, 1940." *Vital Statistics-Special Reports,* Vol. 19, No. 4, June 14, 1944. Crude death rate data for all diseases and by disease category were obtained from F.E. Linder and R.D. Grove: *Vital Statistics Rates in the United States, 1900-1940.* National Office of Vital Statistics, Washington, D.C., 1947; *Vital Statistics of the United States, 1963,* Vol. II, Mortality, Part A. National Center for Health Statistics, Washington, D.C., 1965; and "Annual Summary for the United States, 1976." *Monthly Vital Statistics Report,* Vol. 25, No. 13, December 12, 1977, National Center for Health Statistics, Hyattsville, Maryland.

Figure 3-8. Total Number of Deaths, Selected Years, 1900-2000

     Cancer and other malignant tumors
     Diabetes mellitus
     Intracranial lesions of vascular origin
     Heart disease (all forms)
     Pneumonia (all forms) and influenza
     Nephritis

2. Compute the age-specific death rates for these same diseases and for the same area for the year 1940, the first census year in which the Death Registration Area covered the entire United States.
3. Assume the following relationship:

$$M_{ca}(1900 \text{ U.S.}) = M_{ca}(1900 \text{ DRS}) \frac{M_{ca}(1940 \text{ U.S.})}{M_{ca}(1940 \text{ DRS})}$$

in which M is the death rate; the subscript "ca" represents cause of death "c" in age group "a"; and the parenthetical qualifier signifies the year. (In other words, it was assumed that within an age group for a particular cause of death, the ratio of the death rate in the entire country to the death rate in the DRS was the same in 1900 as it was later found to be in 1940.)

4. Multiply the national 1900 death rates obtained from this equation by the appropriate population counts from the 1900 census to produce estimates of the total numbers of deaths in the United States by age for each of the seven cause-of-death groups.
5. Subdivide the deaths in each of the age-by-cause-of-death cells by sex, assuming that the male-female distribution of the deaths within each cell in the country as a whole was the same as it was in the deaths in the DRA. (The DRA data for 1900 were used instead of the DRS data because the rate volume did not show cause-of-death statistics crossed with age and sex.)
6. Estimate the remaining disease groups by first determining deaths in the entire United States by age and sex for all causes combined, assuming the ratio of the death rate in the entire country to the death rate in the DRS was the same in 1900 as in 1940.
7. Multiply the appropriate 1900 census counts by the death rates as estimated to produce estimates of the numbers of deaths by age and sex in 1900. From these aggregates totals were subtracted for the corresponding age-sex groups resulting from the combination of the figures for the seven major diseases. This provided totals for the country by age and sex for all other causes.

8. Distribute these totals for all-other-causes into the other cause-of-death groupings. Titles of the causes of death, as published in 1900, were reorganized to correspond as closely as possible to the Eighth International Classification of Diseases currently in use. (For the all-other-causes, totaling 53.2 percent of all deaths in the DRS in 1900, the distribution was taken to be the same in the country as a whole as it was within the DRA, within an age-sex total.)

The methodology described above was determined more by the availability of data than by any evident logic. Yet, the underlying assumption is that for general mortality and for seven major causes of death, the ratio within each age group of the death rates in the DRS to the corresponding death rates in the continental United States remained unchanged from 1900 to 1940. Although, in reality, mortality may have occurred differently, we think it is reasonable to suppose that this set of ratios did not change much during the forty years.

It seems, at least, that the estimated figures more accurately picture mortality, by age, at the beginning of the century in the United States than the figures obtained by assuming that the age- and cause-specific rates in the population of the Death Registration States were the same as those in the entire country. There are significant differences between the figures in the numbers of deaths by age and cause. For males aged fifteen to forty-four, the national estimates of deaths are higher by 11 to 27 percent than the death data reported in the Death Registration States. For females aged fifteen to forty-four, national estimates are higher by 12 to 38 percent. Significant differences are also revealed in the projected death totals for various diseases, such as cancer and endocrine, nutritional, and metabolic diseases. Cancer deaths, for example, in the registration states appear to overstate the total for the nation, or, more accurately, the total in view of regional differences in medical care and diagnosis.

The second adjustment in the published statistics is made to achieve greater comparability over the historical period. The need for adjusting counts of death by disease categories results from the changes in disease classification from one period to another in the several codes of the International Classification of Diseases. Throughout, we have attempted to make the death data conform to the latest code, the ICDA-8. We used, with whatever bias this creates, comparability ratios from one code to another developed by the National Office of Vital Statistics. The comparability ratios were developed in each of the periods as a basis for comparing the new code data with data on mortality in the year immediately preceding the revision. Essentially, they were not designed to yield comparability over a long period. However, the choice is between attempting to correct for differences in classification or using mortality data unadjusted. We chose to make the adjustment to reduce biases in analysis as a consequence of misclassification of deaths from a disease.

Some examples may help to clarify the problem. The historical data unadjusted show a sharp decline in nephritis deaths between 1948 and 1949. The National Office of Vital Statistics estimated that 65 percent of the decline is attributable to change in code definition and disease classification. Similarly, 45 percent fewer diabetes deaths were reported when the ICDA was revised from the fifth to the sixth code, a classification change rather than a real difference in deaths.

Adjustments for differences in classification were made from code to code by a chain multiplication process, that is, by multiplying the age-adjusted death rate for a disease category by comparability ratios, one for each change in code. To illustrate, we converted death rates reported for diabetes to the ICDA-8 code classification by multiplying by each of the available comparability ratios. The National Office of Vital Statistics reported that new definitions between the third and fourth and between the fourth and fifth revisions of the ICDA resulted in almost no change in classification of diabetes deaths. From the fifth to the sixth code revision, however, significant changes reduced the reports of death from diabetes. The revision from the sixth to the seventh code increased slightly the number of deaths reported. The next code revision from the seventh to the eighth made no change in the classification of diabetes.

By applying the comparability ratios developed by the National Office of Vital Statistics for a single year over the entire period of each ICDA revision, we have not taken into account many factors that affect cause of death as reported. New knowledge about disease has altered classification of deaths. New diagnostic methods have contributed to these differences, as well as improved education of physicians and attitudes toward reporting cause of death in death certificates. Increased hospitalization has had its effect. Cause of death reporting also is influenced by family requests and sensitivity about certain diseases. Cancer deaths in particular tend to be underreported, but pneumonia or other secondary causes are listed.

The intent is to achieve greater comparability in the historical trend data for all deaths and deaths by cause. Rankings of deaths by cause are changed. As a minimum, spurious historical gains in reduced mortality are avoided (Table 3-3).

Table 3-3.   Change in Age-adjusted Death Rates, by Major Cause, Due to Changing Disease Definitions

Cause of death	Death rates as reported				Death rates adjusted to the eighth ICDA Code				Net change in death rates			
	1900	1930	1963	1975	1900	1930	1963	1975	1900	1930	1963	1975
Influenza and pneumonia	209.5	108.2	27.7	16.6	185.0	95.5	28.9	16.6	−24.5	−12.7	+1.2	0.0
Neoplasms	79.6	116.7	126.7	130.9	75.8	111.1	127.0	130.9	−3.8	−5.6	+.3	0.0
Cardiorenal diseases	287.6	384.7	318.5	243.8	314.5	420.7	317.9	243.8	+26.9	+36.0	−.6	0.0
Cerebrovascular disease	134.4	106.5	76.6	54.5	153.2	121.4	75.9	54.5	+18.8	+14.9	−.7	0.0
Tuberculosis	199.0	74.5	4.3	1.2	189.1	70.8	4.3	1.2	−9.9	−3.7	0.0	0.0
Gastritis, duodenitis, etc.	112.6	23.6	3.4	1.4	74.5	15.6	2.2	1.4	−38.1	−8.0	−1.2	0.0
Appendicitis and hernia	—	25.8	5.0	2.2	—	21.9	4.0	2.2	—	−3.9	−1.0	0.0
Diabetes mellitus	13.0	22.2	13.8	11.6	7.2	12.3	13.8	11.6	−5.8	−9.9	0.0	0.0
Cirrhosis of liver	15.1	8.3	11.2	13.8	12.0	6.6	11.3	13.8	−3.1	−1.7	+.1	0.0
Diphtheria	33.4	4.3	0.0	0.0	27.8	3.7	0.0	0.0	−5.6	−.6	0.0	0.0
Typhoid	31.2	4.7	0.0	0.0	31.2	4.7	0.0	0.0	0.0	0.0	0.0	0.0
Symptoms and ill-defined conditions	117.5	30.4	10.7	12.3	121.0	31.3	10.9	12.3	−3.5	+.9	+.2	0.0
Accidents: Not including motor vehicles	75.3	56.6	26.6	23.5	61.0	45.8	24.6	23.5	−14.3	−10.8	−2.0	0.0
Motor vehicles only	—	28.0	24.3	21.3	—	27.7	24.1	21.3	—	−.3	−0.2	0.0
Suicide	—	—	11.3	12.6	—	—	10.7	12.6	—	—	−0.6	0.0

Sources: See Table 3-2.

A DELPHI EXERCISE FOR YEAR 2000

We have noted the historical gains in improved mortality experience and reported briefly on the expected decline in death rates in the years ahead. Death rates are expected to decline by the year 2000 but at a pace far below the decline since the turn of this century.[1][2] The decline predicted is essentially an extension of the experience of the past decade or so, as reported in a Delphi exercise. Bench scientists, medical administrators, clinicians, and epidemiologists were asked to speculate on death rates in the year 2000 by disease and by age and sex. Persons with national and international reputations in their specialties from leading hospitals, medical schools, and research laboratories participated by stating their opinions about likely mortality rates by the year 2000. Estimates were obtained for men and women separately and by age group for each of seven diseases that are the major causes of death today—heart diseases; cancer; vascular, respiratory, and digestive diseases; cirrhosis; and diabetes.

The responses of the experts indicate that expanded knowledge attributable to current research is not likely to greatly affect mortality rates. Continued research will probably cause only a small change in the death rates of the American people. Importantly, the gains predicted will most likely be concentrated among young age groups. Table 3-4 shows the year 2000 estimate of total deaths by cause of death and age and sex. Table 3-5 compares the distribution of deaths by cause for 1900 and 1975 with the year 2000 projections.

Predictions for Cancer Mortality

Specialists in cancer research were asked to report their expectations on cancer mortality rates for the year 2000, in view of past experience for selected years from 1950 to 1974, the latest year for which vital statistics were available at the time of the inquiry.[14] More specifically, these experts were asked to take account of the ongoing research and the likely products of that research in the years ahead through gains in chemotherapy, immunology, and radiation treatment, as well as new diagnostic methods. In their responses, such potential gains were balanced against increased morbidity from greater hazards, such as lead, asbestos, sodium nitrate, and other substances.

Some gains in reduced cancer death rates are predicted. The median rates forecast by the experts convert to approximately 467,000 cancer deaths for the year 2000, given the census popula-

Table 3-4. Year 2000: Number of Deaths by Age, Sex, and Cause

Cause of death	Total males and females	Males					Females				
		All ages	Under 25	25-44	45-64	65 and over	All ages	Under 25	25-44	45-64	65 and over
Infective and parasitic diseases	20,856	10,829	2,145	1,145	2,744	4,795	10,027	1,709	1,073	1,918	5,327
Neoplasms	467,040	255,769	2,365	11,150	86,281	155,973	211,271	1,753	11,963	67,750	129,805
Endocrine, nutritional, and metabolic diseases	57,672	23,343	584	1,313	5,523	15,923	34,329	405	1,143	5,538	27,243
Diseases of the blood and blood-forming organs	7,271	3,155	424	342	672	1,717	4,116	335	371	728	2,682
Mental disorders	13,268	8,506	774	2,479	3,283	1,970	4,762	205	962	1,277	2,318
Diseases of the nervous system and sense organs	22,736	11,696	2,659	1,658	2,961	4,418	11,040	1,612	1,442	2,877	5,109
Diseases of the circulatory system	1,438,349	659,713	2,049	20,185	151,311	486,168	778,636	1,616	9,341	70,602	697,077
Diseases of the respiratory system	166,062	98,471	3,095	2,710	17,940	74,726	67,591	2,302	1,996	9,306	53,987
Diseases of the digestive system, oral cavity, salivary glands, and jaws	95,054	54,176	937	7,967	23,562	21,710	40,878	717	4,440	12,596	23,125

Diseases of the genitourinary system	38,558	17,285	367	989	3,097	12,832	21,273	279	1,276	3,375	16,343
Complications of pregnancy, childbirth, and puerperium	566	, —	—	—	—	—	566	164	397	5	—
Diseases of the skin and subcutaneous tissue	3,014	1,053	51	76	244	682	1,961	40	129	252	1,540
Diseases of the musculoskeletal system and connective tissue	6,975	2,035	77	205	648	1,105	4,940	141	587	1,272	2,940
Congenital anomalies											
Certain causes of perinatal mortality	38,519	21,717	20,151	581	583	402	16,802	15,249	500	558	495
Symptoms and ill-defined conditions	41,805	22,968	5,357	3,351	5,937	8,323	18,837	3,121	2,253	3,345	10,118
Accidents, poisonings, and violence	189,345	133,142	37,378	46,040	30,439	19,285	56,203	11,960	14,018	12,259	17,966
Total	2,607,090	1,323,858	78,413	100,191	335,225	810,029	1,283,232	41,608	51,891	193,658	996,075

Source: Selma J. Mushkin, et al.: "Cost of Disease and Illness in the United States in the Year 2000." *Public Health Reports* 93:493-588, September-October 1978.

Table 3-5. Distribution of Deaths, by Cause, for 1900 and 1975 with the Year 2000 Projections

	Number of deaths			Percentage distribution		
Disease category	*1900*	*1975*	*2000*	*1900*	*1975*	*2000*
All diseases	1,410,968	1,935,189	2,607,090	100.0	100.0	100.0
Infective and parasitic diseases	428,023	15,715	20,856	30.3	0.8	0.8
Neoplasms	35,917	365,538	467,040	2.5	18.9	17.9
Endocrine, nutritional, and metabolic diseases	6,880	45,684	57,672	0.4	2.4	2.2
Diseases of the blood and blood-forming organs	3,625	5,353	7,271	0.2	0.3	0.2
Mental disorders	4,867	9,595	13,268	0.3	0.5	0.5
Diseases of the nervous system and sense organs	65,433	17,356	22,736	4.6	0.9	0.8
Diseases of the circulatory system	176,170	1,028,415	1,438,349	12.4	53.1	55.1
Diseases of the respiratory system	274,911	109,276	166,062	19.4	5.6	6.3
Diseases of the digestive system, oral cavity, salivary glands, and jaws	54,870	73,189	95,054	3.8	3.8	3.6
Diseases of the genitourinary system	116,846	28,029	38,558	8.2	1.4	1.4
Complications of pregnancy, childbirth, and puerperium	9,209	461	556	0.6	0.0[1]	0.0[1]
Diseases of the skin and subcutaneous tissue	2,159	2,097	3,014	0.1	0.1	0.1
Diseases of the musculoskeletal system and connective tissue	6,897	5,044	6,975	0.4	0.3	0.2
Congenital anomalies	45,470	13,517	38,519[2]	3.2	0.7	1.4[2]
Certain causes of perinatal morbidity and mortality	32,020	28,755	—[2]	2.2	1.5	—[2]
Symptoms and ill-defined conditions	86,794	31,065	41,805	6.1	1.6	1.6
Accidents, poisonings, and violence	60,877	156,100	189,345	4.3	8.1	7.2

[1] Rounds to less than 0.05 percent.

[2] Congenital anomalies and certain causes of perinatal mortality are combined into one category in the year 2000 projections.

Sources: Crude death rate by cause data for earlier years were adjusted to the Eighth ICDA Code by use of the comparability ratios published in "Comparability of Mortality Statistics for the Seventh and Eighth Revisions of the International Classification of Diseases, United States," Series 2, No. 66, National Center for Health Statistics, Rockville, Maryland, October 1975; "Comparability of Mortality Statistics for the Sixth and Seventh Revisions: United States, 1958," National Center for Health Statistics, *Vital Statistics-Special Reports, Selected Studies,* Vol. 51, No. 3, Washington, D.C., March 1965; "Comparability Ratios Based on Mortality Statistics for the Fifth and Sixth Revisions: United States, 1950," *Vital Statistics-Special Reports,* Selected Studies, Vol. 51, No. 3, February 1964; and "Comparison of Cause of Death Assignments by the 1929 and 1938 Revisions of the International List of Deaths in the United States, 1940," *Vital Statistics-Special Reports,* Vol. 19. No. 4, June 14, 1944. Crude death rate data for all diseases and by disease category were obtained from F.E. Linder and R.D. Grove, *Vital Statistics Rates in the United States 1900-1940,*

Table 3-5 continued

National Office of Vital Statistics, Washington, D.C., 1947; *Vital Statistics of the United States, 1963,* Vol. II, Mortality, Part A, National Center for Health Statistics, Washington, D.C., 1965; and "Annual Summary for the United States, 1976," *Monthly Vital Statistics Report,* Vol. 25, No. 13, December 12, 1977, National Center for Health Statistics, Hyattsville, Maryland.

tion projections. If actual 1974 cancer death rates are used in such a conversion, just under 500,000 deaths would be estimated by 2000. The difference is a 6.5 percent reduction in overall cancer deaths. However, this improvement is not uniform for all age groups. The largest gains are expected for the youngest age groups, 42 percent for infants under one year of age and about 30 percent for persons between ages one and twenty-four, perhaps reflecting recent successes in treating Hodgkin's disease and leukemia. Gains of up to 11 percent in mortality are expected for the age groups fifty-five years and over, ages at which the bulk of cancer deaths occur.

However, as one research clinician pointed out, smoking, new chemicals in use, more air pollution, further urbanization, and increased application of toxic substances in agriculture contribute to a potentially higher incidence of cancer in the years ahead that will offset the improvements in care and treatment of cancer. The reports of little overall reduction in death rates in the older age groups add to the separately compiled information reported by the National Cancer Institute that survival rates of those with cancers have shown little change over the past decade.[15]

The experts responding with detailed estimates by age and for men and women for the year 2000 were not unanimous in their views. One research scientist reported that cancer mortality would be virtually wiped out by the year 2000 through improved early detection and treatment of cancer by immunotherapy and chemotherapy and decreased environmental exposure to carcinogens. Other experts were far less optimistic. Marginal improvements were generally expected in cancer of the colon and female genital organ and breast cancer, where earlier detection is increasingly feasible. The major source of disagreement was over the trend in exposure to carcinogens, from smoking and other sources, in the environment. One expert thought that cancer death rates would be 20 to 30 percent higher in 2000 than today because of the large increases in exposure to radiation, chemicals, food additives, and water and air pollution, but another thought the recent increases in knowledge of environmental carcinogens would lead to reduced exposure and substantially reduced death rates by the year 2000. There were similar disagreements about future trends in smoking and lung cancer, but few were optimistic about improvements in early diagnosis and therapy of lung cancer.

Predictions for Other Diseases

Similar inquiries about death rates in the year 2000 to experts in each of the other major diseases produced less divergent responses. Emphasis in their answers differed, however, depending on their particular research interests and concerns. For a number of the diseases, lower mortality, where it is expected, is attributed to improved lifestyles, particularly reduced cigarette smoking and better nutrition, as well as better care due to advances in biomedical knowledge. Pessimism about reduced smoking led the scientists reporting on respiratory diseases to expect higher death rates by the year 2000, and those reporting on cirrhosis of the liver expected increases due to more consumption of alcohol.

Examples from the testimony of the experts help to put the expected gains in perspective. Scientists knowledgeable about heart and vascular diseases see moderate improvements in cardiovascular death rates due to better screening and control of hypertension and arteriosclerosis and moderately more effective operative techniques.[16] They emphasized diet and exercise as preventive measures. Infant death rates are expected to decrease because of better therapeutic techniques. Misreported cases are likely to drop off with more accurate diagnosis. Improvement is also expected because of a decrease in the incidence of rheumatic fever. Lower death rates in the older population will be less noticeable because of the effects of age itself on the myocardium and the increased survival to older ages of persons who are particularly vulnerable to cardiovascular failure.

Favorable to reduced mortality rates from cerebrovascular diseases are improved control of hypertension through early diagnosis and treatment, improved patient compliance, and the recognition of transient ischemic attacks (TIAs), which results in improved detection of stroke-prone individuals.[17] More effective drugs and their more widespread use as well as general improvements in medical practice are factors that lead to a predicted decrease in mortality rates. Several experts specifically mentioned the improved management of subarachnoid hemorrhage and, in particular, the current practice of delaying surgery for hemorrhage so that the patient may become a better surgical risk. Improvement was also noted in the methods for prevention of atherosclerosis.

Experts in respiratory diseases expect influenza and penumonia death rates to decline, especially rates for infants, young children, and those sixty-five years or over.[18] Penumonia deaths, one investigator indicates, should decrease markedly with the development of vaccines for pneumococcal and diplococcal pneumonia and possible mycoplasma penumonia. Another thinks that influenza may well be eradicated by the year 2000 but that improvement in pneumonia mortality reaches an irreducible minimum that reflects the incidence of otherwise dying patients for whom pneumonia happened to be the terminal event.[18]

Better diagnosis and therapy for allergies and fibrotic diseases, pneumonitis, edema, and emboli are cited. Improved treatment is projected for respiratory distress of newborns and for asthmatics. One expert looks to such advances in knowledge of immunology and the disease mechanisms that mortality from asthma may be "almost nil." Advances in enzymatic and tRNA and metabolic pathways may result in the elimination of genetic forms of respiratory disease.

Among those responding to the inquiry on diabetes, several expect that the relationship between viral susceptibility in children and diabetes will be better understood, permitting prevention and early therapy. Most indicated that virtually all of the deaths from diabetes in the younger age groups could be prevented by better management of diabetic ketoacidosis and insulin deficiency. They expect that as progress is made in educating the public and improving health care delivery systems, deaths from diabetes among the younger ages will decrease markedly.[19]

Although the experts generally were more pessimistic about the trends in diabetes death rates among older patients, higher rates are partly attributed to better recognition of the disease as a cause of death. However, real improvements in death rates among the young diabetics result in increased prevalence of diabetics among older age groups. Many specialists reported that death rates could be reduced by proper nutrition, exercise, and improved therapy. One expert thinks it unlikely that the macrovascular complications of this disease will be controlled by 2000. Another, however, indicated that improvements in health care delivery could reduce the complications from large vessel disease, of which diabetes is one, and cut in half the deaths attributed to diabetes.

Scientists working on digestive diseases report means to control gastrointestinal diseases, for which high death rates were reported in the past, by more effective diagnosis and treatment of ulcers, biliary tract problems, peritonitis, intestinal obstruction, enteric and parasitic infections, hepatitis, and dehydration in infantile diarrhea. Progress is also anticipated in detecting the causes and prevention of gallstones, inflammatory bowel disease, and congenital lesions. In part, gains are a result of more widespread availability of medical care and increased public awareness of medical problems.[20]

Cirrhosis deaths are not expected to decline and may even rise slightly owing to the increase in alcoholism, especially among women and teenagers.[20] A few experts predicted a large increase in the incidence of cirrhosis from alcoholism, and only one expressed confidence in a significant control of future alcoholism. The majority agreed that deaths due to cirrhosis resulting from hepatitis will decline when hepatitis is brought under more effective prevention and control. One expert, however, was very concerned about an increasing exposure of large segments of the population to hepatitis B infection, an exposure attributed to increased occupational exposure among hospital personnel, increased drug use, and exposure of patients to infected blood products.

IDENTIFYING PREVENTABLE CAUSES
OF DEATH

Changes in death rates clearly have upper limits, even though those upper limits remain undefined. A basic question is: How long can death be postponed? One approach is to quantify preventable deaths.

The report by Fisher for the National Conservation Commission represents an early major attempt to quantify the number of unnecessary deaths. It was reported, after study, that life in the United States, by the adoption of hygienic reforms then known and entirely practical, could be lengthened by more than one-third—or about fifteen years. It was estimated that at least eight years could be added to life expectancy by reasonably pure air, water, and milk.[9,21]

To arrive at this estimate, in some instances statistical experience of other countries or of selected U.S. cities was used as a guide; for the most part, the figures on preventable or postponable deaths were the educated guesses of eighteen prominent physicians. The physicians were asked to provide conservative estimates of the percentage of deaths from each of almost ninety causes of death that could be prevented and postponed. The percentage of deaths that were judged preventable represented averages of the responses received. A hypothetical condition was selected to define "ratio of preventability": "A ratio of preventability is the fraction of all deaths which would be avoided if knowledge now existing among well-informed men in the medical profession were actually applied to a reasonable extent."[11]

Of the major causes of death reported in 1906, the base year used in computing death rates, the following ratio of preventability was obtained; the causes are shown in the order of the median age of persons who died from the causes.

Cause of death	Percent of all deaths	Percent preventable
Diarrhea and enteritis	7.7	60
Tuberculosis of the lungs	9.9	75
Violence	7.5	35
Pneumonia	7.0	45
Bright's disease	5.6	40
Heart disease	8.1	25
Apoplexy	4.4	35

The causes for which the ratio of preventability exceeded 60 percent included:

Venereal disease
Diarrhea and enteritis
Croup
Meningitis
Diphtheria
Tetanus
Tuberculosis
  (other than lung)
Abscess
Typhoid fever
Puerperal septicemia
Diseases of tubes
Smallpox
Tuberculosis of lungs

Malaria fever
Erysipelas
Alcoholism
Hemorrhage of lungs
Uterine tumor
Chronic poisonings
Dysentery
Cirrhosis of liver
General paralysis of insane
Hydatid tumors of liver
Hernia
Gangrene

Two decades or so later, in the 1930s when the Committee on the Costs of Medical Care reported to the president and the Congress, the concept of preventable or postponable deaths was again applied in formulation of health policy. Preventable deaths, as defined then by the Committee on the Costs of Medical Care, included 88,000 deaths from tuberculosis (1930) and more than 135,000 infant deaths (1931).[22]

Preventable and Manageable Diseases

Many years later, in 1976, a working group on preventable and manageable diseases proposed as a measuring stick of accomplishments in assessment of medical care policies and improvement in science and technology, the use of cases of unnecessary disease, unnecessary disability, and unnecessary untimely death.[2] [3]

The group asked specialists in various fields of medicine to participate in identifying a list of conditions for use as sentinel health events in national and local geographic areas and in individual hospitals. The assumption on which the selection was made was: "If everything had gone well, the condition would have been prevented or managed." For the use of these measuring sticks, the group emphasized that the "chains of responsibility to prevent the occurrence of any unnecessary disease, disability, or untimely death may be long and complex." For example, a patient may become permanently crippled from a chronic disabling disease, such as rheumatoid arthritis, as a result of inadequate instruction and demonstration of an exercise regimen, lack of facilities for physiotherapy, or that patient's unwillingness to cooperate.

In carrying out this work, sets of listings were developed. List A was sufficiently firm, in terms of untimely deaths and unnecessary disabilities, to raise in a clinical setting the question: "Why did it happen?" List B enumerated conditions in which prevention or management is highly effective, but where more than a single case of disease or disability or a single death is required to initiate an immediate clinical inquiry. Specific medical care for the conditions in list B, however, should be associated with a lower rate of incidence of a condition, for example, vascular complications of heart or brain associated with essential hypertension.

The lists show if the disease, disability, or untimely death could have been prevented (P) or treated (T), including a separate designation for treatment that is controversial. In instances where there is a designation of age in a series of notes providing additional guidance, the clinical inquiry would be limited to deaths of persons under sixty-five years of age.

The Crosby Standard

Still a different approach begins with the notion of identifying a "good" death. What standard would we set for a death? Having defined that standard, we could then measure the progress made in reduction of years of life lost and years of sickness before death. Table 3-6 shows the total years of life lost at present as measured from a seventy-five-years-of-life standard. We call this the Bing

Table 3-6. Estimated Total Years of Life Lost up to Age 75
(years remaining to age 75 from midpoint of age group of those who die)
(in millions)

Year	Total	Males	Females
1900	65.8	34.6	31.2
1930	36.1	20.0	16.1
1975	22.9	14.6	8.3
2000	26.4	16.8	9.6

Note: Computed as

$$\Sigma \ (75\text{-}age_i) \ D_i$$

where age_i is the mean age within a 5-year age category (10-year age categories for 1900 and 2000) and D_i is the number of deaths in the age category. Deaths among persons aged 75 and over were not counted.

Crosby standard, even if the years of life have been extended from his age seventy-two at death to age seventy-five.

Clearly, the standard set here is different from the earlier standards on premature death or preventable death. It calls for the development of a set of criteria starting with a target age, a target physical and mental vitality prior to death, and sudden death. It is a standard that calls for death on the golf course while teeing off.

A single standard may not be acceptable, nor will it be appropriate in all instances. Sudden death has its psychological costs for the family, and these costs may be considered too high. Nevertheless, it seems appropriate to ponder the question of setting a standard against which medical progress may be appropriately measured with the full recognition that people are mortal.

REFERENCES

1. Auster, R., Levenson, I., and Sarachek, D.: The production of health: An exploratory study. *In* Essays in the economics of health and medical care, edited by V.R. Fuchs. National Bureau of Economic Research, New York, 1972, pp. 135-158; (a) p. 54.

2. Illich, I.: Medical nemesis. Pantheon, New York, 1976.

3. McKinlay, J.B., and McKinlay, S.M.: The questionable contribution of medical measures in the decline of mortality in the United States in the twentieth century. Milbank Mem Fund Q 55:405-428, summer 1977.

4. Hemminki, E., and Paakkulainen, A.: The effect of antibiotics on mortality from infectious diseases in Sweden and Finland. Am J Public Health 66:1180-1184, December 1976.

5. Kass, E.H.: Infectious diseases and social change. J Infect Dis 123:110-114, January 1971.

6. Dubos R.: Men, medicine, and environment. Pall Mall Press, London, 1968.

7. U.S. Department of Health, Education, and Welfare: Maternal and child health care programs. October 1966. Program analysis 1966-6. Office of the Assistant Secretary for Program Coordination, Washington, D.C., 1966.

8. Howard, L.O.: Economic loss to the people through insects that carry disease. *In* Report of the National Conservation Commission, vol. III. U.S. Senate Document No. 676, 60th Congress, 2d sess. Washington, D.C., February 1909, pp. 752-777.

9. Report of the National Conservation Commission, vol. III. U.S. Senate Document No. 676, 60th Congress, 2d sess. Washington, D.C., February 1909, p. 737.

10. U.S. Department of Labor: Causal factors in infant mortality, a statistical study based on investigations in eight cities. Children's Bureau Publication No. 142. Washington, D.C., 1925.

11. Fisher, I.: National vitality, its wastes and conservation. *In* Report of the National Conservation Commission, vol. III. U.S. Senate Document No. 676, 60th Congress, 2d sess. Washington, D.C., February 1909, p. 652.

12. Mushkin, S.J., and Wagner, D.P.: Expected mortality as a criterion in health policy evaluation. Paper presented at annual meeting of American Public Health Association, session on health status valuation and policy priorities. Washington, D.C., Oct. 15, 1977.

13. Berk, A., Paringer, L.C., and Woolsey, T.D.: Estimating deaths by cause, age, and sex for the United States in 1900. Public Health Rep 93:479-482, September-October 1978.

14. Mushkin, S.J., and Wagner, D.P.: Predicted mortality in the year 2000 due to cancer. Public Services Laboratory, Georgetown University, Washington, D.C., July 1977.

15. National Cancer Institute: Cancer patient survival. Report No. 5. DHEW Publication No. (NIH) 77-992. Bethesda, Md., 1976.

16. Wagner, D.P.: Predicted mortality in the year 2000 due to heart and vascular disease. Public Services Laboratory, Georgetown University, Washington, D.C., August 1977.

17. Wagner, D.P.: Predicted mortality in the year 2000 due to cerebrovascular disease. Public Services Laboratory, Georgetown University, Washington, D.C., September 1977.

18. Wagner, D.P.: Predicted mortality in the year 2000 due to respiratory disease. Public Services Laboratory, Georgetown University, Washington, D.C., August 1977.

19. Wagner, D.P., and Mushkin, S.J.: Predicted mortality in the year 2000 due to diabetes mellitus. Public Services Laboratory, Georgetown University, Washington, D.C., August 1977.

20. Wagner, D.P., and Mushkin, S.J.: Predicted mortality in the year 2000 due to diseases of the digestive system and cirrhosis of the liver. Public Services Laboratory, Georgetown University, Washington, D.C., August 1977.

21. Fisher, I. Economic aspects of lengthening human life. Pacific Med J 53:5, May 1910.

22. Committee on the Costs of Medical Care: Medical care for the American people. Final report of the committee, Publication No. 28. Adopted October 31, 1932. Arno Press, New York, 1972.

23. Rutstein, D.D., et al.: Measuring the quality of medical care, a clinical method. N Engl J Med 294:582-588, Mar. 11, 1976 (tables revised Sept. 1, 1977).

Chapter Four

Biomedical Research and Improved Mortality Rates

Biomedical research is the nucleus of a complex process that generates new information, which is applied to improve the health status of the population. Research has grappled with a significant number of health problems. For example, research efforts related the impurities discovered in water and food to diseases; as a result, public health programs were mounted to purify water and inspect food for contaminants. The control of infectious diseases resulted from research discoveries in vaccines and the use of antibiotics. Polio vaccine has nearly eliminated a dreaded killer and crippler of children and young adults. Current research is struggling with problems of chronic diseases, and it may be years before effective solutions are discovered.

Over the years, biomedical research undoubtedly has led to reduction in mortality. It is difficult, however, to disentangle the factors that account for the historical reduction. Some part of the decline is attributable to advances in medical knowledge (and the health programs—environmental and personal—through which this knowledge is applied); some part is due to factors such as better nutrition, better housing, improved working conditions, and higher income. Isolation of some of the major factors responsible for lower death rates would help to identify the contribution of health programs, as well as the contribution of specific aspects of health programs, such as biomedical research, environmental measures, and personal health care. The question here—What is the relative role of advances in knowledge and of other factors?—is fairly straightforward; the answer is obscured by the complexities of the problem.

The etiology of disease, societal impacts on health and access to care, living habits, personal hygiene, and raw materials used by industry contribute to those complexities.

In this chapter we review briefly the earlier, rather sparse, research that attempted to identify the impact of biomedical research on mortality and life expectancies, present the findings of some case studies in which improved biomedical knowledge and reduced mortality are linked, and outline a model applied in this study that takes the first step toward parceling out the effects of the various determinants of mortality rates. Results of the analysis are presented in terms of the changes in mortality rates associated with changes in biomedical research.

EARLIER STUDIES

Major studies of biomedical advances and mortality rates include those by McKeown, Record, and Turner;[1] Hemminki and Paakkulainen;[2] McKinlay and McKinlay;[3] and the American College of Surgeons.[4] All of these investigators essentially used the same technique, that is, they asked: Is there evidence that a biomedical research intervention has changed the death rate? What has happened to the death rate for identified diseases (or surgical procedures) as a result of a specific new therapy or procedure? A before and after technique of measurement was used. The data were processed in various ways from study to study. To illustrate, Hemminki and his associate used a simple linear regression to measure the effects of antibiotics on death rates from various infectious diseases in Finland and Sweden. The McKinlays essentially used the time trend to compare mortality rates for the years before and after the introduction of a specific therapy to show the effect of biomedical research. McKeown and associates first applied the method that was later used by the McKinlays.

McKeown and associates considered the decline in mortality in England and Wales over a century. They identified specific diseases, mainly infectious diseases whose decline accounted for three-quarters of the reduction in mortality, and attempted to determine the reasons for the decline. One finding was that most of the improvement in mortality took place before a new therapy or procedure was introduced. Nutrition was advanced as the main cause of reduction in overall mortality. These investigators noted changes in death rates by disease after the introduction of one specific measure of prophylaxis or treatment; for pneumonia, it was the introduction of sulphapyridine in 1938. But this procedure failed to allow for all other advances in treatment and prevention that occurred before the introduction of the specific treatment identified. Certainly, advances in knowledge of disease treatment cannot be restricted to a single breakthrough. The conclusion of McKeown and associates that medical measures are not effective in reducing deaths is suspect, because their methodology failed to control adequately for the full range of advances in knowledge about treatment, prevention, and general medical care. Indeed, if, following their general procedure, a straight line trend were drawn for the historical data, the projected death rates would be negative for many diseases.

Hemminki and Paakkulainen assessed the effect of antibiotics by simple linear regression analysis in which slope coefficients (where the vertical axis measures death rates and the horizontal axis measures time) are estimated for each disease before and after the introduction of antibiotics. Their results suggest that the antibiotics did not accelerate the decline in deaths due to selected infectious diseases, but they made several qualifications indicating that no firm conclusion could be drawn from the analysis. They noted that an analysis of mortality rates may fail to capture the impact of antibiotics on functional status because antibiotics relieve disease and hasten recovery.

The McKinlays concluded from their research that medical measures and the presence of medical services are not largely responsible for the marked decline in mortality rates over the century.[3] But their methodology, as pointed out earlier, overlooks the cumulation of knowledge in disease treatment and focuses on only one advance.

For example, the McKinlays considered only one medical intervention for tuberculosis, and mortality rates showed negligible declines after this medical intervention. Figure 4-1, however, presents a chronological sequence of various new drugs that have improved the treatment of tuberculosis. This sequence of medical interventions includes the introduction of penicillin in hospitals, the general distribution of penicillin, the introduction of streptomycin in hospitals, the general distribution of streptomycin, and the introduction of isoniazid, PAS, myambutol, and rifampin. Therefore, the findings shown in Figure 4-1 are quite contrary to the McKinlays' conclusion. We present Figure 4-1 not to suggest an exclusive causal relation between the introduction of a new therapy and death rate reduction but rather to emphasize that medical progress has been a sequential, multifaceted process with not one but many contributions to medical knowledge and new therapies; some are major, and some minor, but all have some impact on mortality or on morbidity. A detailed tracing back of therapies to the first part of the century is included in a separate memorandum.[5]

Measles death rates provide a good illustration of the linkage

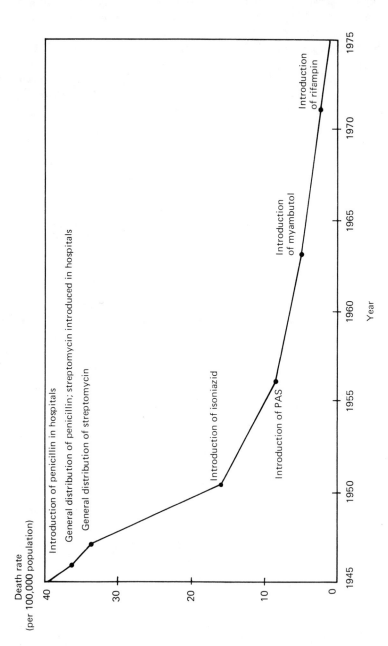

Figure 4-1. Decline in Tuberculosis Death Rate, 1945-75

Source: Death rates from National Center for Health Statistics and drug introductions from *Prescription Drug Industry Factbook '76.* Pharmaceutical Manufacturers' Association, Washington, D.C., 1976, p. 21.

between sickness and deaths because of the close tie between date of introduction of vaccine and measured effect. The McKinlays showed little change in the measles death rate as a consequence of the introduction of the measles vaccine. However, if the number of reported cases of measles is superimposed on the number of deaths, the drop in sickness associated with the vaccine becomes apparent. The reported rate of the disease per 100,000 stood at 204.3 in 1963, dropped to 135.1 in 1965, and to 23.2 by 1970 (Figure 4-2).

The findings of the report on surgical services sponsored jointly by the American College of Surgeons and the American Surgical Association contrast with those of the McKinlays and others. Fifteen contributions to surgical research amenable to analysis were identified; they were selected from a list of sixty-four contributions to surgical research from 1945 to 1970, based on an extensive review of the scientific literature and personal interviews with authorities in each surgical specialty. By use of the ICDA, research contributions were identified according to the diseases they affected.

Age-specific death rates from a base year before the advance in surgical research were used to calculate the number of lives that were saved as a result of the new therapeutic advance. The number of deaths that would have occurred in a year, for example, 1970, when the old therapy was used, was determined and compared with the actual rate for a period when the new therapy was used. The surgical contributions helped save an estimated 78,538 lives in 1970 alone, as indicated in Table 4-1.

The study identifies the numerous assumptions on which the estimates of mortality gains rest:

- The incidence of the disease did not decrease during the period
- The contribution had a direct therapeutic effect on the diseases
- Changes in other factors did not significantly affect mortality

Changes in disease classification over the period required a reduction in the number of surgical processes that could be reviewed in depth. For each surgical procedure, a brief history of the procedure, the effect of its use, and a review of its impact on deaths were presented. Cardiopulmonary bypass, for example, is traced to mid-1953. By the early 1960s, a greatly increased number of patients were receiving cardiac catherization and angiocardiography. Congenital heart disease was being diagnosed with increasing frequency, and open heart surgery techniques were increasingly being mastered by surgeons nationwide. The mortality rates for congenital heart diseases show the effect of the new surgical methods (Figure 4-3).

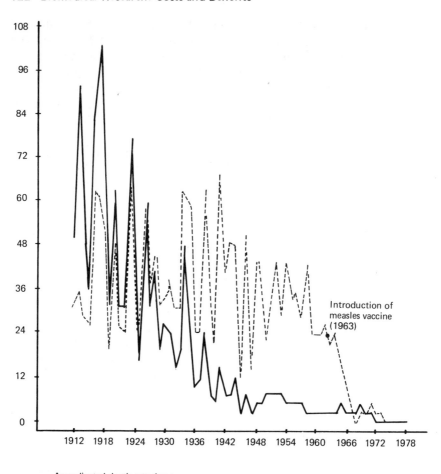

Source: U.S. Center for Disease Control: *Morbidity and mortality, weekly report,* Annual Supplement; U.S. National Office of Vital Statistics: *Vital Statistics-Special Reports,* Vol. 7, No. 9; and U.S. Public Health Service: *Public Health Reports,* various issues for 1912-19 data.

Figure 4-2. Death Rates and Sickness Rates from Measles

The declines in mortality are associated with the specific surgical procedures. But the report by the American College of Surgeons notes: "It is important to emphasize, therefore, that in a number of instances reduction in mortality should not be attributed solely to a surgical advance." Advances in diagnosis, medical therapy, and other

Table 4-1. Estimated Reduction in Deaths in 1970, by Causes of Death Affected by Surgical Advances

Cause of death	Base year for comparison	Total estimated reduction	Deaths in 1970					
			Males			Females		
			Actual	*Projected*	*Reduction*	*Actual*	*Projected*	*Reduction*
Total, all causes		78,538						
Tetralogy of Fallot	1960	260	232	385	153	182	289	107
Ventricular septal defect	1959	400	335	541	206	306	500	194
Atrial septal defect	1957	391	183	343	160	237	468	231
Patent ductus arteriosus	1957	271	110	238	128	100	243	143
Coarctation of aorta	1957	129	142	223	81	82	130	48
Acute nephritis	1950	1,930	513	1,466	953	393	1,370	977
Nephrotic syndrome	1950	1,568	255	1,009	754	193	1,007	814
Chronic nephritis, nephritis unqualified, renal sclerosis unqualified	1950	28,413	4,089	16,156	12,067	3,434	19,780	16,346
Arteriosclerosis	1950	19,620	13,767	20,039	6,272	17,915	31,263	13,348
Duodenal ulcer	1960	2,663	2,771	5,038	2,267	1,145	1,541	396
Disease of mitral valve (rheumatic)	1950	8,605	1,338	5,577	4,239	2,483	6,849	4,366
Disease of aortic valve (rheumatic)	1961	1,051	721	1,502	781	407	677	270
Accidents caused by fire, flames, hot substances	1950	3,011	4,155	5,479	1,324	2,838	4,525	1,687
Heart block	1967	5,508	253	2,935	2,682	254	3,080	2,826
Congenital hydrocephalus	1951	1,120	479	1,077	598	426	948	522
Ulcerative colitis	1950	246	369	426	57	417	606	189
Hypertensive renal disease	1950	3,352	3,079	4,211	1,132	2,682	4,902	2,220

Source: American College of Surgeons and American Surgical Association: *Surgery in the United States: A Summary Report of the Study on Surgical Services for the United States.* Chicago: American College of Surgeons, 1975, p. 162.

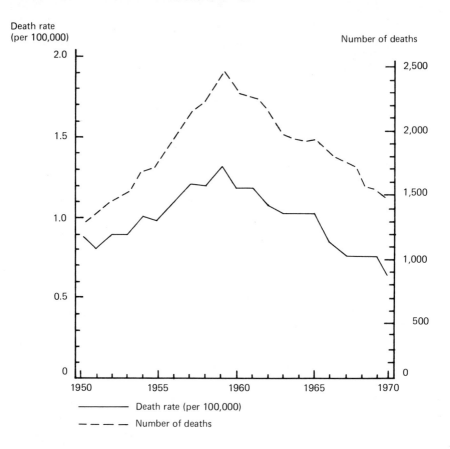

Source: The American College of Surgeons and the American Surgical Association: *Surgery in the United States: A Summary Report of the Study on Surgical Services for the United States.* Chicago: The American College of Surgeons, 1975, p. 158.

Figure 4-3. Mortality Rate and Number of Deaths from Congenital Heart Diseases between 1950 and 1970

improvements in patient care are recognized as factors that affected mortality rates.

CASE STUDIES

The analytical studies just described and another set by Adelman,[6] Auster and associates,[7] Fuchs,[8] Lave and Seskin,[9] Brenner,[10] and Orcutt and associates[11] that are discussed later attempted an overall look at the determinants of mortality. Numerous studies have related a specific medical research finding to reduced mortality. Indeed, the medical literature is replete with such case studies. The drive to understand better the efficacy of therapies and probabilities of success with therapeutic options is leading to more scientific evaluative methods and a better understanding of the probabilities of changes in survival from use of optional treatments.

The National Conservation Commission in 1908 quantified preventable deaths.[1][2] In the course of such quantification, the commission gathered existent data that suggested the extent of preventability of deaths. The commission's compilation recognized the marked and unusual progress toward lengthening life expectancy during the last decades of the nineteenth century, but it did not consider the possibility of new biomedical research in subsequent years. As indicated in Chapter 3, it was estimated that life expectancies could be raised fifteen years by reduction of diseases preventable by the first decade of the twentieth century.

The experience or case materials on which some of the commission's estimates depended are summarized briefly to suggest the types of linkages established between health practices and mortality.

Smallpox: The data are drawn from London and Gloucester. In 1901, the mortality was 34.6 percent among the unvaccinated in London; 10.3 percent where there was protective vaccination.

Diphtheria: Use of the antitoxin in New York City in 1895 is credited with reducing death rates from 37.3 percent to 10.8 percent. In another case, antidiphtheretic serum was reported as having reduced mortality from 50 to 60 percent to 12 to 14 percent.

Alcoholism: Life insurance records show that abstainers have a death rate almost 25 percent below that of nonabstainers.

Yellow fever: In Philadelphia in 1793, within seven weeks, yellow fever caused the death of one-tenth of the city's population. It was found in 1901 that a particular species of mosquitoes (*Aedes aegypti*) transmits the diesase, and when that species was controlled, the disease was almost eradicated. In the southern states in 1887, sixty-two deaths from yellow fever were reported; in 1898, 2,456 cases and 117 deaths; and in 1903, 139 deaths. By 1905, however, during the yellow fever epidemic in New Orleans, application of knowledge about the method of transmission saved 3,500 lives, according to one estimator.

Scurvy: The use of lime juice and fresh vegetables was credited with the eradication of the disease.

Malaria: Discovery of its transmission by the mosquito greatly reduced the death rate from malarial fever in the registration area. In Havana, deaths from malaria dropped from 909 in 1899 to 23 in 1907, when the knowledge about the transmission was applied.

Typhoid: A fall in death rate in registration states is "safely ascribed to improvements in the water and milk supplies of our cities." The reduction in flies and termination of typhoid in certain parts of the city of Washington were attributed to cleaner streets by the displacement of the horse by the automobile (p. 679). The introduction of a water filter in Lawrence, Massachusetts, was followed by a drop of 80 percent in typhoid deaths (p. 650).

Infant deaths: The city of Rochester drew special attention to milk supplies, and the erection of municipal milk stations through which milk in clean nursing bottles could be bought at low prices reduced infant death rates. Death rate experience in a number of cities showed marked declines with provision of milk stations.

Antiseptic surgery: Reduced death rates, illustrated by mortality of those wounded, showed a drop to 5.5 per 1,000 from 15.2 per 1,000 (pp. 629, 688).

Use of tobacco: Several studies from Yale and Amherst are cited, showing that students who were nonusers of tobacco gained more weight, were taller, had larger chest expansion, and far greater lung capacity (p. 712).

More than half a century later, stocktaking centered on new medical therapies and diagnostic methods. The American Medical Association in 1964 undertook a survey of scientific medical advances from 1936 to 1962.[13] The survey was restricted to clinical medicine and to developments being used. A sample of qualified physicians was asked to list ten significant advances in twenty-three areas of medical specialization. The criterion for significance was formulated as follows: "A significant advance is one which medical practitioners would least like to do without in their own practice of medicine." Twenty physicians from each of twenty-two specialties and also from general practice were chosen; an exception was made for the area of experimental medicine and therapeutics from which fourteen physicians were chosen. Illustrations from the list of medical advances are shown in Table 4-2. The full list appears in Table 4A-1 in the appendix at the end of this chapter.

The AMA study does not attempt to examine the mortality consequences of these advances, but certainly one criterion for selection was the lifesaving achieved. The list presents major therapeutic advances. such as antibiotics, antihistamines, antimalarial drugs, tranquilizers, corticosteroids, antituberculosis chemotherapy,

Table 4-2.   Examples of Significant Advances and Technological Developments, 1936-62

Antibiotics for use against bacteria (systemic)
Antihistamines
Antimalarials
Antimetabolics
Antituberculosis chemotherapy
Artificial kidney
Cardiac catheterization
Corticosteroids and ACTH
General anesthetic agents
Improved methods of cardiac resuscitation
Introduction of and improvements in hormonal therapy of cancer
Liver function tests (e.g., BSP)
Modified insulin
Muscle relaxants
Needle liver biopsy
Papanicolaou test for cytodiagnosis of cervical cancer
Perfection of methods for successfully using corneal transplants
Poliomyelitis vaccines
Scanning with radioisotopyes and the development of scanning equipment
Techniques for evaluation of pulmonary function
Tranquilizers
Use of radioisotopes

Source: Reference 13.

anticonvulsants, and antihypertensive drugs. The list also includes a range of diagnostic methods, including needle liver biopsy, esophageal tamponade balloon, use of radioisotopes, and the Pap test for cervical cancer.

The cases of years ago and lists of more recent times underscore the changes in biomedical information that affect mortality. It is frequently stated that 90 percent of the drugs in use today were unknown a decade or so ago. Whether this is factual is less significant than the general concept that the statement conveys, namely, that today's health practices (as applied) tend to be of recent origin. More is being learned each year about diseases, their causes, and the operation of the bodily systems. And much of what is now applied as "good medical practice" is newly understood. Recent advances in biology, physiology, and biochemistry have been enormous, and genetics is now a challenging field of knowledge.

DEVELOPING A MODEL FOR ESTIMATION

To understand what medical advances mean for death rates and for prolonging life, we turn to a model of the factors that determine

mortality rates. The process of formulating this model was complicated and lengthy.

We started with enumerations of factors affecting mortality as
suggested by earlier research. Accordingly, in the initial round, the
following variables were identified: family longevity, nutrition, alcohol consumption, smoking, housing conditions, air standards, age of
water supply systems, worker accidents, automobile usage, crowding,
percentage of population living in urban areas, income levels, unemployment, educational levels, use of health services, numbers of
medical providers, stress, family stability or divorces, illegitimacy,
crime rates, and such characteristics as age, sex, and race. We grouped
the relevant factors into four general types: economic, societal,
environmental, and medical.

We carefully reviewed available data to capture statistically the
characteristics of each of the variables over time. Lack of data posed
a major obstacle. Data selection was based on two criteria: (a)
availability of a consistent (or nearly so) series over the years
1930-75 (and 1900-30), and (b) variance in the data from year to
year. Accordingly, the list of variables that may be hypothesized to
affect mortality rates was scaled down primarily on pragmatic data
grounds. The data characteristics on variables explanatory of mortality rate changes may be grouped into factors for which consistent
yearly data are or are not available or show little variance from year
to year:

Available	*Not available*	*Little variance in year-to-year changes*
Income	Housing quality	Nutrition
Unemployment	Alcohol consumption	Educational levels
Educational levels	Use of health services	Percent of population
Numbers of medi-	Stress	in urban areas
cal providers	Crowding	Family longevity
Crime rates	Family stability or	
Automobile usage	divorces	
Work accidents	Illegitimacy	
Nutrition	Age of water supply	
	systems	
	Air standards	

Biomedical research advance as a factor influencing mortality is
discussed separately in a subsequent section of this chapter.

A second major problem arises from the close correspondence and interdependency of many factors affecting mortality. Income levels, for example, affect nutrition, housing, crowding, use of health services, and educational levels. In turn, income levels are a result of levels of education, adequacy of nutrition, space for privacy, and physical vigor.

Although many important factors have an impact on mortality, the central question that confronts an attempt to use a regression technique is the effective parceling out of the various contributing factors. An ideal measure of the independent effect of each variable would require holding constant each factor, save one, and establishing the relationship of that one factor to mortality rates.

The usual scientific approach to determining how one factor affects another is experimentation. In this case, such experimentation in the laboratory sense with appropriate controls is not feasible. Past biomedical research findings do not lend themselves to experimental design and controls. Such laboratory experimentation, however, is not the only way to find the effect of biomedical research on mortality. Multiple factors in addition to advances in knowledge have an impact on death rates. Multiple regression analysis is frequently used to measure the association of one factor to another as an analogue of a natural experiment.

Multiple regression is a statistical technique designed to estimate the impact of an independent variable on a dependent variable while controlling for the impact of other variables. The "controls" in a regression analysis lie in the explicit inclusion of all important factors influencing the dependent variable in the regression equation.

The simultaneous statistical estimation of the separate effect of each independent variable on the dependent variables enables the social scientist to approximate the laboratory of the natural scientist. There are, however, several caveats that one must bear in mind in using regression analysis: (a) to calculate the "partial" effect of each variable, the independent variables cannot be causally related to each other; (b) all important variables affecting the dependent variable must be included in the regression equation; and finally (c) correlation coefficients obtained from regression analysis can be used to buttress, but not to prove, theoretical arguments about causation.

As suggested, data limitations and interrelationships between the independent variables (for example, income, housing, and nutrition) present difficulties in statistical estimation of the determinants of mortality. Care must be taken in the selection of the variables to be included in the model as well as in the interpretation of the results. Income, for example, may have to stand proxy for a range of variables affecting mortality that are purchased with income. Nutrition, housing, and education are examples of such goods.

The word regression in this statistical context is attributed to Francis Galton, who used the method in treating data on inheritance.[14] When he asked why great fathers do not have great sons, and why great sons do not have great fathers, Galton found that whether he looked forward or backward in time, height regressed toward the average.

A Market Behavioral Model[a]

A model of the interaction among the various determinants of mortality rates may be based on the familiar demand and supply functions for health and health care. In carrying out such a modeling exercise, prices and income are used as standard determinants of a demand analysis. Changes in the environment and changes in various societal variables also are usually considered as factors affecting the demand for health care.

On the supply side, the price and characteristics of providers are important determinants. Providers of health care have kept pace with rising demand through increasing numbers of physicians and other health care personnel as well as building modern plants (hospitals) to supply high-quality services. Another factor, which is particularly important in the field of health, is biomedical research. Research affects the technical effectiveness of much of medical care and also serves as a basis for new initiatives in public health, preventive care, and changes in personal health practices.

Demand and supply functions for health care can be formally written:

$$Q^d = f\,(P, \text{INC, SOC, ENV})$$
$$Q^s = f\,(P, \text{PROV, TECH})$$

where

Q^d, Q^s = the quantity demanded and quantity supplied

P = the price

INC = a vector of economic variables

<hr>

[a]This section has benefited from a lengthy discussion with Teh-wei Hu, who used a similar model in earlier research. See Bernard H. Booms and Teh-wei Hu, "Towards a Positive Theory of State and Local Public Expenditures: An Empirical Example," *Public Finance*, 26, March 1971, pp. 419-436. Earlier iterations of this study used two models. One was a behavioral model, which controlled for institutional aspects of health care. The other was a determinant model, which conceptualized the relationship between health and its determinants as analogous to a production function.

SOC   = a vector of societal variables

ENV   = a vector of environmental variables

PROV = a vector of provider characteristics

TECH = measures of technical advances (biomedical research and development)

The equilibrium condition for the market is

$$Q^d = Q^s = Q.$$

However, the definition of Q poses empirical problems, since health care is a service with various aspects that are not easily quantified. As discussed more fully in Chapters 7 and 15, a major aspect of health care is moving sick people to higher functional states, but data for such measurements are not available fully for one year, and less over time. Another aspect of health care is saving lives or reducing death rates. In this chapter, quantity is defined as the mortality rate (M). Reduced-form equations of the model with price and mortality as endogenous variables can then be estimated as functions of the exogenous variables in the system. Only the reduced-form mortality equation is considered here:

$$M = f \text{ (INC, SOC, ENV, PROV, TECH)}.$$

Because the number of variables for which consistent data are available over the years is limited, the problem of estimation was narrowed to the proxies to be used for each of the vectors of the model. Various proxies were tested, some requiring separate estimation for the period between years for which data were reported with simple linear regressions used for such estimation. The following proxies were selected for the model:

Vector	*Proxy*
Economic variable	Real income per capita (with price adjusted to a base year, 1967)
Societal variable	Stress, as indicated by unemployment rates
Environmental variable	Industrial accident rates
Provider characteristics	Number of nurses and of physicians per 100,000 population
Biomedical advances	(see text)

The measure of health care delivery used deserves more discussion. Although it would be desirable to employ a broad measure of health care delivery, such as per capita health care expenditures, a narrower metric is used. The parameter estimates that result when health expenditures are included in the equation contradict common sense; it is implausible to believe that biomedical research has increased death rates. Rather, the biased estimates result from the multicollinearity among income, health expenditures, and biomedical research. The impact of increased health expenditures appears to be captured in the income and biomedical research variables. In the place of per capita health care expenditures, we used a weighted average of physicians and nurses per capita as a partial measure of health care delivery for the 1930-75 period and nurses per capita in the analysis of the 1900-75 period. Although a more complete physical measure of health care delivery is desirable, the absence of complete historical data sets imposed limitations.

The transmission mechanism between the biomedical research measures and the mortality rate also merits more extensive discussion. It is clear that research advances can be effective only after the increases in biomedical knowledge have diffused into fairly widespread use by the health care delivery system or by changes in the health practices of the population. Provider use determines the application.

The variables used in the present study to measure scientific advances, as indicated in Chapter 2, include the number of new PhD's in the biomedical sciences, patents issued for drugs, patents issued for scientific instruments, new drugs marketed as reported by the pharmaceutical industry, and new biomedical journals. No one variable can capture the whole of what is produced by biomedical research. PhD's in the biomedical sciences essentially are an input into biomedical research work. As an index of personnel inputs it has limitations, because physician researchers and nondoctoral-level researchers are excluded. Drug patents are more likely to reflect the research of industry on biomedical problems than the research of universities and governments. The several measures, then, do not encompass all the sources of contribution to medical knowledge, given the extent of collaboration across nations and the common intellectual community of scientists throughout the world.

New knowledge is a particularly troublesome quantity to measure, especially if quality considerations are taken into account. How does one define a unit of knowledge? Furthermore, since new knowledge does not instantaneously reduce deaths, what is the appropriate time lag? Also, what is the appropriate type of variable? Is a stock variable (the accumulation of knowledge) or a flow variable (a measure of new knowledge) appropriate? In the analyses carried out, flow variables are used—the number of new PhD's, for example—on the theory that many therapeutic procedures in use today are relatively new bits of knowledge.

Each proxy developed to measure biomedical research has advantages and disadvantages. One way to account for the variety of measures is to construct a composite index. We tried this and found the index to be highly correlated with the lagged PhD variable.

Another methodological problem arises in determining the appropriate time lag between development of new inputs to research and reduced mortality or between the invention of a new drug or scientific instrument and reduced mortality. We tested various time lags, drawing on the empirical work done by Battelle for the NIH. The Battelle study[15] examines the characteristics of medical advances from conception to general availability. It found for the twenty-six advances examined that the period ranged from two to sixty-six years, with a median of ten years. The study also found less lag in recent years than earlier. A complex of factors suggests that this is so. The growth of the medical care center that provides care and trains physicians is one such factor. When transmission of new medical knowledge depended on adoption of a therapy by solo practitioners, the process tended to be protracted. In the medical center, far more rapid transfer of new technology takes place. Similarly, in the past, when the costs of care were financed out-of-pocket by the patient and his family, physicians were constrained in their therapy by economic considerations; today, third-party payments for services mean that providers can prescribe on the basis of medical rather than economic judgments.

In the analysis, a lag of ten years was applied in the case of new biomedical PhD's and seven years for new drugs, drug patents, and medical instrument patents. Various other lags were tested, including a distributed lag that called for a statistical procedure proposed by deLeeuw.[16] This procedure is a weighted average of data of previous years, with the weights first increasing and then decreasing in a manner represented by an inverted V.

Tables 4-3 and 4-4 provide the correlation matrices of the biomedical research proxies. Table 4-3 covers the years 1930-75 and includes research expenditures. Table 4-4 covers the years 1900-75, excluding research expenditures, because our estimates of research expenditures for the first forty years of this century are based on the other measures of biomedical research efforts. The following are definitions of the variables used in these tables:

Table 4-3. Correlation Coefficients for the Data for 1930-75

	PHD	DRUG	INST	PHD525	DRUG73	INST73	PHD10	DRUG7	NJR1	OJR1	PHDV14	COJRV12	CNJRV12
PHD	1												
DRUG	.94	1											
INST	.89	.87	1										
PHD525	.97	.97	.84	1									
DRUG73	.97	.95	.89	.97	1								
INST73	.54	.63	.55	.58	.66	1							
PHD10	.91	.95	.80	.97	.95	.65	1						
DRUG7	.96	.93	.84	.95	.98	.65	.92	1					
NJR1	.87	.81	.70	.86	.84	.33	.80	.86	1				
OJR1	.92	.86	.78	.91	.90	.42	.86	.92	.99	1			
PHDV14	.94	.97	.83	.99	.97	.66	.99	.95	.82	.88	1		
COJRV12	.97	.97	.83	.99	.97	.57	.97	.95	.87	.92	.99	1	
CNJRV12	.97	.97	.82	.99	.96	.57	.97	.95	.87	.92	.98	.99	1
RBRE	.96	.96	.84	.97	.97	.64	.96	.96	.82	.88	.97	.97	.97

Table 4-4. Correlation Coefficients for the Data for 1900-75

	PHD	DRUG	INST	PHD525	DRUG73	INST73	PHD10	DRUG7	NJR1	OJR1	PHDV14	COJRV12	CNJRV12
PHD	1												
DRUG	.96	1											
INST	.89	.87	1										
PHD525	.98	.98	.84	1									
DRUG73	.98	.97	.89	.98	1								
INST73	.64	.67	.58	.69	.68	1							
PHD10	.94	.96	.81	.98	.96	.71	1						
DRUG7	.97	.95	.85	.96	.99	.67	.94	1					
NJR1	.91	.87	.74	.91	.88	.60	.88	.90	1				
OJR1	.95	.90	.79	.95	.93	.62	.91	.93	.99	1			
PHDV14	.96	.98	.83	.99	.98	.71	.99	.96	.89	.93	1		
COJRV12	.97	.97	.82	.99	.96	.71	.98	.95	.92	.95	.99	1	
CNJRV12	.97	.97	.82	.99	.96	.71	.98	.95	.92	.95	.99	.99	1

PHD   = the number of new biomedical PhD's

DRUG   = the number of drug patents

INST   = the number of medical instrument patents

PHD525   = an index of the stock of biomedical PhD's

DRUG73 = drug patents cumulated, lagged seven years, and depreciated at 30 percent per annum

INST73   = medical instrument patents cumulated, lagged seven years, and depreciated at 30 percent per annum

PHD10   = the number of new biomedical PhD's, lagged ten years

DRUG7   = drug patents, lagged seven years

NJR1   = new biomedical journals (new SERLINE titles) by initial year of publication, lagged one year

OJR1   = biomedical journals (open SERLINE titles, both new and continuation) by initial year of publication, lagged one year

PHDV14   = the number of new biomedical PhD's, distributed lag (inverted V) over a ten-year period (t-5 to t-14, peak lag = 10)

COJRV12 = open biomedical journals cumulated, distributed lag (inverted V) over a ten-year period (t-3 to t-12)

CNJRV12 = new biomedical journals cumulated, distributed lag (inverted V) over a ten-year period (t-3 to t-12)

RBRE   = expenditures for biomedical research, in constant 1967 dollars

Since all research proxies are highly correlated, the empirical section of this chapter presents the simple lagged and distributed lagged versions of the biomedical PhD variable. In earlier research, carried out as part of this study, we assessed the impact of other proxies and similarly concluded that advances in biomedical research had a significant impact on mortality rate reduction.[17]

The low Durbin-Watson statistic in ordinary least square regressions suggested the need to adjust for first-order serial correlation. A variant of the technique developed by Cochrane and Orcutt was used.[18] Although certain problems arise in adjusting for first-order autocorrelation when the true order of correlation is unknown and the value of rho has to be estimated, a rule of thumb, cited by Rao and Griliches, is that in sample sizes larger than twenty, an adjustment should be made for autocorrelation when the estimate of first-order autocorrelation is larger than three.[19]

THE ESTIMATING EQUATION

The regression analysis employs the market model, using a reduced-form mortality equation in log form:

$$ln\ M = \text{Constant} + e_1\ ln\ \text{INC} + e_2\ ln\ \text{SOC} + e_3\ ln\ \text{ENV}$$
$$+ e_4\ ln\ \text{PROV} + e_5\ ln\ \text{TECH}$$

where the subscripted e's are the estimated elasticity coefficients. The definitions of all variables used are as follows:

M = the age-adjusted mortality rate per 1,000 population

MM44 = the age-specific death rate for men 35-44 per 1,000 population

FM44 = the age-specific death rate for women 35-44 per 1,000 population

INC = real income per capita (in 1967 prices)

INCDL = a linear distributed lag that assigns monotonically declining weights to the current observation of INC and the four previous observations

SOC = a societal proxy, the unemployment rate lagged two years

ENV = an environmental proxy, the industrial work injury rate

PROV = a weighted average of the stock of physicians and nurses per 100,000 population

PROVN = the stock of nurses per 100,000 population

TECHL1 = biomedical PhD's lagged ten years; TECHL2, TECHL3, biomedical PhD's lagged twelve and seventeen years, respectively

TECHDL1 = a de Leeuw-type distributed lag transformation of the biomedical PhD variable. (See reference 16.) This particular transformation is a moving weighted average of inverted V shape with a peak weight at a ten-year lag, declining to zero weights before five and after fourteen years. TECHDL2-TECHDL5 adjusts the ten-year distributed weights from a six- to fifteen-year lag to a nine- to eighteen-year lag.

The double-logarithmic functional form was chosen for conceptual and empirical reasons. It is expected *a priori* that a declining marginal physical product accrues to increments in biomedical research over time. As death rates become lower and lower, it becomes more difficult to achieve equal unit decreases per unit of input. This hypothesis is also consistent with the hypothesis that biomedical research has been rationally allocated over the period, attacking first the causes of death that were most widespread and easiest to solve. The double-log form approximates this nonlinear hypothesis. An additional advantage of this form of the equation is that the estimated coefficients have a simple interpretation. They are elasticity coefficients, which are defined to be the percentage change in the dependent variable associated with a 1 percent change in the corresponding independent variables. Finally, the double-log form of the equation fits the data better than do linear estimates.

FINDINGS

The model, when quantified, indicates that for each 1 percent added input into biomedical research over the seventy-five years, 1900-75, mortality rates dropped about one-tenth of 1 percent (−.10 to −.13). Over the more recent forty-five years, 1930-75, mortality rates dropped one-twentieth of 1 percent for each 1 percent added input, ranging up to one-tenth of 1 percent for each added 1 percent input to biomedical research. As one moves back in time, the elasticities increase. The relative elasticities for each of the periods are summarized briefly here for the several regressions run; the full regression results are shown in Tables 4-5- 4-7. The following summary is presented to indicate the relative stability of the elasticities.

Biomedical research elasticities of mortality rates: summary of regression findings

1900-75		*1930-75*
Uniform time lag	−.10	Uniform time lags
		−.05
		−.08
		−.07

Distributed time lag   −.13   Distributed time lags

−.07
−.09
−.09
−.09
−.10

The estimating equation also permits a parceling out of the relative share of the improvement in mortality that is attributable to biomedical advances and to other factors—economic, societal, and environmental. The relative share of the reduction in age-adjusted mortality rates, as estimated, ranges from 40 to 55 percent for 1900-75 and, depending on the methodology, from 20 to more than 40 percent for 1930-75.

The relative shares attributable to biomedical advances are subject to the many qualifications enumerated earlier, including:

Table 4-5. Empirical Results for 1900-75; Elasticity Coefficients Adjusted for First-Order Autocorrelation

Dependent variable	Mortality	
	Uniform lag Ph.D.'s	*Distributive lag Ph.D.'s*
Constant	3.83	3.90
(*t*)	(8.4)	(6.74)
INC	−.16	
(*t*)	(−2.64)	
% share	23	
INCDL		−.15
(*t*)		(−1.56)
% share		.23
SOC	.02	.02
(*t*)	(1.74)	(1.20)
% share	2	2
ENV	.19	.16
(*t*)	(3.45)	(2.91)
% share	12	10
PROVN	−.07	−.04
(*t*)	(−2.17)	(−1.27)
% share	19	11
TECHL1	−.10	
(*t*)	(−3.50)	
% share	43	
TECHDL1		−.13
(*t*)		(2.85)
% share		55
R^2	.93	.94

Table 4-6.   Empirical Results for 1930-75 with Various Lags and Alternative Death Rates; Elasticity Coefficients Adjusted for First-Order Autocorrelation

Dependent variable	10-year lag	12-year lag	17-year lag	Mortality rate, ages 35-44 Men	Mortality rate, ages 35-44 Women
Constant	3.64	3.26	3.44	2.80	3.82
(t)	(9.59)	(8.39)	(10.37)	(4.72)	(5.41)
INC	−.18	−.11	−.15	−.29	−.47
(t)	(−2.92)	(−1.75)	(−2.63)	(−2.93)	(−4.05)
% share	29	18	24	41	44
SOC	.03	.03	.02	.03	.03
(t)	(2.13)	(2.46)	(1.70)	(1.16)	(1.08)
% share	−1	−1	0	−1	−1
ENV	.27	.28	.26	.44	.58
(t)	(5.25)	(6.04)	(5.88)	(5.41)	(6.02)
% share	16	17	16	24	20
PROV	−.28	−.32	−.25	.13	−.10
(t)	(−1.74)	(−2.36)	(−1.97)	(0.51)	(0.14)
% share	23	26	20	−10	5
TECHL1	−.05			−.09	−.10
(t)	(−1.97)			(2.03)	(1.91)
% share	22			33	24
TECHL2		−.08			
(t)		(−3.43)			
% share		32			
TECHL3			−.07		
(t)			(−3.82)		
% share			.32		
R^2	.92	.92	.94	.86	.91

- The incompleteness of the "count" of biomedical advances
- The extent of multicollinearity of the historical data for each of the variables
- The partial content of the variables other than the count of biomedical advances

The range of figures does not represent the minimum or maximum shares. Quite apart from the basic qualifications, the upper bound shown is a result of the longer lag that reduces the weight of the decade or more when biomedical research was expanded but death rates remained fairly constant. And, as discussed in Chapter 8, the applicability of the distributed lag methodology to assessment of biomedical advances and their contribution is questionable. While the methodology is more precise in some ways than a uniform lag, when applied to analysis of biomedical research, it tends to raise the

Table 4-7. Empirical Results for 1930-75 with Various Distributed
Lags; Elasticity Coefficients Adjusted for First-Order Autocorrelation

Dependent variable: Age-adjusted death rate

Mean lag for TECH	*10 yrs.*	*11 yrs.*	*12 yrs.*	*13 yrs.*	*14 yrs.*
Constant	4.42	4.30	4.21	4.15	4.07
(*t*)	(7.82)	(7.71)	(7.58)	(7.41)	(7.16)
INCDL	−0.33	−0.30	−0.28	−0.27	−0.25
(*t*)	(−3.12)	(−2.89)	(−2.71)	(−2.53)	(−2.31)
% share	51	46	43	42	39
SOC	−.002	−.0002	−.00001	.0004	−0.001
(*t*)	(−0.10)	(−0.01)	(0.00)	(0.03)	(−0.07)
% share	0	0	0	0	0
ENV	.21	.20	.20	.20	.20
(*t*)	(3.93)	(3.93)	(4.02)	(4.07)	(4.08)
% share	13	12	12	12	12
PROV	.08	.08	.07	.05	.03
(*t*)	(0.43)	(0.46)	(0.39)	(0.29)	(0.21)
% share	−7	−7	−6	−4	−2
TECHDL1	−0.07				
(*t*)	(−1.47)				
% share	31				
TECHDL2		−.09			
(*t*)		(−1.83)			
% share		39			
TECHDL3			−.09		
(*t*)			(−2.04)		
% share			39		
TECHDL4				−.09	
(*t*)				(−2.16)	
% share				39	
TECHDL5					−.10
(*t*)					(−2.25)
% share					43
R^2	.93	.93	.94	.94	.94

coefficient for research, lower other coefficients, and increase the instability and lower the significance of the estimates.

A finding of 20 to 40 percent as the share of mortality rate improvement attributable to biomedical research for the period 1930-75 is, in the vocabulary of the econometrician, robust. Repeated manipulation of the historical data with somewhat different models and analytical techniques yielded similar estimates. Estimates for the years before 1930 are weaker. Among other things, the data for the early years of this century are not as adequate as the data for the more recent years.

The relative contributions of the biomedical research measure and the other factors to mortality rate improvement are estimated from the elasticities derived from the regressions combined with average annual growth rates. The following equation is used to divide the total decrease in the mortality rate into portions attributable to each factor:

$$100\% = \sum_{i=1}^{5} \frac{e_i \, \Delta X_i}{\Delta M} + \frac{U}{\Delta M}$$

where the e_i's signify the elasticities from the five independent variables, the Δ's signify average annual percentage changes in the dependent and each of the five independent variables, and U is the unexplained difference.

For the 1900-75 period, the biomedical PhD variable accounts for 43 to 55 percent of the reduction in mortality. Income and providers variables rank second and third, with 23 percent attributed to income and 11 to 19 percent attributed to providers (Table 4-5).

For 1930-75, the biomedical variable accounts for 22 to 32 percent with a uniform lag and a higher percentage, ranging up to 43 percent, with a distributed lag adjusted.

Sensitivity of the Lags

As indicated earlier, one concern in measuring biomedical research effort is determining the appropriate time lag. Three separate time lags seem to be associated with the lapse of time between granting of a doctoral degree and changes in mortality. The first time lag is between graduation and the issuance of biomedical patents or the publication of a major research article. We arbitrarily assumed that the distillation of a dissertation into a patent or a published article takes three years.

The second lag is the period between issuance of drugs or instrument patents and marketing or, alternatively, the lag between publication and widespread diffusion of the initial idea or technique. If we assume that new knowledge is embodied in new MD's as they move into practice, then perhaps a 3- or 4-year lag for time of internship and residency training may be appropriate. The lag between patents and marketing may be estimated from Schwartzman's examination of the time lag between the issuance of a drug patent and approval for marketing by the Food and Drug Administration for all new drugs marketed between 1966 and 1974.[20] His results imply a regulatory lag of three to four years.

The final lag consists of the time necessary for new drugs to become widely used by the medical community. For new knowledge, the time lag is between the widespread diffusion of new ideas and widespread application of these new ideas to actual practices. Again, our only empirical evidence is on the diffusion of new drugs. Peltzman examined the diffusion of a small sample of drug breakthroughs in the 1950s and found the peak effect to be approximately four years after introduction of the drugs.[21] Summing up these lags produces a time lag of ten years between the granting of new PhD's and changes in mortality. Clearly, not all significant biomedical advances are patented, and biomedical scientists probably continue to produce contributions for many years after receiving their terminal degrees. Nevertheless, a ten-year time lag seems reasonable; it also corresponds with the findings of the Battelle study.

For the 1930-75 period, different lags were estimated as a sensitivity test of the assumed ten-year time lag.

Regressions were run in which biomedical PhD's were lagged from one to twenty years. For the early years, the coefficient estimates were small and insignificant, by the tenth year they became significant, and, as the lag was lengthened, they increased in significance. The size of the coefficient was largest with a lag of twelve years, but maintained that order of magnitude for longer lags. Table 4-6 illustrates the simple lagged results for ten, twelve, and seventeen years. The impact of the biomedical variable on mortality was between 22 and 32 percent, depending on the length of the lag.

As a further sensitivity test, the last two columns of Table 4-6 present the results when different dependent variables are used, age-specific death rates for men and women between the ages of thirty-five and forty-four. Income has had the largest impact on the reduced mortality for these narrower age groups. The impact on death rates of the proxy for research effort was computed at 24 percent for women and 33 percent for men. One explanation for the higher share for men might be the difference between men and women in the use of preventive medicine. Men tend to ignore health problems until they reach the stage where lifesaving procedures are more likely to be employed. Women, on the other hand, have more physician visits and more bed-disability days than men, thereby combating illness at earlier stages.

As indicated earlier, it can be argued that a distributed rather than a simple lag is more appropriate. However, the distributed lag smoothes out the data and increases the probability of multicollinearity problems. (Multicollinearity refers to difficulty in obtaining precise estimates of the coefficients due to high correlations among the independent variables.) The distributed lag, an inverted-V-shaped lag spanning a ten-year period, was analyzed over a period in the same way as the simple lag structure. Table 4-7 presents the results for regressions where the peak of the lag ranges from ten to fourteen years. For distributed lags with peaks earlier than ten years, the results were not significant. The results become significant and appear to stabilize for lags with peaks between eleven and fourteen years. The coefficient estimates on the biomedical research variable are slightly higher than in the simple lagged version, and the provider variable becomes insignificant when distributed lags are used. In terms of relative shares, biomedical research, applying a distributed lag technique, accounts for 31 to 43 percent of the decrease in death rates, but this variable may be capturing some of the impact of providers.

In general, the results over both periods indicate that biomedical research contributed importantly to the reduction of death rates. The range of estimates is roughly between 20 and 40 percent, with the higher estimates coming from a version of the model that may be conceptually superior to other versions but fraught with more statistical problems.

Other Validity Tests

We examined other study findings for an explanation of any possible understatement of the coefficients of the specific variables, other than biomedical research, because of the proxy selection. The examination was designed to determine whether there was potential overstatement of the biomedical advance variable. Elasticity coefficients estimated by others for income, providers of care, air pollution, and unemployment were tested.

If, for example, we substitute the elasticities of Auster and associates,[7] for the coefficient found for income or for providers, the share of these variables in determining death rate reductions would go up rather than down. A 1 percent increase in the quantity of medical services was associated in the Auster study with a one-tenth of 1 percent decrease in mortality.

Fuchs[8] analyzed infant mortality data for states of the United States and for developed countries for 1937 and 1965. He regressed mortality rates against income and a dummy variable for time (0 in 1937 and 1 in 1965). Assuming constant elasticities for 1937 and 1965, the coefficient on the time dummy variable indicated improvement in mortality because of advances in knowledge, both in medical sciences and in other areas that impact on mortality. His finding is a somewhat higher rather than lower share for the role of growth in knowledge in reducing death rates (some 40 to 60 percent) over the period 1937-65.

Auster and associates[7] used 1960 age-adjusted death rates for white males across states as the dependent variable in a production function approach. This measure of health implicitly assumes that a constant portion of medical care is allocated to the prolongation of life. Environmental conditions, including income and education, played an important role, and may have offset the advantages of improvement in medical care. Literal predictions, by use of the cross-sectional coefficients on the period 1955-65, implied that technological change reduced mortality during these years by 5.2 percent.

The studies by Lave and Seskin[9] provide estimates of the mortality rate elasticity of air pollution as possible substitutes for work injuries used as a proxy for environmental factors in the present study. Lave and Seskin found that a 1-percent decrease in the minimum concentration of measured particulates would decrease the total death rate by one-twentieth of 1 percent, and a similar percentage decrease in the minimum concentration of sulfates would decrease the total death rate by a somewhat smaller percentage (0.04). The elasticity coefficient assigned to environmental factors in the present study is higher than the sum of these Lave-Seskin estimates, that is, a 1 percent improvement in the environmental proxy is associated with a 0.27 percent drop in the total death rate. Substitution of the Lave-Seskin coefficients would lower the share attributed to the environment and probably raise the share attributable to other factors, including biomedical research.

The coefficients cited are primarily drawn from cross-sectional studies across geographic areas, and the results do not apply to the analyses across time. They are introduced here to help establish validity of the proxies selected. Of course, the specific variables used in the cross-sectional studies are not available for the across-time analyses required to consider directly biomedical advances as a variable.

Although some of these cross-sectional studies attempted to measure indirectly the impact of biomedical research through advances in knowledge or changes in technology, none addressed the problem of direct measurement over time. Fuchs used pooled cross-sectional data with a dummy variable for technology in his regression analysis, but this measure captured more than the direct output from technological change or biomedical research. Auster and associates employed a residual methodology that not only captured technology but also every important factor omitted from the regression.

Brenner examined in considerable detail the relationship between social stress and "pathological indexes including mortality."[10] He found a significant relationship between mortality and social stress. The analyses were carried out both cross-sectionally and across time. If we substitute for the coefficient on societal factors the finding of Brenner that each 1-percent increase in unemployment resulted in about a 0.019-percent increase in deaths, the overall estimated share of the contribution of biomedical research to death rate decline would probably undergo little change. Indeed, the direction of the change, again, would be to lower the share contributed, using Brenner's terminology, to "social pathology" to "social trauma" and likely increase the relative share for biomedical research.

Alternative Measures of Biomedical Advances

We also examined alternative methods for determining the contribution of biomedical research to changes in mortality. We asked, for example: How would the estimates be affected if we used a residual type of analysis in which biomedical research was measured as the difference between the total change that occurred and the change that could be accounted for by demographic, income, environmental, and societal factors?

Using this approach we estimated the residual factor representing the impact of biomedical research and other measures by the following equation:

$$M = \sum_{i=1}^{3} e_i \, \Delta x_i + T$$

where e_i is elasticity; Δx_i is the annual percentage change in real per capita income, societal stress (measured as unemployment rate), and environmental hazards (measured by the work injury rate), respectively; and T is the residual factor representing technological advance and other unexplained variables.

By applying this formula to the 1930-75 average annual age-adjusted death rate decline of −1.488 percent, we obtained a residual factor of −.312 percent annually. In relative terms, the residual corresponds to 21 percent of the mortality change.

We also asked, given a range between a 0.05 percent change in mortality rates for each 1 percent change in biomedical research and a 0.10 percent change in mortality per 1 percent: What would have been the estimated rates for each year from 1930 to 1975?

The impact of biomedical research on the age-adjusted death rates for each year are shown in Figure 4-4. The differences between the

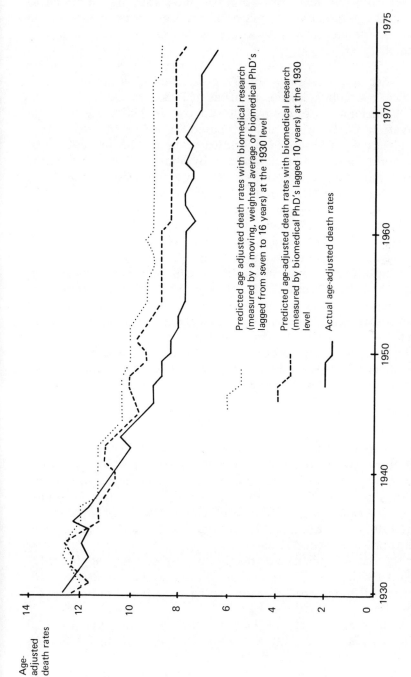

Age-
adjusted
death rates

14
12
10
8
6
4
2
0

1930   1940   1950   1960   1970   1975

Predicted age adjusted death rates with biomedical research (measured by a moving, weighted average of biomedical PhD's lagged from seven to 16 years) at the 1930 level

Predicted age-adjusted death rates with biomedical research (measured by biomedical PhD's lagged 10 years) at the 1930 level

Actual age-adjusted death rates

Source: Actual age-adjusted death rates: *Vital and Health Statistics.*

Figure 4-4. Effect of Biomedical Research on Age-adjusted Death Rates

actual age-adjusted death rates and the rates that are estimated to prevail under alternative assumptions on lags between biomedical research inputs and health status consequences represent essentially the "gap avoided."

By 1975, the age-adjusted death rate would have been 1.3 per 1,000 higher in one estimate and 2.4 per 1,000 higher in the other, if biomedical research had been cut off as of 1930.

Two additional clues were followed up. In 1908, the National Conservation Commission had estimated, as indicated earlier, that the application of knowledge known then to the prevention of deaths could increase life expectancy by almost fifteen years. How does this estimate, made after consultation with experts of that time, compare with what has happened since? Life expectancy at birth today averages seventy-two years; in 1908, it averaged forty-seven years. Thus, the gain of twenty-five years minimally can be factored into application of previous knowledge, fifteen of the twenty-five years, and into new knowledge plus other factors for the remainder. If new knowledge alone accounts for the ten-year extension in lifespan, then 40 percent of the change (10 ÷ 25) would represent the biomedical advances and other contributory factors. The 40 percent contribution represents in this estimate an outside limit for the first three-quarters of the twentieth century.

It is plain that several antibiotics and the development of specifics for a number of diseases ushered in the age of miracle medicine. How much did the antibiotics really contribute to reducing deaths? To approach an estimate, we first cataloged the various antibiotics—a long and impressive list. As a second step, we analyzed the uses of these antibiotics in connection with specific diseases. The list of antibiotics, compiled from the *Physicians' Desk Reference* and *U.S. Dispensatory*, was matched against the diseases for which each drug is used by physicians. *The National Drug and Therapeutic Index* and *Pharmacological Facts and Figures* were used in this matching process. For example, penicillin was matched with meningitis as a preferred drug, according to *Pharmacological Facts and Figures*, and cephaloridine as a second choice.

For the diseases identified, deaths by disease were tabulated for 1930 and 1975 as an approximation of diseases that are treated with antibiotics (differences in disease classification posed familiar problems).

After standardizing by deaths per 1,000, we found that in 1930 4.45 deaths per 1,000 were caused by diseases that in 1975 were treatable with antibiotics, and by 1975, 0.93 deaths per 1,000 were caused by those diseases—a difference of 3.52 deaths per 1,000 between 1930 and 1975. In other words, if the antibiotics available in 1975 had been in use in 1930, 388,000, or 31 percent, of the deaths in 1930 potentially could have been postponed. Biomedical research, through its contribution of antibiotics, may be credited with a partial, if not a major, share of the 31 percent of the reduction in deaths between 1930 and 1975 from these selected diseases.

As we have indicated, we derived estimates suggesting that biomedical research has contributed to reduced death rates. The estimates range from 20 to 40 percent, with a larger contribution indicated for the seventy-five years from 1900 to 1975 than for the forty-five years from 1930 to 1975. As a conservative estimate based on the several checks that have been made, we are using a range of 20 to 30 percent as representing the share of reduced mortality attributable to biomedical research in the forty-five years and a range of 30 to 40 percent for the seventy-five years that have elapsed since 1900.

APPENDIX

Table 4A-1.   Significant Medical Advances and Technological Developments

Acceptance of widespread immunization programs:
  For poliomyelitis, measles, influenza
  Tetanus toxoid
Access to cardiac chambers, e.g., mitral commissurotomy
Acid and alkaline phosphotase levels with associated connotations
ACTH
Adrenal corticosteroids
Advances in delineation of etiologies of contact dermatitis (e.g., cosmetics)
Advances in fracture reduction
Advances in hand surgery
Advances in manipulative treatment (i.e., cervical or lumbar traction)
Advances in medical rehabilitation:
  Development of the concept of total medical rehabilitation care
  Widespread establishment of rehabilitation centers
  Development of pre-vocational evaluation techniques
  Development of rehabilitation nursing
  Technical advances in speech therapy
Advances in neuro-physiology, neuro-psychopharmacology and neuro-biochemistry
Advent of practical telecobalt therapy for general cancer treatment (cobalt bomb)
Advances in prevention of hearing loss:
  Industrial use of ear plugs
  Conservation of hearing programs in industry
Advances in prostatic surgery by both open and endoscopic use
Advances in psychotherapy
Advances in reconstructive and restorative surgery, especially surgical care of arthritic joints, hands, elbows, knees, and feet
Advances in renal vascular surgery, renal transplantation in identical twins, and progress toward success in other transplantations
Advances in repair of maxillofacial injuries
Advances in surgery of trauma, e.g., skin grafting, internal fixation of fractures

Advances in transplantation and homotransplantation of tissues along with a better understanding of host immune reaction
Advances in treatment of retinoblastoma
Advances in urinary diversion procedures and the use of intestinal segments as substitutes for ureters, bladder, or urethra
Alpha-chymotrypsin in cataract surgery
Amebicides (e.g., chloroquine)
Anatomy of the lungs—recognition of importance of bronchopulmonary segment made definite surgical and medical therapy possible
Angiocardiography, angiography, arteriography
Development of new concentrated vascular radiopaque media of low toxicity
Development of rapid film sequencing equipment, automatic injectors, and arterial catheters for cardiovascular roentgenology
Antibiotics
  For use against bacteria, fungi, for intestinal tract sterilization
Anticonvulsants
Antihistamines
Antihypertensive drugs
Antimalarial drugs
Antimetabolics
Antiparkinson agents
Antituberculosis chemotherapy:
  Isoniazid (INH)
  Para-aminosalicyclic acid (PAS)
  Streptomycin
Artificial kidney
Audiometry and associated developments and improvements in audiometers
Automatic X-ray film processing and exposure control
Automation in the laboratory
Better equipment for pediatric anesthesia:
  Digby-leigh valve and other unidirectional valves
  Improved endotracheal equipment

Cancer chemotherapeutic agents, e.g., mechlorethamine HCL
Cardiac catheterization
Cardiac resuscitation
Cardiac surgery
  Open heart surgical procedures using extracorporeal circulation and hypothermia
Cerebral angiography
Changing attitudes toward mental disease, illustrated by:
  Teaching of emotional problems in medical schools
  Use of the halfway house
  Open door policies of large mental hospitals
  Psychiatric units in general hospitals
Chemotherapy for central nervous system
  Syphilis and bacterial meningitis
Cholangiography and cholecystography
Chromium tagged red blood cells
Chromosome counts and mapping
Clinical management of fluid and electrolyte imbalance, especially for diabetic coma
Closure of patent ductus
Collection and handling of blood and blood products
Community and public health advances:
  Community health centers
  Sanitation procedures and laws
  Use of public health units in rural areas
Control of increased intracranial pressure (intravenous urea, hypotension, positive-negative respiration)
Controlled cardiac arrest during surgery
Correction of Meniere's disease
Corticosteroids
Cranioplasty with alloplastic materials, e.g., tantulum, plastics, stainless steel
Cytodiagnosis in gastric carcinoma
Delineation of etiologies of contact dermatitis
Delineation of inborn errors of metabolism
Delineation of patterns of normal growth and development (child development)
Dermatomes (Reese, Padgett, Barker, and Brown)

Development and improvement of various intracutaneous tests (histoplasmin, tuberculin)
Development and increasing use of operating room monitors (flowmeter, electro-cardiogram, cardiac monitor)
Development and more general uses of vaccines, e.g.: Influenza; poliomyelitis; smallpox (newer types); tetanus-diphtheria-pertussis (newer types); yellow fever
Developments in cleft lip and cleft palate repair
Developments in electroencephalography
Developments in telemetering of physiological data and application of this knowledge to aerospace travel
Development of blood banks with subsequent improvements in collection, processing, storage, and administration of blood and its derivatives
Development of cerebral angiography
Development of child psychiatry
Development of drains in hydrocephalus
Development of electrocardiography of the fetus prior to and during delivery
Development of electromyography
Development of electroshock treatment
Development of exchange transfusions in erthroblastosis fetalis
Development of exfoliative cytology
Development of fractional pneumoencephalography
Development of functional orthetic devices and splints
Development of hypothermia
Development of improved agencies in control of carcinoma, including: Electrocautery; chemotherapy; radiation and radioactive isotopes; radical surgical techniques
Development of inert synthetic materials for use in reconstructive surgery:
  Implantation at surface depths
  Sub-cutaneous implantation to restore form and contour
Development of insecticides, e.g., DDT
Development of modern ventilators, assistors, and improved methods for artificial respiration, e.g., Ambu respirator
Development of myelography
Development of programs emphasizing early auditory and speech training in children with impaired hearing

Table 4A-1 continued

Development of safe, effective antimicrobial, antifungal, and antituberculosis agents for control of virtually every significant pathogenic organism encountered in the genito-urinary tract

Development of stereotactic surgery

Development of techniques for hemodialysis and peritoneal dialysis

Development of Treponema pallidum immobilization test

Diagnosis and management of congenital heart defects by cardiac catheterization, angiocardiography, and surgical correction

Diagnosis and treatment of protruded cervical discs, including myelography, discography, and anterior fusion

Diet:
Knowledge of need for vitamins
Better awareness of dietary needs

Discovery and identification of many viruses, e.g.: Respiratory, myxoviruses, ECHO, adenovirus, etc.

Discovery of idoxuridine in the treatment of herpes simplex keratitis

Discovery of the relationship of prostatic carcinoma, and certain other neoplasms, to hormone balance with the development of orchiectomy, androgen, and estrogen therapy as control measures

Discovery of role of excessive oxygen as a cause of retrolental fibroplasia when administered to premature infants

Effective oral diuretics

Electrolyte determination

Electromyography, nerve conduction velocity determination and other electrodiagnostic techniques

Electroretinography

Enzyme determination, e.g.: SGOT, amylase, alkaline, acid phosphatase

Esophageal tamponade balloon

Establishment of tissue banks (blood vessels, bones, skin, etc.)

External cardiac massage

Fenestration surgery

Fluorescent antibody technique

Fluoridation of public drinking water

Fractional pneumoencephalogram

Functional extremity splints

Gait training

General anesthetic agents:
Fluothane (Halothane)
Cyclopropane
Trichlorethylene

Goldmann applanation tonometry

Hormone determination

Hypothermia

I^{131} in diagnosis and treatment of thyroid abnormalities

Identification of the trachoma virus with potential for developing a successful vaccine

Improved anesthetic agents and techniques

Improved artificial limbs

Improved esophagoscopes

Improved gastroscopes

Improved identification, understanding, and rehabilitation of intersex problems

Improved methods of cardiac resuscitation

Improved methods of treating detached retina, including scheral buckling with encircling plastic bands and photocoagulation

Improved pre- and post-operative care:
Blood banks; controlled or assisted respiration; early ambulation; fluid and electrolytes; heparin and dicumarol; plasma, serum albumin and fibrinogen; vitamin K

Improved status and development of mental hygiene programs (assistance of psychopharmacology)

Improved treatment of burns

Improved understanding of wound management

Improvements and developments in fluoroscopy:
Image intensifier
Cine-radiography
Use of television circuits in fluoroscopy

Improvements in and miniaturization of hearing aids

Improvement in areas of dressing materials, tapes, and cleansing agents

Improvements in bronchiography

Improvements in bronchiogram

Improvements in bronchoscopy

Improvements in cell, tissue, and organ culture for basic investigations in cell biology and for practical clinical research in microbiology, biochemistry, and chemotherapy

Improvements in contact lenses and their use for a wide variety of visual problems

Improvements in gonioscopy

Improvements in intravenous pyelography, angiography, and cineradiography

Improvements in microscopy (phase contrast, electron)

Improvements in myelography

Improvements in oral and mechanical contraceptives

Improvements in planigraphy

Improvement in prenatal care leading to decreased incidence of toxemia in pregnancy

Improvements in prosthetic devices

Improvements in radiation therapy and equipment:
Supervoltage therapy; teletherapy units (Co-60 and Ce); rotational therapy; refinements in dosimetry; oxygen as a radiosensitizer; BUDR sensitization of DNA

Improvement in radical hysterectomy and node dissection techniques

Improvements in respirators

Improvements in tonometry

Improvement of treatment of diabetes in pregnancy

Improvements in use of blood and blood components:
Blood banking; blood substitutes; refined transfusion techniques

Increased community-doctor interest in:
Accidents; athletic injury control; health maintenance programs; poison control; pre- and post-natal care

Increased emphasis on health of employees:
Improvements in care of handicapped and injured worker
Physical examinations in industry
Pre-employment examinations and matching of jobs to capabilities
Progress in understanding of sickness absence
Study and treatment of alcoholism

Improvements in industrial hygiene engineering, e.g., lighting ventilation

Increased recognition of systemic diseases and syndromes manifested in the skin

Increasing knowledge of etiologies of sterility

Increasing knowledge of Rh and ABO incompatibilities

Increasing number of routine examinations of breast and pelvic organs

Inhalation therapy, including the ventilatory aid IPPB (intermittent positive pressure breathing)

Introduction of and improvements in hormonal therapy of:
Lymphomas; leukemias; breast cancer; prostate cancer

Introduction of and improvements in hormone replacement therapy of:
Diabetes; hypothyroidism; hypoadrenalism

Isolation and identification of many viruses

Isolation and perfusion of tumors

Isoproterenol

The Kuntscher and other types of intra medullary nails for fractures of long bones

Liver function tests, e.g., BSP

Local anesthetic agents:
Lidocaine; mepiracaine

Major exploratory, resective, extirpative pulmonary surgery

Mass diagnostic surveys:
Blood pressure tests on a mass screening basis
Detection of diabetes mellitus
X-ray for tuberculosis and other chest lesions
Papanicolaou smears for cytodiagnosis of cancer

Medullary prostheses to replace head and neck of femur following trauma and arthritis

Metabolic and genetic information about mental deficiency and certain diseases of the nervous system

Miniaturized surgical instruments

Modified insulin

More frequent physical examinations

More widespread psychiatric counseling and understanding of the mentally ill

Mucosal biopsy capsules

Table 4A-1 continued

Muscle relaxants:
  Succinylcholine; turocurarine; gallamine
Myringoplasty and tympanoplasty
Needle liver biopsy
New and improved optical, electrical, and mechanical instruments for diagnostic and therapeutic use
Oral hypoglycemic agents
Organ transplantation
Papanicolaou test for cytodiagnosis of cervical cancer
Penicillins and broad spectrum antibiotics
Perfection of methods for successfully using corneal transplants
Perfection of prefrontal and fractional lobotomy
Perfection of rhizotomy
Perfection of spinothalamic tractotomy
Pin index safety system for gas cylinders
Pitocin
Plastic and metal implants
Poliomyelitis vaccines
Progestational hormones
Psychomotor stimulants
Quantitative and qualitative colormetric procedures:
  Liver and kidney function tests
Radioisotopes for diagnosis and treatment of:
  Thyroid disease; kidney function and diseases; protein metabolism; brain tumors; pancreatic insufficiency; plasma and blood volume and determination of blood circulation; metabolic studies (fat absorption); malignant diseases; polycythemia; pituitary tumors; B-12 absorption studies
Radiology:
  Arteriography; radiopaque myelography with the use of iophendylate and other safe contrast media for radiological diagnosis
Ready availability of very fine atraumatic suture materials
Recognition and delineation of pneumonoconiosis
Recognition of chromosomal abnormalities in certain genetic diseases, e.g., mongolism
Recognition of etiology of retrolental fibroplasia
Recognition of fibrinogen deficiency

Recognition of maternal infections as bases for congenital malformations (e.g., rubella) and infections (e.g., toxoplasmosis)
Recognition of nutritional abnormalities as etiologies of disease:
  Vitamin deficiency
  Essential amino acid deficiency
  Relation of diet to hepatic pathology
Recognition of toxoplasmosis as a cause of uveitis
Recognition of value and standard use of recovery room
Reconstructive nasal surgery
Refined technique and equipment for therapeutic exercise:
  Cervical and lumbar traction
  Progressive resistive exercises
  Proprioceptive facilitation techniques
  Neuromuscular re-education
Refinements in anticoagulants
Refinements in pneumonectomy (recognition of the bronchopulmonary unit as a surgical unit)
Refinements in soda lime CO_2 absorption
Resection of coarctation
Scanning with radioisotopes and the development of scanning equipment
  Scintillation scanning
Serum and urinary hormone levels in relation to endocrine disorders
Serum electrolyte determinations
Shortwave, microwave, and ultrasonic diathermy
Standardization of anesthetic equipment
Stapes surgery
Studies in stress reaction (isolation, cold, heat, noise, fatigue, anoxia, etc.)
Sulfa drugs, e.g., sulfadimethoxine, sulfapyridine, sulfisoxazole
Sulfonamides
Sulfones for leprosy and dermatitis herpetiformis
Surgical correction of aortic aneurysms
Surgical microscope
Surgical plastic and metal implants
Surgical treatment of malignancies of larynx and pharynx

Surgical treatment of vascular lesions of brain (e.g., aneurysms)
   and angiomatous malformations
Techniques for evaluation of pulmonary function
Tracheostomy for extensive brain surgery
Tranquilizers
Treatment of the thyroid with radioiodine:
   Hyperthyroidism; thyroid malignancies
Use of carbonic anhydrase inhibitors, such as acetazolamide, in
   treatment of glaucoma

Use of extracorporeal circulation
Use of hypothermia in neurosurgical procedures
Use of preserved bones (bone banks)
Use of ultraviolet light in diagnosis of fungal infections
Vagotomy
Valvular and arterial prostheses
Vascular prostheses and homografts
Vascular surgery

Source: Reference 13.

REFERENCES

1. McKeown, T., Record, R.G., and Turner, R.D.: An interpretation of the decline of mortality in England and Wales during the twentieth century. Population Studies 29:391-422, November 1975.

2. Hemminki, E., and Paakkulainen, A.: The effect of antibiotics on mortality from infectious diseases in Sweden and Finland. Am J Public Health 66:1180-1184, December 1976.

3. McKinlay, J.B., and McKinlay, S.M.: The questionable contribution of medical measures to the decline of mortality in the United States in the twentieth century. Milbank Mem Fund 55:405-428, summer 1977.

4. American College of Surgeons and American Surgical Association: Surgery in the United States; A summary report of the study on surgical services for the United States. American College of Surgeons, Chicago, 1975.

5. Dwork, D.: TB therapies 1900-1975. Public Services Laboratory, Georgetown University, Washington, D.C. (processed), 1978.

6. Adelman, I.: An econometric analysis of population growth. Am Econ Rev 53:314-339, June 1963.

7. Auster, R., Leveson, I., and Sarachek, D.: The production of health, an exploratory study. J Human Res 4:411-436, fall 1969.

8. Fuchs, V.: Some economic aspects of mortality in developed countries. *In* The economics of health and medical care, edited by M. Perlman. John Wiley & Sons, Inc., New York, 1974, pp. 174-193.

9. Lave, L., and Seskin, E.: Air pollution and human health. Johns Hopkins University Press, Baltimore, Md., 1976.

10. Brenner, H.M.: Health costs and benefits of economic policy. Int J Health Serv 7:581-623, April 1977.

11. Orcutt, G.H., et al.: Does your probability of death depend on your environment? A microanalytic study. Am Econ Rev Papers and Proceedings 67:260-264, February 1977.

12. Report of the National Conservation Commission: Vol. III, U.S. Senate Document No. 676, 60th Congress, 2d session, Washington, D.C., February 1909.

13. American Medical Association: Report of the Commission on Cost of Medical care. Vol. III, Significant medical advances. American Medical Association, Chicago, 1964.

14. *Cited in* On equality of educational opportunity, edited by F. Mosteller and D.P. Moynihan. Vintage Books, New York, 1972, p. 34.

15. Leininger, R.I., and Levy, G.W.: Further analyses of the characteristics of research resulting in clinical advances from inception to clinical usage. Battelle Columbus Laboratories, Columbus, Ohio, February 1977.

16. de Leeuw, F.: The demand for capital goods by manufacturers: a quarterly time series. Econometrica 30:407-423, July 1962.

17. Chen, M., and Wagner, D.: Gains in mortality from biomedical research 1930-1975: an initial assessment. Soc Science and Medicine 12:73-81, November 1978. (Although, in general, alternative proxies show a significant impact of biomedical research on mortality, the partial aspects of the output proxies make

them less robust than alternative formulations of the more comprehensive input measures, biomedical research PhD's.)

18. Cochrane, D., and Orcutt, G.H.: Application of least squares regressions to relationships containing autocorrelated error terms. J Am Stat Assoc 44:32-61, 1949. (The version used in this report is included in S.A.S. 76 described in A users guide to S.A.S. 76. S.A.S. Institute, Releigh, N.C., 1976.)

19. Rao, P., and Griliches, Z.: Small-sample properties of several two-stage regression methods in the context of autocorrelated errors. J Am Stat Assoc 64:253-272, March 1969.

20. Schwartzman, D.: Innovation in the pharmaceutical industry. Johns Hopkins University Press, Baltimore, Md., 1976, pp. 162-181.

21. Peltzman, S.: The diffusion of pharmaceutical information. *In* Drug development and marketing, edited by R.B. Helms. American Enterprise Institute, Washington, D.C., 1975, pp. 15-26.

✳ *Chapter Five*

Biomedical Research and Savings in Cost of Death

In the preceding chapter, biomedical advances are shown to account for 20 to 40 percent of the historical reduction in mortality. What do these reductions mean in terms of economic costs saved? In this chapter, we examine the economic cost of premature death and the contribution of biomedical advances to the historical reduction in such costs.

The cost of death, or valuation of human life, is of greater significance than it was in the past because estimates of this cost are being applied to programming decisions. Indeed, the pursuit of the contribution of biomedical research to saving in economic cost as a consequence of improved mortality stems from the current concern about program analysis as a means toward greater efficiency in the allocation of resources.

PRICING A HUMAN LIFE

Despite the moral question involved in valuing a human life, such valuation is frequently performed. Individuals and governments place a value on human life and the avoidance of deaths and disablement, even though the notion of attaching a material worth to life is abhorred. Some years ago, Thedié and Abraham[1] stated the issue of choice in resource allocations that gives rise to this valuation: "A cross-road is laid but a sharp turn remains. Some hospitals are built, why not more? Certain sums are spent on medical research. Why not larger or smaller amounts?"

Despite any misgivings about the notion of pricing a life, current practices explicitly or implicitly call for this price. Courts, by their awards in liability cases, for example, place a value on life lost. Workmen's compensation agencies pay benefits that call for valuation of life, as do insurance companies. Many agencies carry out activities that require such valuation, and the list of those agencies and programs that apply human life valuations has grown as governmental activity has expanded. Today, among the agencies that call for valuation as part of their routine program operations are the Department of Transportation, OSHA, EPA, and the new Energy Department. In some program decisions, the valuation is implicit; in others, an effort is made to put a value on human life for purposes of making decisions about whether to spend additional resources for added safety.

A wide range of costs are incurred by several federal agencies in lifesaving activities. In planning the construction of nuclear energy plants, upward of $4 million is spent to save a life.[2] Outlays for construction of these plants so that they will be safe, however, represent more than "lifesaving;" the program of nuclear energy production is at stake because of the public's grave concern about nuclear accidents, and this public concern is made known to government. Government is responsible for public safety, and the possibility exists for scaling the amount of safety because nuclear plant engineering permits sequential reduction of probabilities of accidents. Reductions in hazards are often obtained at only a substantial increase in cost. Other agencies that have no similar hazard problems set the value of a human life at a substantially lower amount. No uniform, governmentwide practice exists.

Measuring Human Capital

Human capital valuation is the traditional method used to estimate the value of a human life. The value, as measured, represents the added production that results as a consequence of a life saved or through investment in people, or both.

Human capital valuation requires determination of future earnings of those whose lives have been saved. Earnings for this purpose, in concept, are marginal wages or the earnings of the additional workers. The computation essentially requires a determination of the number of productive years of work added by the lifesaving measures and added product per added worker during those additional years. Despite the imperfections in the labor market and the unreality of marginal wages, measurement necessarily is based on equating earnings to marginal product.

Accepting earnings as the basic measurement requires calculation of each year's earnings into the future on a comparable basis. To arrive at comparability, it is important to bear in mind that today's earnings are more valuable than tomorrow's same earnings. A dollar today has a greater value than it will have a year from now—today, it can be deposited and it will earn interest. At an interest rate of 10 percent, this year's dollar will be worth more than $2.50 in ten years. Similarly, the discount process is such that for each year in the future, earnings are reduced to reflect that the dollar is not received this year and interest is lost. For example, a dollar to be received in ten years would be worth only 38.6 cents today at a 10 percent discount rate.

With r standing for the interest rate, 10 percent in the preceding examples, the present value of $\$X$ earned n years in the future is $\$X/(1 + r)^n$. In a present value analysis, at a discount rate of 10 percent, a stream of dollar earnings are computed (X_0, X_1, X_2 ... X_t) that have a present value of:

$$X_0 + \frac{X_1}{(1 + .10)} + \frac{X_2}{(1 + .10)^2} + \cdots \cdot \frac{X_t}{(1 + .10)^t}$$

As indicated in Chapter 1, professionals essentially disagree on the appropriate discount rate to be used in determining present values of future earnings for purposes of measuring human capital. The literature on this subject is rich. Eckstein,[3] Hirschleifer,[4] Hitch and McKean,[5] Feldstein and Summers,[6] and Baumol,[7] among others, have contributed to it. Various concepts have been used, ranging from a rate that represents a pure time preference rate to a rate equivalent to the interest rate on borrowing for commercial purposes, corrected, perhaps, for a variety of factors—tax-exempt equivalency, transaction costs, or differences in risk. As a consequence, the convention now is to apply alternative discount rates in calculating the values of human capital. By such alternative computations, the sensitivity of values derived to the choice of a discount rate can be shown.

In computing the value of lives saved as a consequence of reduced mortality over the past three-quarters of a century, we applied a single rate for each of the years of the study to reflect the rate of pure time preference. But we also applied alternative rates to the estimates for the more recent period to suggest the disparity in findings attributable to differences in the discount rate.

However, we did not follow another convention in the valuation of human life saved as a potential consequence of a health program; namely, we did not use a discount rate of 4 or 6 percent (except as an additional display). These rates may be traced to the early studies of Weisbrod,[8] Fein,[9] Klarman,[10] and others. Since the time of these studies, however, commercial interest rates that reflect the productivity of funds in private investment have climbed considerably. Even the 10 percent rate applied here as one alternative may be low by today's investment returns, given the inflationary pressures experienced. The 10 percent rate essentially derives from the rate selected several years ago by the Office of Management and Budget as the before tax return on capital in private investment.[11]

We also did not apply recent experimental research on personal discount rates that points to variation in such rates by age and other characteristics. Gilman[12] found that discount rates by age and other characteristics ranged from about 36 percent to about 6 percent; they declined with age and income but were higher for females than males and higher for nonwhites than whites. In other words, young persons, women, lower income groups, and blacks prefer more than others current consumption over delayed consumption—this year's income to later income. If applied to the computation of values in Table 5-1, the valuation for young persons would be reduced significantly as would the valuation for women. At the same time, the values for older persons would be somewhat increased.

The Worth of A Life

What is the value of a life saved, assuming average wages, by age, can be used as a proxy for marginal earnings? Table 5-1 shows the present value of future earnings for 1975 and 1976, by age and sex, and at alternative discount rates. Table 5-2 shows the present value of future earnings for earlier years and year 2000; illustrative figures for selected age groups of males for 1976 follow:

Selected age groups (males)	2.5 percent discount rate	10 percent discount rate
1-4	$493,131	$ 40,715
10-14	517,653	87,846
20-24	525,538	162,506
30-34	440,669	186,965
40-44	307,337	165,624
65-69	16,594	13,481

As these estimates indicate, a wide difference occurs in the value of human life at each of the selected ages according to the discount rate used. At ages twenty to twenty-four and a 2.5 percent discount

Table 5-1. Present Value of Future Earnings, by Age and Sex, 1975 and 1976

Age group	1975				1976			
	Discounted at 2.5 percent		Discounted at 10 percent		Discounted at 2.5 percent		Discounted at 10 percent	
	Male	Female	Male	Female	Male	Female	Male	Female
Average, all ages	$350,024	$235,564	$102,631	$ 70,853	$369,046	$246,268	$109,480	$ 74,511
1-4	465,698	337,872	38,036	30,223	493,131	354,319	40,715	31,678
5-9	475,743	345,144	55,705	44,285	503,736	361,902	59,630	46,416
10-14	488,017	354,078	82,066	65,164	517,653	371,274	87,846	68,301
15-19	499,514	359,329	117,367	91,810	528,581	376,362	125,331	95,799
20-24	497,478	349,965	152,964	113,891	525,538	366,780	152,506	118,793
25-29	469,209	318,545	173,868	119,888	494,934	334,744	184,040	125,872
30-34	418,195	276,359	176,882	114,057	440,669	290,450	186,965	119,900
35-39	357,392	233,413	170,362	105,802	376,263	245,669	179,914	111,628
40-44	292,064	191,253	156,719	95,489	307,337	201,184	165,624	100,925
45-49	223,887	150,486	134,756	83,230	234,990	157,870	142,229	87,630
50-54	156,964	111,124	105,213	67,962	163,993	116,212	110,576	71,385
55-59	96,840	74,360	72,093	59,846	100,556	77,283	75,598	51,937
60-64	47,175	43,023	38,439	30,676	47,825	44,536	39,670	31,816
65-69	17,715	22,536	14,048	16,238	16,594	23,232	13,481	16,792
70-74	8,025	12,298	6,580	9,351	6,825	12,579	5,706	9,580
75-79	3,557	6,197	3,018	4,981	2,749	6,310	2,368	5,075
80-84	1,595	2,995	1,410	2,565	1,124	3,038	1,002	2,604
85+	610	1,183	610	1,183	402	1,191	402	1,191

Note: Dollar figures represent asset values of expected future earnings at 1975 and 1976 price levels.

Source: Computed from unpublished Bureau of Labor Statistics data on earnings and work experience rates by age and sex, based on life expectancy as calculated by the Office of the Actuary of the Social Security Administration.

Table 5-2. Present Value of Future Earnings, Discounted at 2.5 Percent, by Age and Sex, Selected Years, 1900-2000

Age group	Males				Females			
	1900[1]	1930	1963	2000[1]	1900[1]	1930	1963	2000[1]
Average, all ages	$4,662	$33,776	$172,565	$1,387,483	$1,578	$19,887	$105,828	$867,288
1-4	4,085	39,994	228,307	1,471,000	2,288	25,489	139,079	1,019,000
5-9		41,649	234,849			26,521	142,930	
10-14	5,680	43,106	241,308	1,551,000	2,377	27,398	146,843	1,074,000
15-19		44,394	245,096			28,192	147,147	
20-24	5,904	44,437	240,310	1,583,000	2,057	27,762	140,868	1,067,000
25-29		44,227	223,795			25,231	130,056	
30-34	5,530	38,671	199,221	1,423,000	1,292	22,850	118,100	905,000
35-39		33,971	170,495			18,871	105,544	
40-44	4,360	28,525	139,965	1,051,000	782	15,226	92,440	657,000
45-49		22,849	109,639			11,736	78,789	
50-54	2,841	17,319	81,788	623,000	496	8,661	65,286	414,000
55-59		12,104	56,873			5,905	52,483	
60-64	1,425	7,384	34,032	249,000	268	3,323	40,359	213,000
65-69		4,059	18,011			1,310	30,120	
70-74	499	2,351	10,785	49,000	121	276	21,920	69,000
75-79		1,224	6,047			[2]	14,697	
80-84	175	542	3,231	11,000	[2]	[2]	7,448	23,000
85+	39	115	221	2,000	[2]	[2]	1,180	6,000

[1] Ten-year age categories were used for 1900 and 2000.

[2] Comparable data not available.

Sources: A. Berk and L.C. Paringer: "Cost of Illness and Disease, 1900." Public Services Laboratory, Georgetown University, Washington, D.C., 1977; A. Berk and L.C. Paringer: "Cost of Illness and Disease, 1930." Public Services Laboratory, Georgetown University, Washington, D.C., 1977; J.S. Landefeld: "Economic Cost of Illness, 1963." Public Services Laboratory, Georgetown University, Washington, D.C., 1978; and S.J. Mushkin, et al.: "Cost of Disease and Illness in the United States in the Year 2000." Public Health Reports 93:493-588, September-October 1978.

rate, the value of a male life is $525,538; at a 10 percent rate, the estimate is $162,506. The figures cited include imputed value of household services of men as well as the value of earnings received as fringe benefits. Both discount rates, moreover, are adjusted for an assumed rise in productivity of 2 percent per annum in the years ahead.

Perhaps most important in understanding the measured consequences of biomedical research or other health programs applying a human capital valuation is the wide difference in value of future earnings of young persons; here, the differences are greatest in worth as assessed by present value of earnings or of consumption postponed for a long time, and conversely, the higher the rate of discount, the smaller that value.

In deriving these figures, we discounted earnings, as indicated earlier. But other assumptions were made. One such assumption is the work-force participation rate in the future for men and women if death had not occurred. Three assumptions about the possible work-force participation if death had not come prematurely were: (1) the rates of work-force participation would remain at 1975 levels; (2) the rates would decline, following the trends of the past decade or so; or (3) the decline would be reversed, as indicated by the long-term growth of the aged population and the mounting social costs of early retirement.

In making these computations of attachment to the work force, we adjusted the population to reflect the expected improvement in mortality experience. Estimates from the Office of the Actuary of the Social Security Administration were used to estimate the number of survivors for each year of age from thirteen to ninety-five in each year from 1973 to 2049.[13] For younger persons in 1975, who would be expected to live beyond the year 2050, no further change in life expectancy was assumed. All age groups expected to survive beyond 2050 were computed to have the same survivorship by age and sex as in 2050.

The work experience rates used are for 1975, as shown in Table 5-3. Corresponding rates for the selected study years 1900-2000 are given in Table 5A-1 in the appendix to this chapter.

The value of a life saved, or of a death postponed, in the context of the concept of human capital depends not only on the amount of earnings but also on the activity of persons in a given age group in the work force. In the prime age groups, fewer than 5 percent of the men are not in the work force during a year, but by ages fifty-five to fifty-nine this percentage triples to 15 percent, with sharp increases as age increases so that almost six out of every ten males sixty-five to sixty-nine years old do not have work experience in a given year.

Table 5-3. Work Experience Rates,[1] by Age and Sex, 1975

	Percent	
Age group	Males	Females
15-19	66.9	57.9
20-24	88.9	73.5
25-29	93.9	66.8
30-34	95.5	59.8
35-39	95.2	62.1
40-44	94.3	62.3
45-49	92.4	60.3
50-54	89.6	57.1
55-59	84.8	51.9
60-64	72.4	40.5
65-69	40.9	20.6
70-74	23.1	10.5
75-79	13.0	5.4
80-84	7.4	2.7
85+	4.2	1.4

[1] Percentage of population in each age category having some work experience during a year.
Source: Derived from unpublished Bureau of Labor Statistics data; ages over seventy were extrapolated.

The concept of human capital relates human worth to economic product and earnings. But in the standard economic accounts, housekeeping is not counted as a contribution to economic product. Conventional modification of the concept involves assigning, somewhat arbitrarily, a value for housekeeping services, as indicated in Chapter 1. One modification made is the assignment of a value for housekeeping equal to one-half of men's earnings,[14] to the earnings of domestics,[15] or to the value of time spent in various household tasks on the same basis as such time is priced in the marketplace.[16] Another modification, based on age and education, assigns a value for housekeeping equal to the market earnings forgone because of household tasks.[17] In the estimates of present value of future earnings shown here, the modifications in concept or addition of a value for unpaid work at home have been extended. Household earnings were calculated for each married woman who was not in the labor force, according to her age and number of children, by assigning a price to each of the services performed by the married woman based on market prices. However, household earnings also were added for women in paid employment who do household chores as well and for men who help with household work. Data limitations prevented extending those adjustments to single persons.

The present values of future earnings (work place and household) for each of the selected study years are shown in Tables 5-1 and 5-2.

The values of future earnings for 1900 and 1930 were computed as if the estimates were made in each of these years, that is, without knowledge of the future experience. To have done otherwise, that is, to reflect the actual experience in wages between 1900 and 1975 and between 1930 and 1975, would make for less comparability in the estimates of worth of a life and the gains attributable to the reduction in mortality over the first seventy-five years of the twentieth century.

The value of a life in 1900 dollars is considerably less than the 1975 or 1976 value and a small fraction of the projected year 2000 values. For men thirty to thirty-four years old, the relative values at the price and wage levels of each of those years are compared in Figure 5-1. This age group is selected as illustrative of a prime-age earner group (with adjustment to use data for the age group twenty-five to thirty-four for 1900 and year 2000 due to lack of data).

SAVINGS IN THE COST OF
PREMATURE DEATH

The total number of deaths and the decline in mortality rates, discussed in Chapter 3, can be converted now to values in dollar terms by applying the estimates of present value of future earnings by age and sex. They can also be converted to the savings in cost that have resulted from improved life expectancy.

Trends in Cost of Death

Despite the drop in death rates, total deaths have increased as the population has grown, but this increase in number is dwarfed by the growth in cost per death. While the number of deaths in the population increased by one-third from 1900 to 1975, the total cost of premature death rose almost fortyfold, and from 1930 to 1975, about sevenfold. Higher earnings levels, greater labor force participation by women, and the postponement of death for the very young increase the cost of premature death as computed (Table 5-4).

From one perspective, the economic cost of a death at constant values is the same for all persons and all years. We use average earnings in each of the years as an adjustment factor. Adjusted for differences in earnings levels but not for the differences in work-force participation rates, the cost of premature death in 1930 exceeds that of 1975; however, the 1900 cost is below the 1975 level.

The adjustment corrects for differences in average earnings but

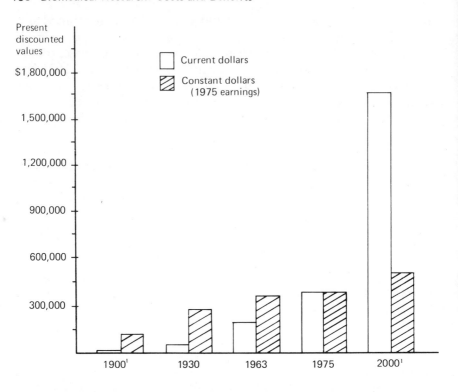

[1] 1900 and 2000 values are for 25- to 34-year-old males.
Sources: A. Berk and L.C. Paringer: "Cost of Illness and Disease, 1900." Public Services Laboratory, Georgetown University, Washington, D.C., 1977; A. Berk and L.C. Paringer: "Cost of Illness and Disease, 1930." Public Services Laboratory, Georgetown University, Washington, D.C., 1978; L.C. Paringer and A. Berk: "Costs of Illness and Disease, Fiscal Year 1975." Public Services Laboratory, Georgetown University, Washington, D.C., 1977; and S.J. Mushkin, et al.: "Cost of Disease and Illness in the United States in the Year 2000." *Public Health Reports* 93:493-588, September-October 1978.

Figure 5-1. Present Discounted Values (at 2.5 Percent) for Men 30 to 34 Years Old, Selected Years, 1900-2000

does not take account of the lifetime pattern of earnings by age relative to the age profile of deaths. In 1900, a substantial share of all deaths was among infants and young children whose economic value in terms of expected future earnings, even when discounted by an interest rate as low as 2.5 percent, was less than that of a young adult. The economic cost per premature death at constant average earnings levels does not, accordingly, adjust the figures for the variation in distribution of earnings by age relative to the age distribution of the deaths. The cost per death has declined from the

Table 5-4. Estimated Economic Cost of Premature Death, Selected Years, 1900-2000

Premature deaths	1900	1930	1963	1975	2000
Total cost, all deaths (in billions):					
Current	$ 3.6	$ 20.1	$ 85.0	$146.2	$715.2
Constant average earnings	85.6	147.9	161.5	146.2	174.8
Cost per death (in dollars), at constant average earnings	60,643	112,706	89,099	75,530	67,044
Total number of deaths	1,410,968	1,312,287	1,812,921	1,935,789	2,607,090
Number of deaths at under age 65	1,174,362	836,163	713,330	694,911	800,986

Sources: Computed from A. Berk and L.C. Paringer: "Cost of Illness and Disease, 1900." Public Services Laboratory, Georgetown University, Washington, D.C., 1977; A. Berk and L.C. Paringer: "Cost of Illness and Disease, 1930." Public Services Laboratory, Georgetown University, Washington, D.C., 1977; J.S. Landefeld: "Economic Cost of Illness, 1963." Public Services Laboratory, Georgetown University, Washington, D.C., 1978; L.C. Paringer and A. Berk: "Costs of Illness and Disease, Fiscal Year 1975." Public Services Laboratory, Georgetown University, Washington, D.C., 1977; and S.J. Mushkin, et al.; "Cost of Disease and Illness in the United States in the Year 2000," *Public Health Reports* 93:493-588, September-October 1978.

1930 high owing to the postponement of death to later ages and in part to the trend toward earlier retirement.

By 1975, cost per death stood at thirty times the 1900 level and five times the 1930 level. Adjusted to a constant average earnings basis, the economic cost of premature death per death amounted to $60,000 in 1900, increased to almost $113,000 in 1930, and dropped to less than $76,000 by 1975. The movement of these cost figures mirrors the improvements in mortality characteristic of the intervening periods. Between 1900 and 1930, much of the gain in reduced mortality was concentrated among the young; between 1930 and 1975, substantial gains were made in increased life expectancy for persons in their middle years.

Cost of Death, by Cause

In 1900, infective and parasitic diseases and diseases of the respiratory system accounted for $1.3 billion of the $3.6 billion economic cost (Table 5-5). By 1975, the single cause-of-death category responsible for the greatest economic cost, $44 billion, was accidents, poisonings, and violence—30 percent of the total cost. Disease as an economic cost is of a far lower order than accidents. At one extreme, infective and parasitic disease and diseases of the

Table 5-5.   Cost of Death, in Millions, by Cause of Death, Selected Years, 1900-75

Disease category	1900 — Current earnings levels	1900 — 1975 earnings levels	1930 — Current earnings levels	1930 — 1975 earnings levels	1975 — Current earnings at 1975 levels
All diseases	$3,594	$85,561	$20,110	$147,868	$146,227
Infective and parasitic diseases	1,317	31,353	3,432	25,232	2,121
Neoplasms	33	791	991	7,287	21,704
Endocrine, nutritional, and metabolic diseases	14	340	422	3,100	2,527
Diseases of the blood and blood-forming organs	8	194	152	1,117	546
Mental disorders	14	327	124	912	2,143
Diseases of the nervous system and sense organs	179	4,255	523	3,846	3,185
Diseases of the circulatory system	238	5,673	2,584	18,998	32,819
Diseases of the respiratory system	689	16,404	2,641	19,419	6,277
Diseases of the digestive system, oral cavity, salivary glands, and jaws	139	3,321	2,046	15,042	6,839
Diseases of the genitourinary system	195	4,640	979	7,198	1,299
Complications of pregnancy, childbirth, and puerperium	14	327	352	2,589	223
Diseases of the skin and subcutaneous tissue	6	143	43	317	116
Diseases of the musculoskeletal system and connective tissue	17	409	49	361	374
Congenital anomalies	152	3,620	449	3,303	5,006
Certain causes of perinatal morbidity and mortality	107	2,547	1,874	13,779	11,938
Symptoms and ill-defined conditions	248	5,897	512	3,768	4,991
Accidents, poisonings, and violence	223	5,318	2,938	21,600	44,118

Note: Cost is computed at a 2.5 percent discount rate after taking account of a 2 percent rise in productivity.

Sources: A. Berk and L.C. Paringer: "Cost of Illness and Disease, 1900." Public Services Laboratory, Georgetown University, Washington, D.C., 1977; A. Berk and L.C. Paringer: "Cost of Illness and Disease, 1930." Public Services Laboratory, Georgetown University, Washington, D.C., 1977; and L.C. Paringer and A. Berk: "Costs of Illness and Disease, Fiscal Year 1975." Public Services Laboratory, Georgetown University, Washington,

respiratory system accounted for only $8.4 billion, or about 6 percent of total cost. Even diseases of the circulatory system and neoplasms together accounted for $54 billion, or only $10 billion more than accidents. Indeed, about two-thirds of the cost of premature death in 1975 can be attributed to accidents, poisonings, and violence; diseases of the circulatory system; and neoplasms.

At the turn of the century, concentration of public activities on the communicable and infectious diseases was fruitful in terms of reductions in deaths and in cost of premature death. By 1930, infectious and parasitic diseases and diseases of the respiratory system declined in relative importance. The share of economic cost of disease attributable to these two categories of disease was 56 percent in 1900, 30 percent in 1930, and less than 6 percent in 1975.

The mid-1970s posed a different set of health problems and potential for corrective action. As indicated earlier, the primary causes of death underlying the high 1975 costs were mainly either social or environmental in origin. The problems tend to be intractable, basic etiological information is lacking, and the persons affected tend to be middle-aged or older.

Table 5-6 shows the economic cost of death in current dollars and adjusted to constant dollars, with average earnings used as the adjustment. The approximately $76,000 average cost per death in 1975, when computed on the basis of disease category, shows a wide range around that average. Of the major causes of death—those that account for approximately three-fourths of the total—the highest economic cost per death is for deaths attributed to certain causes of perinatal mortality. Cost per death from congenital anomalies ranks second, and accidents, poisonings, and violence, third. For diseases of the circulatory system, the economic cost per death is relatively low, below the average. Cost per death in 1975 was particularly high for those disease categories that have relatively low death rates, but the deaths occur primarily among young adults. Costs of death, as measured, tend to be relatively low per death when persons afflicted with terminal disease are advanced in age.

The contrast between mental illness and neoplasms sharpens the factors underlying the variation. For 1975, the cost of premature deaths attributable to mental disorders was $223,000 per death. The cost per cancer death was $59,000, or about 26 percent of the mental illness cost. For cancer, the cost per death reflects the high proportion of all deaths from cancer and the older age groups affected. However, much of the cost of both mental illness and cancer is the cost of illness and hospitalization or nursing home care, rather than the cost of death.

Divergence in cost by disease category, even at constant earnings

Table 5-6.   Estimated Economic Cost per Death, Discounted at 2.5 Percent, by Major Causes of Death, Selected Years, 1900-2000[1]

	At 2.5 percent discount rate									
	1900		1930		1963		1975		2000	
Cause of death	Current	Constant[2]	Current	Constant[2]	Current	Constant[2]	Current	Constant[2]	Current	Constant[2]
Infective and parasitic diseases	$3,077	$73,262	$25,419	$186,904	$73,592[3]	$139,909[3]	$132,559[3]	$132,559[3]	$ 561,996[3]	$137,322[3]
Neoplasms	923[3]	21,976[3]	8,259	60,728	42,162	80,156	59,301	59,301	243,786	59,575
Diseases of the circulatory system	1,354	32,238	6,964	51,206	25,363	48,219	31,926	31,926	126,231	30,840
Diseases of the respiratory system	2,505	59,643	19,000	139,706	52,142[3]	99,129[3]	57,590	57,590	183,377[3]	44,814[3]
Diseases of the digestive system	2,536[3]	60,381[3]	21,533	158,331	56,263[3]	106,964[3]	93,689	93,689	404,023[3]	98,733[3]
Diseases of the genitourinary system	1,666	39,667	8,024	59,000	41,934[3]	79,722[3]	46,377[3]	46,377[3]	195,679[3]	47,824[3]
Congenital anomalies	3,341	79,548	32,082[3]	235,897[3]	171,927[3]	326,857[3]	370,813[3]	370,813[3]	1,552,065[3],[4]	379,293[3],[4]
Certain causes of perinatal morbidity and mortality	3,343[3]	79,595[3]	32,310	237,574	186,571	354,698	411,644	411,644	—	—
Symptoms and ill-defined conditions	2,847	67,786	14,475[3]	106,434[3]	63,740[3]	121,179[3]	161,005[3]	161,005[3]	643,822[3]	157,326[3]
Accidents, poisonings, and violence	3,662	87,190	23,883	175,610	116,730	221,920	281,006	281,006	1,076,115	262,980
Average cost per death[5]	2,547	60,643	15,328	112,706	46,866	89,099	75,530	75,530	274,344	67,044

[1] "Major" indicates that the causes of death listed here account for approximately three-fourths of the total number of deaths.
[2] Constant 1975 prices adjusted by average earnings index.
(average earnings index = 1900 1930 1963 1975 2000
            .042 .136 .526 1.0 4.092).

[3] Not a major category for that year.
[4] Also includes certain causes of perinatal mortality in the year 2000.
[5] Average of all causes.

Sources: A. Berk and L.C. Paringer: "Cost of Illness and Disease, 1900." Public Services Laboratory, Georgetown University, Washington, D.C., 1977; A. Berk and L.C. Paringer: "Cost of Illness and Disease, 1930." Public Services Laboratory, Georgetown University, Washington, D.C., 1977; J.S. Landefeld: "Economic Cost of Illness, 1963." Public Services Laboratory, Georgetown University, Washington, D.C., 1978; L.C. Paringer and A. Berk: "Costs of Illness and Disease, Fiscal Year 1975." Public Services Laboratory, Georgetown University, Washington, D.C., 1977; and S.J. Mushkin, et al.: "Cost of Disease and Illness in the United States in the Year 2000." Public Health Reports 93:493-588, September-October 1978.

level, yields some insight into the progress made in reducing death rates (Table 5-7). The cost of cancer per cancer death, when computed as an index with 1930 as a base year, is declining to some degree. The 1975 cost was 98 percent of the 1930 level. Almost a threefold rise occurred in cost per cancer death from 1900 to 1930. The pattern of progress by disease category is better illustrated by Figure 5-2.

The relative progress made toward reduction in deaths is evident in the cost estimates. When biomedical science and medical therapies lowered death rates appreciably, economic cost even at constant earnings level did not uniformly decline. Indeed, between 1900 and 1930 cost of death increased as more persons lived to young adulthood. By 1975 the postponement of death to the older age groups began to lower costs.

Economic cost per death from accidents, poisonings, and violence nearly doubled between 1900 and 1930 and continued upward through 1975. Certain cases of perinatal mortality, mental disorders, and diseases of the nervous system followed a similar pattern, although with greater disparity between the years. Costs of other diseases of concern in most current policy debate are more similar to cancer costs, that is, costs were higher for 1930 than in 1900 but dropped off since 1930. Most of the disease categories fit into this class.

The major question is whether the progress toward death rate reduction can be accelerated for those in their productive years of life. A great burden falls on policymakers to identify areas where economic costs can be reduced the most and where past trends can be accelerated to achieve this cost reduction.

A Future Perspective

For the future, another approach to policy formulation is to assess the savings in economic cost of premature death in the extreme case of a successful attack on a disease, eliminating that particular cause in the years ahead. When a particular disease is understood and cured or prevented, persons who would have died earlier from that specific cause, of course, die of another. The resulting figures, accordingly, are highly stylized.

The National Center for Health Statistics periodically publishes estimates of the number of years that would be added to life expectancy if deaths from selected diseases were eliminated. The maximum economic benefit from such reductions are reflected in the estimates of the economic cost of death (Table 5-8). If 2.5 years of life expectancy were added as a result of a cure or a preventive of cancer, the economic costs of deaths due to cancer would fall by $21.7 billion (based on the particular set of economic assumptions

Table 5-7. Index of Economic Costs per Death by Cause of Death, Selected Years, 1900-2000, Base Year 1930

Disease category	1900	Base year 1930	1963	1975	2000
Infective and parasitic diseases	39.2	100.0	74.9	70.9	73.5
Neoplasms	36.2	100.0	132.0	97.7	98.1
Diseases of the circulatory system	63.0	100.0	94.2	62.3	60.2
Diseases of the respiratory system	42.7	100.0	71.0	41.2	32.1
Diseases of the digestive system	38.1	100.0	67.6	59.2	62.4
Diseases of the genitourinary system	67.2	100.0	135.1	78.6	81.1
Congenital anomalies	33.7	100.0	138.6	157.2	160.8[1]
Certain causes of perinatal morbidity and mortality	33.5	100.0	149.3	173.3	[1]
Symptoms and ill-defined conditions	63.7	100.0	113.9	151.3	147.8
Accidents, poisonings, and violence	49.6	100.0	126.4	160.0	149.8
All causes	53.8	100.0	79.1	67.0	59.5

[1] Congenital anomalies and certain causes of perinatal morbidity and mortality are combined into one category for the year 2000.

Sources: A. Berk and L.C. Paringer: "Cost of Illness and Disease, 1900." Public Services Laboratory, Georgetown University, Washington, D.C. 1977; A. Berk and L.C. Paringer: "Cost of Illness and Disease, 1930." Public Services Laboratory, Georgetown University, Washington, D.C., 1977; J.S. Landefeld, "Economic Cost of Illness, 1963." Public Services Laboratory, Georgetown University, Washington, D.C., 1978; L.C. Paringer and A. Berk: "Costs of Illness and Disease, Fiscal Year 1975." Public Services Laboratory, Georgetown University, Washington, D.C., 1977; and S.J. Mushkin, et al.: "Cost of Disease and Illness in the United States in the Year 2000." *Public Health Reports* 93:493-588, September-October 1978.

used in developing the estimate). The added savings in economic cost, or the outside limits of the benefits to be derived by achieving successful cures or preventives, are arrayed in Figure 5-3. To put the estimates in a longer time horizon, the savings are shown for costs in 1975 and in 2000.[18]

These outside limit numbers lend some perspective to the development of measures of resource allocation based on economic cost. In the economic cost of death calculations, we did not assume a uniform value for all deaths without regard to age, occupation, or sex. On the contrary, we restricted the count of economic cost of death to premature death in the sense of death before full retirement

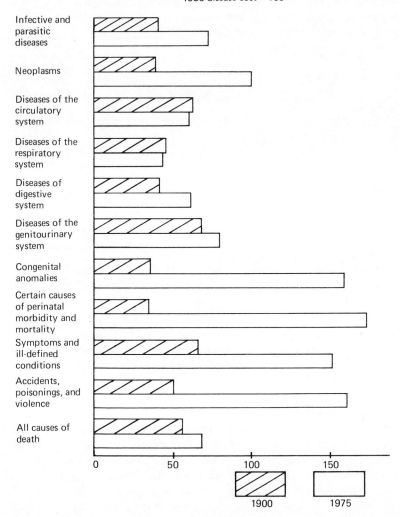

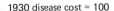

Figure 5-2. Index of Economic Costs per Death, for Ten Causes of Death, 1900 and 1975 (Constant Earnings Levels)

Sources: A. Berk and L.C. Paringer: "Cost of Illness and Disease, 1900." Public Services Laboratory, Georgetown University, Washington, D.C., 1977; A. Berk and L.C. Paringer: "Cost of Illness and Disease, 1930." Public Services Laboratory, Georgetown University, Washington, D.C., 1977; and L.C. Paringer and A. Berk: "Costs of Illness and Disease, Fiscal Year 1975." Public Services Laboratory, Georgetown University, Washington, D.C., 1977. Discounted present values of deaths in 1900 price levels were adjusted to 1975 earnings by dividing by an index of average earnings, which is .042 for 1900 and 1.00 for 1975.

Table 5-8. Increases in Life Expectancy Due to the Elimination of Particular Diseases, Gains in Years of Life, and Maximum Economic Benefits of Such Elimination

	Years of life added		Maximum economic benefits (in billions)	
Disease	*At birth*	*At age 40*	*1975*	*2000*
Cancer	2.47	2.38	$21.7	$113.9
Diabetes	.24	.23	[1]	[1]
Heart	5.86	6.10	32.8[2]	181.6[2]
Acute myocardial infarction	2.43	2.53	[1]	[1]
Arteriosclerosis	.13	.14	[1]	[1]
Diseases of the respiratory system	.83	.61	6.3	30.5
Influenza and pneumonia	.47	.30	[1]	[1]
Cirrhosis of the liver	.28	.25	[1]	[1]

[1] Estimates included in broader disease classification.
[2] Represents estimated cost of mortality of diseases of the circulatory system.
Source of estimate of years of life added: National Center for Health Statistics: *U.S. Life Tables,* 1969-71, Vol. I, No. 5.

from the work force. On ethical grounds, such a count of the value of life has been appropriately challenged. The outside limits as computed require this important qualification.

Measuring Past Performance

The data on changes in life expectancy that could be achieved by wiping out particular diseases lend a perspective to future potential outlook. These data show, for example, what could be achieved by a successful combination of environmental, personal, and medical advances. The record of the past in economic costs of disease may be approached by analyzing the question: What would the 1975 economic costs have been if death rates of earlier years existed rather than the actual rates of 1975? The difference between the actual experience and that which would have prevailed at death rates for earlier years (when valued separately for each age at death and for men and women by applying the present value of future earnings figures shown in Table 5-1) represents the savings in cost of death as a result of the historical improvements in mortality.

The estimates assume that the 1975 population is held constant by age and sex, that earnings are constant, and that work experience is also unchanged.

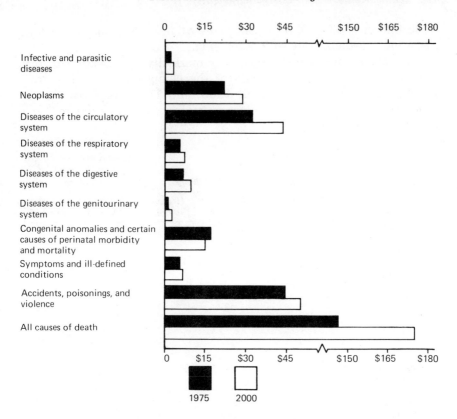

Sources: L.C. Paringer and A. Berk: "Costs of Illness and Disease, Fiscal Year 1975." Public Services Laboratory, Georgetown University, Washington, D.C., 1977; and S.J. Mushkin, et al.: "Cost of Disease and Illness in the United States in the Year 2000." *Public Health Reports* 93:493-588, September-October 1978. Discounted present values at 2000 prices were deflated to 1975 earnings levels by dividing by 4.092.

Figure 5-3. Total Economic Cost of Death by Disease Category, Ten Major Causes of Death, 1975 and 2000, at 1975 Earnings Levels, Discounted at 2.5 Percent, in Billions

Had 1930 death rates prevailed in 1975, total deaths would have been higher by more than 1 million—3.2 million instead of 1.9 million. Economic savings as a consequence of the gains in mortality would approach $221 billion at the 1975 present value of future earnings levels (and assuming a discount rate of 2.5 percent). Had 1900 death rates prevailed in 1975, total deaths would have been 4.7 million or 2.4 times the 1975 actual experience. The economic savings as a consequence of the improved mortality would approach

$725 billion at the 1975 present value of future earnings levels (and assuming a discount rate of 2.5 percent).

The savings in economic cost vary markedly by disease category. The major savings (in billions) for the changes in mortality from selected diseases between 1900, 1930, and 1975 are shown in the following table.[19] (The detailed estimates are presented in Table 5A-2 in the appendix.)

Diseases	Total cost of death (in billions)			Savings in economic cost of death (in billions) Contrast	
	1975 at 1975 death rates	1975 at 1930 rates	1975 at 1900 rates	between 1930-75	between 1900-75
All diseases	$146	$367	$871	$221	$725
Infective and parasitic diseases	2	63	321	61	319
Diseases of the respiratory system	6	47	162	41	156
Diseases of the genitourinary system	1	18	55	17	54
Complications of pregnancy, childbirth, and the puerperium	(0.2)	7	7	7	7
Cost increases: neoplasms	22	19	4	−3	−18

Mortality losses due to pregnancy would have risen thirty-two times in 1975 if 1930 mortality rates had prevailed, and infectious and parasitic diseases would have risen thirty times. Genitourinary diseases would have caused fourteen times as great a mortality loss in 1975 had 1930 rates prevailed; this disease category includes many infections of the genitourinary system that were treatable with antibiotics in 1975 but were often fatal in 1930. Similarly, respiratory diseases, which would have gone up almost seven times, were no longer usually fatal in 1975.

Neoplasms, as indicated earlier, would have caused less mortality loss in 1975 had 1930 rates of cancer mortality prevailed in 1975. In 1975, the death rate from neoplasms was 171.7 per 100,000, while in 1930 that rate was 97.4 per 100,000. Therefore, cancer deaths were fewer per 100,000 population in 1930 than in 1975. Our computations do not show as large a decrease in 1975 had 1930 rates applied, because of the aging of the population. However, mortality losses from cancer, computed on the basis of the present value of future earnings at 2.5 percent, would have been $19 billion had 1930 death rates from cancer been applied in place of $22 billion as the estimated experience of 1975.

Several qualifications should be noted. First, as we mentioned before, because cancer often was not reported as a cause of death in years past, the reported death rate from this disease was lower than was actually the case. Second, the much higher incidence of overall cancer-caused deaths between 1930 and 1975 is not reflected in the estimates of cost of the mortality losses in 1975; these costs rose much more modestly than did the overall cancer death rate, because cancer deaths now occur at a later age than they did in 1930. Thus, mortality losses in 1975 from cancer were lower than would have been the case had cancer caused death at the same age in 1975 as it did in 1930. The changing sex distribution of cancer victims also should be noted.

Further, the overall rise in cancer deaths obscures the decline in several kinds of malignancies. Digestive system malignancies, for example, declined from 48.9 per 100,000 in 1930 to 46.8 per 100,000 in 1975. The major cause in the increase of cancer deaths comes from respiratory system malignancies—up from 3.2 per 100,000 in 1930 to 39.5 per 100,000 in 1975.

In the context of the total cost of premature death, savings in costs since 1930 are about equal to $1.50 on each $1.00 of the remaining 1975 cost (at a 2.5 percent discount rate). And savings since 1900 are about equal to $5.00 on each $1.00 of the remaining 1975 cost.

In effect, the actual economic cost factors—demographic, social, and economic—applied in constructing a cost figure weight the 1900 and 1930 death rates by the value of discounted earnings of 1975, by age and sex. The calculations have an artificial meaning. Death rates of 1900 or 1930 are incompatible with the value of earnings in later years. Death rates of 1900 and 1930, moreover, would have produced a different population by 1975 than existed. Years of labor force participation would be fewer. Economic trends, including shifts from agriculture to industry since the turn of the century, have contributed to a larger paid female labor force and a high retirement rate, including part-time retirement of men at ages forty-five and over. Even setting aside the interaction of sickness and deaths, productivity and the numbers of persons in the work force might well be affected. Life expectancies, both for a worker and particularly for his or her children, have a good deal to do with the worker's production and the amount of resources he or she is willing to set aside from today's production to enhance future consumption.

Obviously, this highly artificial computation does not attempt an answer to the query: What would have happened in 1975 if 1930 or 1900 death rates had prevailed unchanged over the forty-five- to seventy-five-year period?

As a way of measuring the change in economic costs of death over the period, the calculations permit useful statements about the significance of those changes.

- Four major causes of death show the largest drop in economic costs of death under 1975 demographic, social, and economic conditions.
- Considering all causes, the overall reduction in mortality rates since 1930 has cut the cost of premature death by $221 billion and since 1900 by $725 billion.
- Two causes, cancer and mental disorders, were more costly in 1975 than they would have been if death rates of 1930 had prevailed.

ASSET VALUE OF LIFESAVING

Still another method may be used to assess the economic impact of the reduction in mortality rates during the seventy-five-year period, 1900-75.[20,21] In the preceding section, the savings in economic costs of premature death due to postponement of death were calculated on the basis of the difference between what the cost would have been in 1975 at 1975, 1930, and 1900 death rates. This estimate of the economic impact of postponement of death may be made by asking: What is the asset value of the postponement of death that occurred over the seventy-five years? If death rates of 1900 had prevailed over the whole period without improvement, what would have been the labor force of 1975 in contrast to what it actually was, and what would have been the future earnings equivalents of those lost workers?

The starting point for this estimate is the actual labor force of 1975, by age and sex. For each age cohort in 1975, computation of the difference in survival is based on a comparison of the survival rates of 1900 and the actual cohort experience. Based on this comparison, the changes are derived from the number of workers on a full-time equivalent basis. Estimates are made for each decade beginning with 1900 death rates. Major assumptions are called for in estimating the asset value of death postponed. It is assumed that births, immigration, family composition, rate of technological change, and productivity per worker are unaffected by changes in mortality rates. Although the assumptions are unrealistic, the simplifications mostly impart a downward bias to the estimates and yield conservative values for the economic gains attributable to reduced mortality.

The added workers or work years are represented by the difference between the actual labor force in 1975 and a projected (hypothetical) labor force if survival rates of earlier years had prevailed.

As Table 5-9 shows, a total of 27 million workers and an equivalent number of work force years would have been lost to the economy in 1975 if death rates had remained unchanged at 1900 rates throughout the period 1900 to 1975. If 1930 death rates had prevailed throughout the forty-five-year period, the work force in 1975 would have been smaller by 9 million, or 10 percent below the actual level.

The hypothetical labor force, or added work force years, is an illustrative figure derived as the product of the ratio of period survival rates in each decade to cohort survival rates each year and the present labor force for each age and sex group. For example, the ratio for the 1900 computation would be as follows:

$$\frac{\text{Projected (1900) period survival population}}{\text{Actual cohort survival population}}$$

$$\times \text{ actual labor force } 1975 = \text{hypothetical labor force } 1975$$

This ratio of projected to actual survival rates will be less than one, since improvement in mortality experience results in actual survival rates exceeding those projected by period survival rates of earlier periods.

The result of this computation is an approximation of what the labor force would have been in 1975, if mortality rates had remained constant from the earlier period or benchmark year to 1975 and if it is assumed further that other factors influencing the size of the population had remained unchanged, that is, that births and immigration had followed their actual historical path. The mortality experience of the labor force is assumed to be the same as that of the general population at each age group.

Reduction in mortality not only adds persons to the work force but also enlarges the asset value of human capital created by those additional workers. Just as the stream of benefits in the form of annual income from a security or piece of physical equipment is valued by capitalization of the annual income flow of that security

Table 5-9.   Gains in Work-Force Years in 1975 Due to Improvements in Mortality Rates between Benchmark Year and 1975

Mortality rates of benchmark years	Hypothetical increase (in millions) in 1975 work-force years	Percentage of 1975 labor force	Increase (in millions) in work-force years, by sex	
			Males	Females
1900	27.4	29	16.6	10.7
1910	20.6	22	12.6	8.0
1920	15.1	16	8.6	6.5
1930	9.1	10	5.3	3.8

Source: Reference 21.

or equipment, the earnings of labor can be valued. Capitalization is essentially a calculation of the value of a given income payment over time, reflecting that the lower the value, the further off in time the actual receipt of the income. A person's stock of human capital or asset value is simply the present value of his or her future earnings discounted to take account of years elapsing before receipt and the length of time over which the earnings are received.

Again, moral issues are involved in this type of calculation, but the benefits of improved mortality over the decades may be viewed as assets or human capital stock values resulting from the lower mortality. Except for the improvement in death rates from earlier years, the size of the labor force in 1975 and the future earnings of the labor force would be reduced.

Table 5-10 shows the changes in human capital stock values. The figures represent the present discounted value of earnings forgone by workers (in each age-sex group) who would have died before 1975 had death rates of earlier periods prevailed. The earnings streams include market earnings and the value of household production. At a 10 percent discount rate, the increase in human capital assets attributable to improvements from 1930 death rates is $1 trillion; at a 2.5 percent discount rate, $2.3 trillion. The improvement in mortality rates since 1900 has yielded additional workers and earnings equivalent to an asset value of $7.2 trillion at a 2.5 percent discount rate and $3.1 trillion at a 10 percent rate.

These asset estimates are consistent with an overall model of economic growth. A 10 percent rise in the number of workers also requires an increase in the physical capital stock. In the familiar Harrod-Domar model of economic growth, changes in the supply of labor need to be accommodated by changes in the rate of saving so that the effective ratio between physical capital and labor returns can remain constant as indicated by long-term GNP trends. Thus, the

Table 5-10. Capital Asset Value of Workers in 1975 Attributable
to Improvements in Mortality Rates since 1900 and 1930, Alternative
Discount Rate Estimates in Trillions

	10 percent discount		*2.5 percent discount*	
Workers	*1900*	*1930*	*1900*	*1930*
All[1]	$3.1	$1.0	$7.2	$2.3
Males	2.2	.7	5.2	1.7
Females	.9	.3	2.0	.6

[1] Harrod-Domar Model—variable savings rate.
Source: Reference 21.

Harrod-Domar model, which assumes a constant effective labor to capital ratio, would imply that a 10-percent increase in the current period labor force would be matched by a 10-percent increase in the stock of physical capital. From 1930 to 1975, the improvement in death rates since 1930 levels means an estimated $219-billion increase in the physical capital stock. The increase in life expectancies from 1900 to 1975 would imply a 1975 physical capital stock increase of $656 billion.

It is plausible to model the economic growth patterns differently, in a way that would lower the gains in output attributable to the additional workers. Physical capital could be substituted for labor so that the economic benefits resulting from the additional workers would be less. We applied a neoclassical model that substitutes capital for labor. The estimated gains (in trillions) as a consequence of the improved mortality since 1900 and 1930 are somewhat lowered, as indicated in the following table:

	Amounts in trillions			
	10 percent discount		*2.5 percent discount*	
Model	*1900*	*1930*	*1900*	*1930*
Harrod-Domar model (constant labor-capital ratio)	$3.1	$1.0	$7.2	$2.3
Neoclassical model (substitution of capital for labor)	2.4	0.9	5.7	2.0

CONTRIBUTIONS OF BIOMEDICAL RESEARCH TO ECONOMIC GAINS

In Chapter 4, we cautioned that not all gains in mortality reduction can be attributed to biomedical advances. Analyses carried out over a two-year period of the effect of biomedical advances on reduction of deaths indicate that 20 to 30 percent of the mortality decline in the period 1930-75 is attributable to these scientific advances with a larger percentage, 30 to 40 percent, over the seventy-five-year period.

By combining the earlier estimates with the estimated gains attributable to past progress in biomedical advances, we can place a value on those advances. The value of the contribution of biomedical research to postponement of death is summarized in the following table:

Gains	*Total*	*Share attributable to biomedical research, 1900 base*	*Total*	*Share attributable to biomedical research, 1930 base*
Savings in cost of single year premature deaths, in billions (at a 2.5 percent discount rate)	$725	$218-$290	$221	$44-$66
Asset value of postponed death, in trillions (at a 2.5 percent discount rate)	$5.7-$7.2	$1.7-$2.9	$2.0-$2.3	$0.4-$0.7

Improvements in life expectancy achieved through biomedical advances since 1930 have generated additions to the work force that are the equivalent of about a half-trillion dollars in present values of future earnings in the economy and a 1975 saving in cost of death of $44 to $66 billion. Over the seventy-five years from 1900 to 1975, the gains attributable to biomedical research have been larger—about $1.7 to $2.9 trillion in asset values generated and a $218- to $290-billion saving in the 1975 cost of death.

In subsequent chapters, the contribution of biomedical research to the improved well-being of the population is examined.

APPENDIX

Table 5A-1. Labor Force Participation Rates, by Age and Sex, Selected Years, 1900-2000

Age group	1900[1]	1930[1]	1963[1,2]	2000[1]
Males				
5-14	8.3	—	—	—
15-19	76.1	40.1	47.5[3]	74.4
20-24		88.8	87.8	
25-29	94.9	95.8	97.3	94.1
30-34		96.1		
35-39	94.5	95.9	97.9	95.6
40-44		95.4		
45-49	92.8	94.7	96.5	91.5
50-54		92.8		
55-59	86.1	89.6	88.5	76.8
60-64		82.7		
65-69	68.0	63.0		29.8
70-74		58.1		
75-79	63.1	53.6	40.0	9.1
80-84		49.5		
85+	58.5	45.7		
Females				
5-14	3.0	—	—	—
15-19	29.2	22.8	31.8[3]	58.3
20-24		41.8	46.3	
25-29	19.4	30.2	35.4	57.2
30-34		23.6		
35-39	15.0	22.3	43.1	57.3
40-44		21.1		
45-49	14.2	20.3	45.5	56.3
50-54		19.0		
55-59	12.6	16.5	34.9	40.5
60-64		13.9		
65-69	9.3	11.0		14.8
70-74		9.2		
75-79	8.3	7.8	10.8	3.5
80-84		6.6		
85+	7.3	5.5		.6

[1] Labor force participation rates were used for 1900, 1930, 1963, and 2000, in the absence of data on work experience rates by age and sex.

[2] The labor force participation rates used for 1963 and 1956 rates to adjust for unemployment.

[3] The age group used in 1963 was 14-19.

Sources: A. Berk and L.C. Paringer: "Cost of Illness and Disease, 1900." Public Services Laboratory, Georgetown University, Washington, D.C., 1977; A. Berk and L.C. Paringer: "Cost of Illness and Disease, 1930." Public Services Laboratory, Georgetown University, Washington, D.C., 1977; J.S. Landefeld: "Economic Cost of Illness, 1963." Public Services Laboratory, Georgetown University, Washington, D.C., 1978; and S.J. Mushkin, et al.: "Cost of Disease and Illness in the United States in the Year 2000." *Public Health Reports* 93:493-588, September-October 1978.

Table 5A-2. Mortality Losses: Actual 1975 Losses Compared to Losses Had 1930 or 1900 Mortality Rates Prevailed in 1975 (Earnings Discounted at 2.5 Percent)

Cause of death	Actual 1975 mortality losses (millions)	1975 losses if 1930 mortality rates had prevailed (millions)	1975 simulated losses (1930 rates) over actual 1975 losses (percent)	1975 losses if 1900 mortality rates had prevailed (millions)	1975 simulated losses (1900 rates) over actual 1975 losses (percent)
All causes	$146,227[1]	$367,427[1]	251	$870,798[1]	596
Infective and parasitic diseases	2,121	62,870	2,964	320,532	15,113
Neoplasms	21,704	19,408	89	13,164	61
Endocrine, nutritional, and metabolic diseases	2,527	8,362	331	3,991	158
Diseases of the blood and blood-forming organs	546	2,810	515	2,305	422
Mental disorders	2,143	2,036	95	3,165	148
Diseases of the nervous system and sense organs	3,185	9,372	294	40,970	1,286
Diseases of the circulatory system	32,819	47,868	146	66,477	203
Cerebrovascular diseases[2]	5,080	10,405	205	—	—

Diseases of the respiratory system	6,277	47,442	756	161,847	2,578
Diseases of the digestive system, oral cavity, salivary glands, and jaws	6,839	36,789	538	35,657	521
Diseases of the genitourinary system	1,299	18,243	1,405	55,015	4,237
Complications of pregnancy, childbirth, and puerperium	223	7,183	3,218	7,465	3,344
Diseases of the skin and subcutaneous tissue	116	796	686	1,554	1,339
Diseases of the musculoskeletal system and connective tissue	374	924	247	4,489	1,201
Congenital anomalies	5,006	8,086	162	30,197	603
Certain causes of perinatal morbidity and mortality	11,938	33,853	284	21,261	178
Symptoms and ill-defined conditions	4,991	9,211	185	53,153	1,065
Accidents, poisonings, and violence	44,118	52,176	118	49,557	112

[1] Totals may not add up due to rounding.
[2] Also included in previous category.

Sources: A. Berk and L.C. Paringer: "Economic Costs of Illness, 1930-1975." Public Services Laboratory, Georgetown University, Washington, D.C., 1977, and unpublished work done by Cynthia Resnick and Stephen Sheehy, Public Services Laboratory, Georgetown University, 1978.

REFERENCES

1. Thedié, J., and Abraham, C.: Economic aspects of road accidents. Traffic Engineer Control 2:589-595, February 1961.

2. Based on discussion at Conference on the Measurement of the Costs of Illness. Public Services Laboratory, Georgetown University, Washington, D.C., October 17, 1975.

3. Eckstein, O.: Statement. *In* U.S. Congress, Joint Economic Committee, Economic analysis of public investment decisions: interest rate policy and discounting analysis. Report of the Subcommittee on Economy in Government, Washington, D.C., 1968, pp. 50-57.

4. Hirschleifer, J.: Investment decisions under uncertainty: applications of the state preference approach. Q J of Econ 80:252-277, May 1966.

5. Hitch, C.J., and McKean, R.N.: The economics of defense in a nuclear age. Harvard University Press, Cambridge, Mass., 1960.

6. Feldstein, M., and Summers, L.: Inflation, tax rules and the long-term interest rate. *In* Brookings papers on economic activity. The Brookings Institution, Washington, D.C., 1978, vol. 1, pp. 61-99.

7. Baumol, W.J.: On the social rate of discount. Am Econ Rev 58:788-803, September 1968.

8. Weisbrod, B.A.: Costs and benefits of medical research: a case study of poliomyelitis. J Pol Econ 79:527-544, May-June 1971.

9. Fein, R.: Economics of mental illness. Basic Books, New York, 1958.

10. Klarman, H.E.: Syphilis control programs. *In* Measuring benefits of government investment, edited by Robert Dorfman. The Brookings Institution, Washington, D.C., 1965, pp. 367-414.

11. Stockfish, J.A.: Measuring the opportunity cost of government investment. Institute for Defense Analyses, Arlington, Va., March 1969.

12. Gilman, H.: Determinants of personal discount rates (valuation of future income) and their implications for social and economic policies. Address to the National Economists Club, Washington, D.C., October 1977.

13. U.S. Social Security Administration, Office of the Actuary. Unpublished data, 1976.

14. Malzberg, B.: Mental illness and the economic value of a man. Ment Hyg 582-591, October 1950.

15. Rice, D.P.: Estimating the cost of illness. Health Economics Series No. 6. Public Health Service Publication No. 947-6. U.S. Government Printing Office, Washington, D.C., 1966.

16. Cooper, B.S., and Rice, D.P.: The economic cost of illness revisited. Soc Sec Bull 39:21-36, February 1976.

17. Acton, J.P.: Measuring the monetary value of lifesaving programs. Law Contemp Problems 40:46-72, autumn 1976.

18. Mushkin, S.J., et al.: Cost of disease and illness in the United States in the year 2000. Public Health Rep 93:494-588, September-October 1978.

19. Berk, A., and Paringer, L.C.: The economic costs of illness 1930-1975. Public Services Laboratory, Georgetown University, Washington, D.C., March 1977.

20. Mushkin, S.J.: Health as an investment. J Pol Econ 70:129-157, October 1962.

21. Mushkin, S.J., and Landefeld, J.S.: The economic benefits of improvements in mortality experience, 1900-1975. Public Services Laboratory, Georgetown University, Washington, D.C., 1978.

Chapter Six

Biomedical Research Priorities and Mortality

For more than three-quarters of a century, death statistics have guided research in the biomedical sciences. In summary form, we review the major issues facing policymakers concerned with biomedical research, and present some findings drawn from an assessment of priorities in biomedical research.

PRESENT TARGETING OF RESEARCH FUNDS

We reviewed the present allocation of expenditures as part of a special study of biomedical research expenditures to determine if the funds are going where the health problems are.[1]

Congressional interest in 1976 and 1977 in fund allocations for biomedical research led to the special review. As indicated earlier, pending legislation presumably would allot the largest sums for the diseases with the highest mortality and morbidity rates and with the greatest adverse effect on the health and productivity of persons and on the economy.

An initial round of testing was carried out applying mortality and morbidity allocations among eight research institutes of the National Institutes of Health. The indexes for the examination of the relationship between mortality and morbidity data and resource allocation were (a) number of deaths; (b) number of days of hospital care; (c) number of restricted activity days; (d) number of bed-disability days; (e) number of work-loss days; and (f) number of visits to physicians and dentists. Several of these indicators are shown in Table 6-1 for fiscal year 1976.

The review showed a significant correlation between the number of deaths from a disease and congressional funding for the National Institute concerned with that disease, as suggested by method V in Table 6-2. Congress seems to view Institute activities in terms of the Institute name, and the appropriations made to an Institute are directed toward reduction in deaths in the disease group identified with that Institute.

A major deviation from this correspondence is in the relative position of funds for the Heart and Cancer Institutes. Heart disease accounted in 1975, for example, for almost 38 percent of the deaths, whereas cancer accounted for 19 percent. However, funds allocated to the Cancer Institute far outranked funds allocated to the Heart Institute. This exception to the allocation of funds in relation to numbers of deaths probably reflects congressional perception about the relative burdens on patient and family of the two diseases. It may also reflect congressional sensitivity to the public's perception of the relative threat of cancer and heart disease to well-being.

A 1976 Gallup poll showed cancer to be the most feared affliction.[2] Cancer was named by 58 percent of respondents as "the worst thing" that could happen to them, whereas only 10 percent named heart disease—the leading cause of death. Blindness, clearly not a death-related state, was named by 21 percent. Burdens of illness—pain, disfigurement, or dysfunctionality—seem to underlie fear of disease.

Even taking into account the break in pattern when the Cancer Institute and the Heart Institute are included, a rank order correlation between appropriations and deaths shows that causes of death are a critical decisionmaking factor in Institute funding (Table 6-2).

These data, as initially developed, were meaningful only for the eight disease-specific Institutes of NIH. They did not apply to the National Institute of General Medical Sciences, the National Institute on Aging, or the National Institute of Environmental Sciences. If, however, the National Institute of General Medical Sciences were included in an appropriations scale for all Institutes, it would rank third, exceeded only by the Cancer and Heart Institutes. This high rank indicates congressional concern for fundamental biomedical research, because the Institute of General Medical Sciences is primarily charged with funding basic research which may or may not be relevant to a particular disease or to several diseases.

RESEARCH MISSIONS OF THE INSTITUTES

The allocation of funds among Institutes is now identified with deaths. But the mere correspondence between Institute name and research mission within the Institute is far too simplistic. The Institutes are complex research organizations with diverse orientations and a mix of biomedical science concerns that overlap extensively. The legislatively determined central mission and scope of the Institutes also vary. Some missions are disease-linked; that is, the Institute deals with a particular disease wherever it appears in the body. For example, the National Cancer Institute is concerned with all neoplasms, whether in the respiratory system, the digestive system, the blood, or the bladder. Some Institutes are concerned with systemic functioning of some body system rather than a disease or group of diseases. For example, the Lung Division of the National Heart, Lung, and Blood Institute deals with lung and breathing functions; its interest concerns both pulmonary tuberculosis and malignant neoplasms of the lung. Two Institutes are concerned with particular age groups; the National Institute on Aging is interested in the general process of aging, and the National Institute of Child Health and Human Development is concerned with the full range of diseases that affect the young. The National Institute of Environmental Health is concerned with a wide range of morbidity and mortality problems caused by or aggravated by exposure to environmental agents—its research concerns range, for example, from bladder cancer to silicotuberculosis.

Each Institute has research mandates that span the research approaches just detailed. The National Institute of Arthritis, Metabolic, and Digestive Diseases has a clearly mixed research approach. It deals with disease-specific research for diseases such as arthritis and system-specific research for digestive diseases. In its concern with metabolism, this Institute deals with research on diseases that involve bodily processes.

Some research within the Institutes is directed toward particular processes that affect various body systems and is linked to several diseases. One example is genetic research; another is basic research on cell division throughout the body.

Moreover, the National Cancer Institute researches all neoplasms, but cancer is a disease that affects many body systems. Thus, malignant neoplasms of the respiratory system are of concern to the National Heart, Lung, and Blood Institute; malignant neoplasms of

Table 6-1. Appropriations, Fiscal Year 1976, and Indicators of the Impact of Diseases for Eight Research Institutes at the National Institutes of Health

Institute[a]	Appropriation ($ millions)	Deaths (thousands)	Short-term hospital bed days (millions)	Restricted activity days (millions)	Bed disability days (millions)	Work-loss days (millions)	Visits to physicians and dentists (millions)
NCI	$ 762.6	366	23.4	79.0	42.9	4.6	50.6
NHLI	370.3	804	42.4	648.8	248.1	55.0	230.8
NIAMDD	179.8	109	69.8	985.7	352.9	77.0	373.4
NINCDS	144.7	209	13.3	304.7	128.3	17.1	80.3
NICHD	136.6	43	26.3	156.8	72.0	8.0	78.7
NIAID	127.2	100	20.4	1,182.0	570.9	149.7	174.8
NIDR	51.4	[1]	1.4	22.0	8.2	4.7	328.4
NEI	50.3	[1]	3.0	64.1	13.7	4.0	59.4
Subtotal	1,822.9	1,631	200.3	3,443.1	1,437.1	320.1	1,376.3
Not allocated[2]	374.9	306	44.9	843.2	272.6	127.1	613.7
Total	$2,197.8	1,937	245.2	4,286.3	1,709.7	447.2	1,990.0

[1] Less than 0.5 thousand deaths are not allocated.
[2] Includes NIGMS ($187.4), NIEHS ($37.8), NIA ($19.4), and DRR ($130.3). Mortality and morbidity data cannot be allocated to these institutes.

Source: J. Perpich: NIH funding in relation to mortality and morbidity. NIH memorandum from the Office of the Director, May 10, 1976.

a. NCI   – National Cancer Institute
NHLI   – National Heart and Lung Institute
NIAMDD – National Institute of Arthritis, Metabolism, and Digestive Diseases
NINCDS – National Institute of Neurological and Communicative Disorders and Stroke
NICHD – National Institute of Child Health and Human Development
NIAID   – National Institute of Allergy and Infectious Diseases
NIDR   – National Institute of Dental Research
NEI   – National Eye Institute
NIGMS – National Institute of General Medical Sciences
NIEHS – National Institute of Environmental Health Sciences
NIA   – National Institute on Aging
DRR   – Division of Research Resources

Table 6-2. **Kendall Rank Order Correlations between Alternative Rankings of Institute Interest and 1976 Institute Funding**

		Disease measure	
Method	*Deaths*	*Short-term hospital days*	*Practitioner visits*
I	.27	−.02	.20
II	.38	−.05	.24
III	.45	−.02	.27
IV	.53	−.02	.31
V	.97	n.a.	n.a.

Methods

I – Double counting. All Institutes expressing interest in a disease are given full credit for each of the disease measures in that category.

II – Overlapping interests are shared equally among all interested Institutes.

III – Primary interests are given a weight double that given to secondary interests.

IV – Secondary interests are shared equally among all interested Institutes but are multiplied by one-half to indicate the secondary nature of their interests; primary interests share the residual.

V – One Institute, one disease category.

n.a.–not available.

Source: Reference 1.

the brain are within the scope of the National Institute of Neurological, Communicative Disorders and Stroke; and malignant neoplasms of the digestive system are within the mission of the National Institutes of Arthritis, Metabolism, and Digestive Diseases. And the National Institute of Environmental Health Sciences necessarily has a research interest in environmentally caused cancers.

LIMITATIONS OF MORTALITY AS AN ALLOCATOR

As pointed out earlier, one example of the limitations of mortality as an allocator is the public's fear of blindness, ranking second only to cancer, even though the disease is not associated with premature death.

Indeed, the appropriate measurement of health status is critical to the way in which the concerns and interests of the Institutes are set forth. For example, if death were the only major measure of burden of illness, few resources would go to the National Institute of Dental Research. Dental diseases, in terms of cost of illness, are far from inconsequential. In terms of numbers of visits to practitioners, the National Institute of Dental Research ranks second among the Institutes. Critical variables are omitted in most of the currently available measures of burden of illness. Pain, disfigurement, and economic impacts of debility, including the common cold, are among the factors not yet quantified, but they bear on any calculus of determining research priorities. Moreover, the variables do not assess some of the factors that influence individual preferences for action, such as risk aversion or family responsibilities.

Measurement, in terms of health status, is made more difficult by the complexity of Institute orientation and mission definition. Significant detail about diseases is required. For the present study,[1] a round of allocations was made in which only three health status measurements were used as the only series available on a three- or four-digit code basis compared to the six available regularly on a two-digit code basis. The three illness measurements used were deaths, hospital bed days, and visits to practitioners; these are the only health status measures available in sufficient disease detail to match Institute research concerns. Even this limited list of measures is not problem-free. (Considerable data problems hamper actual application of the data in a statutory distribution formula.)

Officials of the Institutes, working through an ad hoc committee at NIH, outlined their perceptions about the research mandates within which they were working. They defined the disease interests by using the third and fourth digits of the International Classification of Disease.

Allocations based on the defined Institute interest in disease categories were computed by quantifying a number of algorithms (methods I-V). Table 6-3 shows the percentage distribution of funds under three allocations based on the algorithms tested. The two algorithms with sharply variant results are those labeled method I and method V. Method V is a revision of the initial round of study, which, for simplicity, assigned diseases to single Institutes based on the assumption of a simplistic link of research mission to the name of the Institute. The "one Institute, one disease" ranking of deaths is well correlated with the ranking of congressional funding, as indicated earlier. Method I goes to the opposite extreme, and allocates indicators of research interest to any Institute with a defined mandate to carry out research in some aspect of the disease assigned; for this series, there is far less correspondence between death and funding.

The allocation by short-term hospital days differs from that of visits to physicians as an indicator of use of health services, and each of these differs in turn from the allocations based on deaths—underscoring the difficulties of priority setting by reference to particular indicators.

The following observations summarize the results of the allocations. They give little encouragement to any automatic formula designs.

- Death rates stand out as the most important criterion used by the Congress in the allocation of research funds to Institutes.
- There is no one correct way to allocate burden of illness measures to Institute. In all, five algorithms classified by three alternative disease indicators were computed—a total of fifteen different rankings of relative shares. *A priori*, there is some rationale, medical or economic, for each, but, again, no obvious or consistent link between diseases and scientific concerns of the Institutes is apparent.
- Even if there were agreement on a particular allocation, there is no way to select the proper illness measure or to devise a common denominator for combining the various measures.
- The three morbidity and mortality measures, which can actually be employed in this sort of allocation by four-digit code, fall far short of representing a rounded picture of the impact of diseases on health status.

CLASSIFICATION OF HEALTH RESEARCH EXPENDITURES, BY DISEASE

For years, the question has been raised: How is the nation's bill for health research divided among disease categories? For years, there has been no ready answer.

A beginning toward a response was made in 1974 when a contract was given to Orkand Corporation to determine the feasibility of developing a methodology by which funds for national health research could be classified by disease problem.[3]

The task was defined as twofold: (*a*) to select an appropriate disease classification system, and (*b*) to develop a pilot program to test the feasibility of collecting funding data to match the disease classification system. After reviewing these tasks, Orkand concluded that it is feasible with some gaps and some omissions to classify health research expenditures (or obligations) according to the disease problems to which they relate. Furthermore, the study recommended that, unless a decision is made to require detailed data by disease for basic research, the current ongoing estimating procedure should continue to be used to develop the information on basic research in place of detailed reporting and coding.

For the pilot program, national health research expenditures were

Table 6-3. Percentage Shares[1] of Total Allocations According to Various Indicators and Algorithms

Institutes	Deaths I	Deaths II	Deaths III	Deaths IV	Deaths V	Funding Fiscal year 1976
NIAMDD	25.06	25.42	20.80	16.57	8.87	8.70
NIDR	.25	.24	.25	.26	–	2.49
NIEHS	27.68	25.92	19.07	13.08	n.a.	1.83
NHLBI	25.01	26.52	34.42	41.43	49.26	17.91
NINCDS	6.72	5.59	6.37	6.51	12.56	7.00
NIA	.02	.02	.01	.01	n.a.	.94
NIAID	3.66	4.24	4.46	4.54	4.70	6.15
NCI	7.37	7.58	10.71	14.25	22.11	36.89
NEI	.71	.42	.30	.21	–	2.43
NIGMS	.16	.36	.36	.36	n.a.	9.06
NICHD	3.37	3.70	3.26	2.79	2.39	6.61
Total[2]	100.00	100.00	100.00	100.00	100.00	100.00

Institutes	Short-term hospital days I	STHOSP II	STHOSP III	STHOSP IV	STHOSP V	Funding
NIAMDD	28.56	32.60	33.24	33.16	35.59	8.70
NIDR	.44	.51	.52	.53	.45	2.49
NIEHS	19.89	16.27	12.29	9.32	n.a.	1.83
NHLBI	15.39	13.93	16.34	18.39	22.24	17.91
NINCDS	7.76	7.22	7.35	7.40	6.80	7.00
NIA	.05	.03	.02	.02	n.a.	.94
NIAID	10.15	8.90	9.14	9.26	8.93	6.15
NCI	5.21	4.59	5.84	7.26	12.20	36.89
NEI	1.58	1.28	1.28	1.25	1.41	2.43
NIGMS	1.64	2.21	2.14	2.09	n.a.	9.06
NICHD	9.34	12.45	11.82	11.32	12.34	6.61
Total[2]	100.00	100.00	100.00	100.00	100.00	100.00

Institutes	Physician visits I	PHYSV II	PHYSV III	PHYSV IV	PHYSV V	Funding
NIAMDD	21.50	20.29	20.85	20.92	27.35	8.70
NIDR	12.07	24.48	24.50	24.51	24.45	2.49
NIEHS	15.89	11.54	8.47	6.28	n.a.	1.83
NHLBI	15.00	11.79	13.90	15.57	15.73	17.91
NINCDS	8.04	6.25	5.87	5.62	5.97	7.00
NIA	.03	.02	.02	.01	n.a.	.94
NIAID	15.18	12.66	13.77	14.63	13.30	6.15
NCI	2.06	1.81	2.17	2.60	3.65	36.89
NEI	3.40	4.10	4.07	4.02	4.55	2.43
NIGMS	0.00	0.00	0.00	0.00	n.a.	9.06
NICHD	6.82	7.07	6.39	5.84	4.97	6.61
Total[2]	100.00	100.00	100.00	100.00	100.00	100.00

[1] Percentages calculated from unrounded figures.
[2] Totals may not add to 100 percent due to rounding.

Table 6-3 continued

Methods

   I – Doublecounting. All Institutes expressing an interest in a disease are given full credit for each of the disease measures in that category.

   II – Overlapping interests are shared equally among all interested Institutes.

   III – Primary interests are given a weight double that given to secondary interests.

   IV – Secondary interests are shared equally among all interested Institutes but are multiplied by one-half to indicate the secondary nature of their interests; primary interests share the residual.

   V – One Institute, one disease allocation.

Source: Reference 1.

divided among the several types of research agencies, for example, NIH, other federal agencies, industry, state and local governments, private foundations, and so forth. The major effort was addressed to a pilot test of NIH operations and more particularly to NIH extramural contracts and grants. Two samples were drawn of contracts and grants and verified; together, the drawn samples consisted of 405 procurements.

While a NIH-wide taxonomy is useful in that it provides a breakdown of extramural expenditures by disease and health-related activities, even more useful is a methodology that provides information by Institute, by disease, and health-related activities. It was difficult, however, to identify the samples with specific diseases. For example, in the test, approximately 18 percent of the grant sample could not be classified into one of the disease or health-related categories and were grouped as "other." The methodology again underscores the wide-ranging concerns of the separate Institutes among disease problems, which we discussed earlier in the attempt to associate morbidity and mortality data to Institute.

Cost Per Death and Research

Given the preliminary pilot test data on grants and contracts for extramural research and a parallel set of figures on the voluntary agencies, the issues of allocation may be clarified further from a cost or obligations perspective.

At one extreme, it might be argued that priority should be given to those diseases that have the highest cost per death. When the cost per death is high, it follows that deaths tend to occur at the peak years of economic productivity and for those who are actively attached to the work force. At the other extreme, a reasonable argument can be made that priority should instead be given to those diseases in which costs per death are relatively low primarily because a large portion of those deaths occur during the early years of life. They may also be low because they occur after retirement but with years remaining of possible active participation in society through other than gainful employment.

In rank order, the cost per death, by disease, in 1975 was as follows:

Average cost, all deaths	$ 75,530
Diseases of the circulatory system	31,926
Diseases of the genitourinary system	46,377
Diseases of the respiratory system	57,590
Neoplasms	59,301
Diseases of the digestive system	93,689
Infective and parasitic diseases	132,559
Symptoms and ill-defined conditions	161,005
Accidents, poisonings, and violence	281,006
Congenital anomalies	370,813
Certain causes of perinatal morbidity and mortality	411,644

If funds were allocated in terms of highest cost per death, more would go toward research on perinatal mortality and congenital diseases and less for diseases of the circulatory system. However, as indicated earlier, allocations in terms of number of deaths that influence aggregate cost, rather than cost per death, would give greatest priority to the diseases of the circulatory system.

Alternatively, the aggregate cost of death estimates can be used to compare the preliminary test findings on research outlays with such costs. These figures are shown below for selected disease categories.

Disease category	Rank in extramural contracts and grants	Rank in voluntary health agency funding	Total cost of death	
			Rank	Amount (in millions)
Neoplasms	1	1	3	$21.7
Diseases of the circulatory system	2	2	2	32.8
Diseases of the digestive system, oral cavity, salivary glands, and jaws	3	less than .1%	5	6.8
Diseases of the respiratory system	4	8	6	6.3
Endocrine, nutritional, and metabolic diseases	5	11	9	2.5
Diseases of the genitourinary system	6	9	10	1.3
Congenital anomalies	7	12	7	5.0

The allocation of research and development funds is heavily concentrated on two diseases, neoplasms and circulatory diseases. While accidents, poisonings, and violence account for the largest share of the total cost of death, neoplasms and diseases of the circulatory system are costly as well.

Of the pilot test findings on extramural contracts and grants, a substantial share of the total went for the two major killers, neoplasms and diseases of the circulatory system. Similarly, of the funds of the voluntary agencies, according to data provided to Orkand by NIH, Division of Resources Analysis, almost $6 out of each $10 went to the two major killers.

Table 6-4 shows the rankings for seventeen categories of disease by the pilot test amount of extramural grants and contracts, and by deaths, disability days, and total economic cost of illness and disease. The rank order correlations between the pilot amount of extramural funding by disease and the selected criteria indicate that not one of the Kendall rank order correlations is high. Deaths come closest to an association with extramural funding, followed by total economic cost of disease. Kendall rank order correlations of pilot results on expenditures for extramural grants and contracts of NIH and three selected criteria are the following:

Deaths	.52
Disability days	.35
Total economic cost (direct and indirect)	.46

We have attempted some crude applications of the partial and incomplete data on health research expenditures by disease class to suggest the uses that might be made of the data if complete information were at hand.

Deaths stand out as the statistics that primarily guide expenditure decisions. Those administrators and secretaries of DHEW who were concerned in the early days of the department that research concentrations had not appropriately shifted from acute diseases to chronic diseases to meet current problems could be reassured by even the partial information available.

The given concentration on deaths, over a decade of almost stationary death rates, naturally raised doubts about the efficacy of the expenditures being made for research. However, the issue of what the research outcome really is surfaced sharply, leading to the development of new directions. At the same time, the recent decline in death rates takes the pressure off the defense of health research and permits more orderly consideration of the product expected.

In some ways, NIH lives in the best of political-scientific worlds. It is funded by the Congress in relation to deaths with the mission to

Table 6-4.   Disease-by-Disease Rankings of NIH Extramural Grants and Contracts as Contrasted with Rankings by Death, Disability, and Economic Cost

Extramural grants[1]	Deaths[2]	Disability days[3]	Total economic cost[4]
1. Neoplasms	1. Diseases of the circulatory system	1. Diseases of the circulatory system	1. Diseases of the circulatory system
2. Diseases of the circulatory system	2. Neoplasms	2. Diseases of the respiratory system	2. Accidents, poisonings, and violence
3. Diseases of the digestive system	3. Accidents, poisonings, and violence	3. Mental disorders	3. Neoplasms
4. Diseases of the nervous system	4. Diseases of the respiratory system	4. Diseases of the musculoskeletal system and connective tissue	4. Diseases of the digestive system
5. Endocrine, nutritional, and metabolic diseases	5. Diseases of the digestive system	5. Diseases of the nervous system and sense organs	5. Diseases of the respiratory system
6. Diseases of the respiratory system	6. Endocrine, nutritional, and metabolic diseases	6. Accidents, poisonings, and violence	6. Mental disorders
7. Diseases of the genitourinary system	7. Symptoms and ill-defined conditions	7. Infective and parasitic diseases	7. Diseases of the nervous system and sense organs
8. Congenital anomalies	8. Certain causes of perinatal morbidity and mortality	8. Diseases of the digestive system	8. Diseases of the musculoskeletal system and connective tissue
9. Diseases of the blood and blood-forming organs	9. Diseases of the genitourinary system	9. Endocrine, nutritional, and metabolic diseases	9. Certain causes of perinatal morbidity and mortality
10. Mental disorders	10. Diseases of the nervous system and sense organs	10. Symptoms and ill-defined conditions	10. Symptoms and ill-defined conditions
11. Diseases of the musculoskeletal system and connective tissue	11. Infective and parasitic diseases	11. Diseases of the genitourinary system	11. Diseases of the genitourinary system
12. Accidents, poisonings, and violence	12. Congenital anomalies	12. Neoplasms	12. Endocrine, nutritional, and metabolic diseases
13. Symptoms and ill-defined conditions	13. Mental disorders	13. Congenital anomalies	13. Congenital anomalies
14. Infective and parasitic diseases	14. Diseases of the blood and blood-forming organs	14. Diseases of the skin and subcutaneous tissue	14. Infective and parasitic diseases
15. Certain causes of perinatal morbidity and mortality	15. Diseases of the musculoskeletal system and connective tissue	15. Diseases of the blood and blood-forming organs	15. Complications of pregnancy, childbirth, and puerperium

16. Diseases of the skin and subcutaneous tissue	16. Diseases of the skin and subcutaneous tissue	16. Diseases of the skin and subcutaneous tissue
17. Complications of pregnancy, childbirth, and puerperium	17. Complications of pregnancy, childbirth, and puerperium	17. Diseases of the blood and blood-forming organs
	16. Complications of pregnancy, childbirth, and puerperium	
	17. Congenital anomalies	

Sources:

[1] The Orkand Corporation: "A feasibility study to develop a methodology to classify national expenditures for disease and health-related research and development." (Excludes nondisease or system-oriented grants, i.e., environmental health and expenditures by NIMH.), 1974, p. 62.

[2] L.C. Paringer and A. Berk: "Costs of illness and disease, fiscal year 1975." Public Services Laboratory, Georgetown University, Washington, D.C., 1977.

[3] Disability days are the sum of work-loss days, bed-disability days for housewives and children under six, school-loss days, and disability days for those in institutions and unable to work. Derived from L.C. Paringer and A. Berk, ibid., National Center for Health Statistics data from Series 10, and Employment and Earnings, January 1976, from the Bureau of Labor Statistics.

[4] L.C. Paringer and A. Berk, ibid., p. 24.

reduce those deaths.[4] But the funds are used by the scientific community to assess the next scientific steps required, including basic research. The Wooldridge Report of 1965 stated it this way:

> Its [NIH's] internal structure continues to suggest that it is almost exclusively concerned with waging a series of campaigns against specific disorders like cancer, heart disease, or mental illness. Its position within the government suggests that it is regarded as the research arm of the United States Public Health Services. . . . It is in fact much the largest and most significant single institution for the promotion of the life sciences in the world.[5]

REFERENCES

1. Mushkin, S.J., and Landefeld, J.S.: Allocation of morbidity, mortality, and physician services, by institute (NIH): Report no. A9. Public Services Laboratory, Georgetown University, Washington, D.C., March 1978.

2. Gallup Poll: Most feared diseases. American Institute of Public Opinion, Princeton, N.J., 1975.

3. The Orkand Corporation: A feasibility study to develop a methodology to classify national obligations for disease and health-related research and development. Final report. The Corporation, Bethesda, Md., July 1975.

4. Lambright, W.H.: Governing science and technology. Oxford University Press, New York, 1976.

5. The Wooldridge Report to the President: Biomedical science and its administration. U.S. Government Printing Office, Washington, D.C., 1965. Cited in Lambright, W.H.: Governing science and technology.

Chapter Seven

Sickness As a Criterion of Research Program Need and Outcome

Health of the population has long been a public policy goal. Although efforts have been made to assess health in positive terms of vitality, both physical and mental, negative indexes of sickness are still being applied as indicators of a population's health.

Incidence of disease in a population or its prevalence and mortality rates are the measures being applied to assess need and to judge a program intervention's success. Accordingly, the numbers of persons afflicted with various diseases or the numbers of new cases of those diseases are frequently used. Standards are formulated based on relative disease rates in a community or a state—cross-sectional at a given time. For example, cancer incidence rates in various sections of the United States or rates in different geographic regions or countries, according to age and sex of the population, are used to define health problems. Other morbidity data and indexes are used: disability days, percentage of persons with limitations, restricted activity days, bed-disability days, work-loss days, and days absent from school. To estimate the economic cost of sickness in the population, other counts of disability related to work loss are used, that is, the adult institutionalized population and the numbers not in the work force because of sickness; bed-disability days are applied as a proxy for work loss of housewives. Although these morbidity counts are an improvement over mortality rates alone as a measure, these broad categories of disability have proved deficient for many policy evaluation purposes because the variables are too gross to reflect the way people value reduced disability even if they cannot return to full health.

Recent research on health status has proceeded along two lines, one toward a new composite measure, the other toward a set of selected evaluation criteria. Disability levels or functional states have been defined, with values attached to different states in a scaling process; they have been combined into a single index. Bush and co-workers, as indicated in Chapter 1, formulated measures of "functional years," or "well years," or value-adjusted life expectancies. The combined measure is derived by weighting the functional level expectancies for which scalar values were obtained.[1,2] Similarly, Zeckhauser and Shepard adopted the concept of quality-adjusted life years as an evaluation criterion.[3] Wylie and White[4] developed the Maryland Disability Index for measuring effectiveness of rehabilitation services. The disability scores correspond to the usual clinical judgments of a patient's condition. Katz and co-workers similarly developed an Index of Independence in Activities of Daily Living for measuring functional status of the elderly and chronically ill.[5]

Still another approach is a classification system that identifies levels of symptom severity.[6] In one such functional state formulation, emphasis is given to functionality, despite the presence of a diseased condition, to suggest that maintaining persons with disease in a fully functioning position serves a public program objective, even though the persons affected are not well and the disease has not been prevented or cured by health intervention measures.[6] Earlier, Karnofsky and Burchenal proposed a comprehensive set of disability levels to which they assigned arbitrary intervals from zero to one hundred for use in evaluating cancer chemotherapy.[7] More recently, the Sickness Impact Profile was applied in analyses of clinical trials of cancer therapies.[8]

Essentially, functional states are being advanced as measures for assessing the condition of a population's health, instead of the more traditional classification of morbidity. The purpose is different, and the criteria required are accordingly different. Partially in response to evaluation needs, the National Center for Health Statistics is classifying conditions by the extent to which they bother people—a "great deal," "some," "very little," or "other."[9] Also, statistics are being reported on persons with some limitations and on those with severe limitations in activities. Table 7-1 shows major categories of diseases by degree of bother to suggest the advance being made toward understanding disease severity. Some diseases, such as emphysema, bother frequently; other diseases, such as hypertension, often bother little or infrequently.

Table 7-1. Health Conditions by Degree of Bother for Ten Major Classes of Chronic Illness

Disease, in order of numbers chronically limited	Frequency of bother				Degree of bother			
	All the time	Often	Once in a while	Not bothered	Great deal	Some	Very little	Not bothered
	Percentage of those with the disease							
1. Arthritis	24	17	50	2	30	46	17	2
2. Heart disease	16	10	37	34	21	26	15	34
3. Impairment of back and spine	14	16	49	7	32	37	8	7
4. Mental disorders	Data not available from NCHS							
5. Hypertension without heart involvement	6	5	37	49	9	22	17	49
6. Impairment of lower extremities and hip	15	11	36	16	19	30	13	16
7. Diabetes	15	5	29	46	12	22	14	46
8. Asthma	14	21	52	2	43	36	11	2
9. Paralysis (complete or partial)	29	4	13	14	20	19	7	14
10. Emphysema	44	11	23	10	32	32	13	10
11. Cerebrovascular disease	44	6	20	27	32	24	11	27
12. Hernia	10	(15)	20[1]	37	14	31	15	37
13. Neoplasms	Data not available from NCHS							
14. Ulcer	11	(76)	[1]	12	30	41	15	12
15. Gall bladder	8	(64)	[1]	27	26	32	13	27

[1] The sum of "some of the time" and "other" percentages.

Source: Reference 9.

Individuals also have been asked to rate themselves according to how they perceive their state of health. This rating method is used in a number of different surveys, including the following: Health Interview Survey,[10] Survey of Economic Opportunity,[11] and National Longitudinal Study.[12]

These relatively sophisticated approaches to health status measures and improved survey instruments should provide useful data for future analyses. If consistent measures of health status had been obtained regularly since 1900 to 1930, it would now be relatively simple to summarize the results and understand the changes that have taken place. The health status of the population could have been traced over time, and the effects of medical research and medical care (including preventive public health measures) could have been documented in a reasonably direct manner. However, such health status measures are not available.

Surprisingly, even with available statistics, it is difficult to answer the simple, straightforward question, "Is there less sickness now than earlier in this century?" We attempt to answer the question in a somewhat different way, by systematically examining different sources of information. A great many ambiguities and contradictions remain, and wisdom dictates a certain skepticism in regard to the assumptions and conclusions. Nevertheless, our answer is that the population suffers less sickness today than the same population would have suffered in 1900 or in 1930. In the remainder of this chapter, we examine the difficulties with concepts and data that we had to overcome, at least partially, to reach our conclusion, and we indicate the discernible shift in disease patterns.

SOURCES OF SICKNESS DATA

Sickness itself is conceptually difficult to define. Examination by a physician may indicate either existence or nonexistence of a pathological condition. However, a person's decision to visit a physician in the first instance is based on his or her perception of the seriousness of the symptoms and of the cost in terms of other demands on the family and its budget constraint.

Data on physician visits by disease category are currently available from the National Disease and Therapeutic Index[13] and the National Ambulatory Medical Care Survey.[14] Unfortunately, however, there are inconsistencies between the two series and neither covers an extended period of time. (The NDTI extends back to 1956 and the Ambulatory Medical Care Survey, to 1973.)

The only information from physicians about disease conditions over any substantial historical period comes from records of notifiable diseases that physicians were asked to report to their public health departments. Reporting, even for this limited category of diseases, is not uniform from year to year and there is known to be considerable nonreporting. More recently, registries have been set up for specific diseases, for example, cancer and heart, and since 1957, the NCHS has been carrying out the Health Examination Survey for a sample of the population.

Most of the historical data on health conditions come from household surveys in which reports of health conditions are based on the respondent's perception of illness and his or her access to care. Under the best of conditions, the diagnosis of illness reported is likely to be of uncertain reliability. Two persons at a given time may have different responses to and understanding of disease symptoms. Over the decades, the responses to and understanding of symptoms have changed markedly. Physicians' diagnoses of diseases also have changed as medical knowledge has expanded. Some diseases, such as syphilis and cancer, are no longer shrouded in mystery. Indeed, some public programs, such as the permanent disability benefit program, brought the disabled "out of the woodwork."

Comparable data on sickness in the population are rare for the years before 1957. The few sickness surveys in the first decades of the twentieth century provide essentially little guidance—they were taken in a few localities or were limited to certain groups in the working population.[15-18] Some special surveys were made, such as the 1928-31 survey of about 9,000 white families for the Committee on the Costs of Medical Care,[19] the National Health Survey of 1935-36,[20] and the earlier surveys of more than half a million persons by the Metropolitan Life Insurance Company, from 1915 to 1917, to determine prevalence of illness on a given day.[17]

The tenth decennial census of the United States for 1880 included a query on the number of persons "so sick or disabled as to be unable to pursue their ordinary occupations on the day of Census enumeration." Rates of sickness or disability by age and sex are given for persons at age fifteen or older, based on a total of twenty million persons in this age group in nineteen states. No data were published, however, on the causes of illness.[21] The eleventh decennial census for 1890 continued the question on morbidity, but responses for only twelve states were compiled. For three states, the rates for disability due to acute or chronic diseases on June 1, 1890, were reported.[22]

During 1908, when the National Conservation Commission report was being prepared for the president and the Congress, Fisher emphasized the lack of current sickness data.[23] Although an estimate was prepared for that presidential report, it was crude—derived by applying a ratio to mortality rates. Another estimate prepared for the American Association for the Advancement of Science in 1906 established a figure of nine days of average illness per annum per person.[24]

Historical data on disability among workers were gathered by companies concerned with costs of disability protection because they were either direct providers of disability benefits or insurers. Such data also were gathered in some of the surveys mentioned above. Studies by Edison Electric Illuminating Company of Boston,[18] U.S. Rubber,[25] and Metropolitan Life[17] provide some relevant historical information about loss of work due to sickness. A record of all absences for one full working day or longer because of disability among its employees, for example, was kept for some years by the Edison Electric Illuminating Company of Boston beginning in January 1913.

Serious qualifications exist about the comparability of the survey data gathered before 1957. Such surveys were not comparable to each other or to recent NCHS Health Interview Surveys. A sketching of the data from NCHS Health Interview Surveys that are most comparable yields the findings of increasing rather than decreasing restricted-activity days, some growth in bed-disability days, and a small dropoff of work-loss days. The year 1957 was an influenza year and thus distorts the numbers to some degree (Figure 7-1). The figures shown for 1930 are from the CCMC study,[19] which is the primary source of earlier-year sickness data. It was not essentially a national sample survey because it was limited to about 9,000 white families in eighteen states. Information was collected from a single informant, usually the housewife. A substantial memory recall was required about illness and services used; families were interviewed periodically for twelve months at intervals of two to four months. Few multiple illnesses were reported (4.3 percent of cases were designated as due to more than one cause), suggesting that mostly serious illnesses were reported. Of the 33,547 illnesses reported for the entire survey population, nearly 80 percent were attended by physicians. The diagnoses of 61 percent of these attended illnesses were verified by physicians. The large proportion of attended cases contrasts with the low average number of physician visits—less than three per person per year during the period of the survey, 1928-31.

As indicated earlier, the 1880 and 1890 censuses were point prevalence surveys, i.e., for a given date, June 1. The 1880 census reported: "These figures are no doubt too small for each state, but

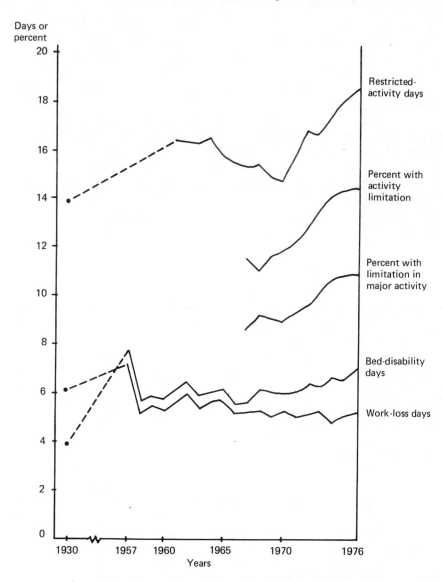

Figure 7-1. Changes in Measures of Disability

they are larger than any that have been heretofore reported as a result of inquiries of this kind, and furnish therefore probably the best data with regard to the morbidity of a large, general population which have heretofore been obtained."[2][1] The observation made about the 1880 morbidity survey also applies to the 1890 survey, that is, the census was taken at a time of year when there was probably the least amount of sickness and disability among adults. From the perspective of enumeration experts at the time, and from our current perspective, the 1890 reported morbidity rates are almost certainly too low.

The Metropolitan Life Studies represent a compilation of widely separated surveys, over a period of three years, limited to selected cities. Other regional health surveys were made. Important in this context are the Hagerstown studies by Sydenstricker[16] and the studies in the Eastern Health District of Baltimore.[15] Disease categories in these surveys are not comparable, and although much effort was made to convert 1928-31 CCMC data to greater comparability with the Eighth ICDA Code and the NCHS data, in the case of the Metropolitan Life Studies, the required detail for conversion was not available. Reporting by disease category did change, however, partly in response to improved diagnoses by physicians, to different attitudes toward disease, to a better understanding of disease as a consequence of more education, to improved financial access to medical care owing to higher earnings and third-party payments, and to changes in disease classification.

The kinds of sickness data collected in the several early studies differed. The National Conservation Commission number was a type of prevalence count. The Metropolitan Life Insurance studies also reported a prevalence of disease defined essentially as the counts of numbers (and rates) of persons who on the single day of the survey had the reported disease or illness. The CCMC data relate to case rates per 1,000, that is, the number of cases of disease or illness reported over a twelve-month period, which is not exactly comparable to either incidence or prevalence. The NCHS household survey data are reported on a prevalence basis for chronic diseases and on an incidence basis for acute illnesses. A count of illnesses on a particular date or over a specified brief period, such as two weeks, yields information on the existence of those illnesses in the population. Persons with diabetes report diabetes, those with asthma report asthma, and so forth. However, persons with infectious diseases and many respiratory illnesses may be symptom-free on the date of the survey. Only if new cases of influenza or colds, for example, are counted during a given time can sufficient data be gathered to permit an estimate of the number of episodes or conditions in the population.

How many persons were sick earlier in our history and how many are sick now depend on how people regard themselves, how they view sickness in general, what they understand about specific sickness, and what it costs them to cope with it. A respondent in Koos's study of the health of Regionville[26] makes this observation: "I wish I really knew what you meant about being sick. Sometimes I felt so bad I could curl up and die, but had to go on because the kids had to be taken care of and besides we didn't have the money to spend for the doctor. How could I be sick?"

Sickness itself is a heterogeneous phenomenon. It includes dysfunction attributable to diverse pathological conditions and of highly varying severity and duration. Beyond these problems, a historical study must contend with changes in survey techniques and instruments. Specific measures, such as restricted-activity days, are subject to the responses in terms of the definition being used. Each of the measures responds to societal and economic factors and these have changed over time, as indicated more fully in a subsequent section of this chapter.

When acute illnesses take a heavy toll in a family, both in deaths among children and protracted periods of fever and discomfort with uncertain outcomes in terms of life or death, minor illnesses, especially for workers, are likely to be understated. Also, notions of minor ailments and even statements about diseases of aging change. The National Conservation Commission poses the issue of morbidity that does not cause a person to stay home from work or compel him or her to stay in bed as follows:

> The extent of these milder ills is not generally appreciated. They are often carefully guarded secrets. . . . Once you penetrate beneath conventional acquaintance, there will almost invariably be found some functional impairment of heart, liver, kidneys or bladder; or dyspepsia, gastritis, jaundice, gallstones, constipation, diarrhea; or insomnia, neurasthenia, nervousness, neuritis, neuralgia, sick headache; or tonsillitis, bronchitis, hay fever, catarrh, grip, colds, sore throat; or rupture, hernia, phlebitis, skin eruption; or rheumatism, lumbago, gout, obesity; or decayed teeth, baldness, deafness, eye ailment, spinal curvature, lameness, broken bones, dislocations, sprains, bruises, cuts, burdens, or other troubles.[23]

The concept of aging and illness in old age has changed, as has the notion of "female troubles," and both changes have altered attitudes toward reporting diseases. These differences, along with the aging of the population and the large numbers of women at work, tend to contribute to the factors that account for differences in morbidity. It is thus clear that the resulting unadjusted morbidity rates give a confusing, contradictory, and imcomplete picture of long-term trends in the nation's health.

COMPARISONS, BY DISEASE

When we look at specific diseases some of the problems in making comparisons across time become plainer. The principal causes of illness and injury in the Metropolitan Life Insurance Study,[17] the most extensive of its kind for the first part of the twentieth century, were, in the rank order of prevalence among workers, influenza and pneumonia, accidents, diseases of the nervous system, diseases of the respiratory system, diseases of the digestive system, and rheumatism, as shown in Table 7-2.

The relative order of importance of diseases has changed. The respiratory diseases and mental disorders continue to outrank the others. Accidents, as represented by industrial accidents, and tuberculosis are down in relation to population size. Tuberculosis does not appear on a list of the fifteen most prevalent diseases in 1975, and the relative ranking of rheumatism has changed.

In 1908, a few years earlier than the Metropolitan Life study, it was estimated that more than half a million workers were killed or crippled each year as a result of occupational injuries. Also, about half a million workers were estimated to be suffering from tuberculosis, and half of this number were incapacitated while the remaining group was able to earn only half of its usual wage.[27] Syphilitics were estimated in 1908 at two million; it was assumed that they accounted for half of the institutionalized population.

The annual case rates per 1,000 persons over the period 1930-75 also show the difficulty of recording changes in illness in the

Table 7-2. **Metropolitan Life Insurance Data, 1915-17, on Persons Sick and Unable to Work, Ranked by Frequency of Causes of Illness or Injury**

Causes of work loss or injury	*Persons unable to work, per 1,000 workers*
Influenza and pneumonia	2.2
Accidents	1.8
Diseases of the nervous system	1.7
Other diseases of the respiratory system	1.7
Diseases of the digestive system	1.7
Rheumatism	1.6
Tuberculosis	0.9
Cerebral hemorrhage, apoplexy, paralysis	0.7
Organic diseases of the heart	0.6
Childbirth	0.5
Cancer	0.2

Source: Reference 19.

population. The highest case rates in the CCMC study for 1930 were for influenza and colds, followed by accidental injuries and childhood diseases, such as measles, tonsillitis, and whooping cough. Otitis media also ranked among the top illnesses. Rheumatism, at the bottom of this top-disease listing, is unlike the other short-term acute illnesses reported. A number of diseases that were important causes of sickness in the 1930s have been practically eliminated, including the following:[2][5]

Disease	*Case rate per 1,000*
Malaria	3.35
Smallpox	.39
Scarlet fever	6.02
Diphtheria	1.82
Poliomyelitis	.18
Erysipelas	.67
Salpingitis and pelvic abscess	.83

In other instances the extent of sickness has been significantly reduced. Respiratory tuberculosis, widespread in the early 1900s, was reported in the Metropolitan Life surveys at 0.7 per 1,000; it stood at 3.9 per 1,000 in 1930. In 1975, the rate (reflecting the impact of better diagnosis) was 1.5 per 1,000 on a prevalence count. Venereal diseases as reported are down from rates of 1 per 1,000 in 1930, and this reduction occurs despite the greater openness about social diseases, which would be expected to increase prevalence as reported.

INDICATORS OF IMPROVED HEALTH

Despite the sickness data that point to stability, if not growth, in sickness, the decline in mortality is a major indication that health status has improved. There are also other indicators of improved health status. Reportable communicable diseases have declined sharply, with only a few exceptions. Young people mature earlier and obtain greater height, factors generally regarded as indicating better nutrition and health. The duration of disability due to various diseases has been reduced. The illness rates in the U.S. Army and Navy, as indicated in Table 7-3, have declined almost continuously since 1900—the exceptions being periods of war.[28][29] For these and reasons mentioned previously, we believe that the health status of the U.S. population is higher now than it was in 1900 or in 1930.

Table 7-3. **Noneffective Rates on Account of Disease Condition per 1,000 Average Strength of the Army and Navy, Selected Years, 1904-74**

Selected years	Noneffective rate		Period	Percentage change	
	Army[1]	Navy[2]		Army	Navy
1904	39.1	26.8[3]	1904-11	−32.5%	−11.6%
1911	26.4	23.7[3]	1911-27	−5.3	+21.1
1927	25.0[4],[5]	28.7	1927-37	−3.6	−25.4
1937	24.1[4]	21.4	1937-53	−40.2	−42.5
1953	14.4[4]	12.3	1953-60	−32.8	−31.0
1960	9.7[4]	8.5			
1971	10.3[4]	6.7			
1973	11.3[4]	5.7	1960-73	+16.0	−33.0
1974	n.a.	5.6	1960-74	−	−33.0

[1] Annual Reports of the Surgeon General, U.S. Army in Continental U.S., 1911, 1919, 1938, 1953, 1961, 1973.
[2] M. Horton: "Economic analysis of progress in the medical care of the U.S. Navy and Marine Corp personnel," Appendix, 1966, table 2.
[3] The rate of disease was calculated by assuming that the disease rate was the same percentage of the combined disease and injury rate as it was in 1926.
[4] Total army instead of continental U.S. enlisted personnel. War evacuees are included in some of the data, raising such rates.
[5] Estimated under the assumption that the ratio of disease to injury is the same as the 1937 experience.
Sources: References 28, 29.

Notifiable Diseases

Notifiable, or communicable, diseases have largely been brought under control. Table 7-4 shows the rate per 100,000 of notifiable diseases.[30] As indicated, measles, diphtheria, smallpox, malaria, and typhoid have been successfully combated by preventive measures, vaccination in some instances and environmental measures in the case of typhoid and malaria. No cases of smallpox have been reported in the United States since 1950. In 1930, some 6.8 million cases of malaria were reported,[31] but malarial infection in the United States today is largely attributable to contraction abroad. For the most part these diseases, that were so costly in terms of work capacity and childhood illnesses, have been wiped out. Several other diseases that caused much debility, but not mortality, have been virtually eliminated. Hookworm was eliminated partly through the efforts of the Rockefeller Sanitary Commission to educate and treat people in rural areas affected by the disease. Pellagra has also been controlled following the work of Joseph Goldberger in isolating the "pellagra preventive" factor.[32] Diseases such as pellagra, hookworm, and malaria made people sick, often lessening vigor and efficiency, but did not affect death rates to any sizable extent.

Table 7-4. Rates per 100,000 Population for Specified Reportable Diseases, 1915-17 (Rate per 100,000 Population Enumerated as of April 1 for 1940, 1950, 1960, and 1970, and Estimated as of July 1 for All Other Years)

Year	Syphilis and its sequelae[4]	Gonorrhea	Malaria	Typhoid and paratyphoid fever[1]	Scarlet fever and streptococcal sore throat[2]	Hepatitis[3]	Diphtheria	Whooping cough	Measles	Acute poliomyelitis	Smallpox	Tuberculosis
1977	30.0	465.47	0.25	0.18	n.a.	26.2	0.04	1.0	26.5	0.01	n.a.	13.9
1976	33.7	470.47	0.22	0.20	n.a.	26.2	0.06	0.5	19.2	0.01	n.a.	15
1975	38.0	472.91	0.18	0.18	n.a.	25.5	0.14	0.8	11.4	0	n.a.	16
1970	43.8	285.2	1.5	0.2	239.2	32.0	0.2	2.1	23.2	(Z)	n.a.	18.3
1965	59.7	163.8	.1	.2	204.3	17.7	.1	3.5	135.1	(Z)	n.a.	25.3
1960[4]	68.0	139.6	(Z)	.5	175.8	23.4	.5	8.3	245.4	1.8	n.a.	30.8
1955	76.0	149.2	.3	1.0	89.8	19.5	1.2	38.2	337.9	17.6	n.a.	46.9
1950	154.2	204.0	1.4	1.6	42.8	2.5	3.8	80.1	210.1	22.1	n.a.	80.4
1945	282.3	225.8	47.4	3.7	140.1	n.a.	14.1	101.0	110.2	10.3	.3	86.8
1940	359.7	133.8	59.2	7.4	125.9	n.a.	11.8	139.6	220.7	7.4	2.1	78.0
1935	205.6	130.8	108.1	14.4	211.0	n.a.	30.8	141.9	584.6	8.5	6.3	87.9
1930	185.4	135.5	80.0	22.1	144.5	n.a.	54.1	135.6	340.8	7.5	39.7	101.5
1925	181.2	149.3	86.8	40.0	161.9	n.a.	82.1	131.2	194.3	5.3	34.2	n.a.
1920	145.3	175.4	173.0	33.8	151.6	n.a.	139.0	n.a.	480.5	2.2	95.9	n.a.
1915	n.a.	n.a.	n.a.	74.0	108.6	n.a.	132.7	n.a.	254.1	3.1	50.2	n.a.

Z Less than 0.05.
[1] Beginning 1950, excludes paratyphoid fever.
[2] 1912-19, excludes streptococcal sore throat.
[3] 1950-52, infections only; thereafter, infections and serum. Reporting incomplete. 1975-77 includes unspecified cases.
[4] Denotes first year for which figures include Alaska and Hawaii.
n.a.- not available.

Sources: 1915-70 figures: U.S. Bureau of the Census: "Historical Statistics of the United States, Colonial Times to 1970"; 1975-77 figures: unpublished data from U.S. Center for Disease Control.

Age at Maturity and Height

The average age at menarche has declined from 14.2 years in 1900[33] to 12.8 years in 1960-62.[34] The reduction in the average age at menarche is at least partly the result of being healthier during youth. Attaining a greater height can also be attributed in part to better health and nutrition. The following cross-section of height by age shows declining height in 1960-62 by age for both men and women.[34]

Age group	Height in inches	
	Men	Women
All	68.2	63.0
18-24	68.7	63.8
25-34	69.1	63.7
35-44	68.5	63.5
45-54	68.2	62.9
55-65	67.4	62.4
66-74	66.9	61.5
75 and over	65.9	61.1

This table suggests that young men and women attain greater height today than they did at the turn of the century, and study results suggest that bigger is better.[35] However, the aging process also contributes to the differences in the height of a twenty-year-old person and a seventy-year-old person.

When the 1960-62 survey results were compared to a life insurance study during the period 1895-1900, it was found that the average height of men had increased by 1.2 inches, or 1.8 percent. This comparison required adjustment for height attributable to shoes, and age differences in the population. Comparison of the 1960-62 results with the height of Army recruits in 1910 showed an increase in height of 1.3 inches, or 1.9 percent, between 1910 and 1960. A similar comparison for women found that their average height increased 1.3 inches, or 2.1 percent, from 1910 to 1960.

Duration and Severity of Sickness

The duration of sickness has been markedly lowered for many types of illness and impairment. New medical knowledge on early ambulation as well as advances in surgical techniques and the gains from antibiotics are contributing factors. In the early 1930s, for example, persons who developed appendicitis were hospitalized for 13.8 days as compared with 6.1 days today. Normal deliveries meant 12 days in the hospital instead of the 3.7 days mothers spend today.

The common cold or minor respiratory diseases far outrank many other causes of illness in the population, as reported in household surveys. But this rank in all years for which survey data are available does not completely tell the story of the predominance of minor respiratory conditions. In a family survey, colds are likely to be considerably underreported because of memory gap. Moreover, definitions of illness in such a survey may omit minor symptoms of a cold. Collins,[36] in discussing this tendency to underreport minor acute illnesses, observed that special respiratory studies have found illness rates as high as ten times the rates reported in household surveys in the 1930s (see Chapter 10).

From one perspective, the serious illness defined in terms of extent of dependence on others, pain, degree of impairment, duration, cost of treatment, and prognosis is of special concern in health policies. From another perspective, the minor diseases may create more immediate loss in production or GNP. Respiratory ailments, for example, from 1922 to 1924 accounted for approximately half of all absences and 40 percent of all the time lost because of sickness, among men. Colds and related diseases incapacitated, on the average, four of every ten men annually and seven of every ten women. Frequency of occurrence of the illness, that is, the relative numbers affected, may be a criterion; still another might be a composite of frequency, duration, and severity. Certainly, reduction in illness-caused deaths is a major, but not the only, goal of any national health program.

A number of important causes of death are comparatively infrequent causes of illness. Because of persistent linking of sickness rates and death rates in many discussions, we correlated the incidence rates for sickness by disease with death rates for those same diseases using both 1930 and 1975 data. Using mortality rates by disease category as the dependent variable in a simple regression analysis, we found no significant positive or negative correlation for the years 1930 and 1975. If the sign on the regression coefficient had been significantly positive, this would have indicated that diseases with high sickness levels produce the most fatalities. If the sign had been significantly negative, this would have indicated that diseases with high sickness levels are mainly nonfatal. Since the results were not statistically significant, there seems to be little association between disease-specific sickness and death rates. Hence, we cannot say that sickness has declined because the death rate has declined. We need to look at data other than death rates to determine the overall level of sickness. Nevertheless, it is true that the reduction in the death rate from sickness and the decline in the duration of illness contribute substantially to a higher level of well-being in the population.

The Military Experience with Illness

The Army and the Navy have experienced an impressive reduction in the loss of time from illness and disease since the early 1900s and the years before.[28,29] There has been a decline in hospital admissions and in "noneffective" rates for military personnel that indicates improved health in terms of both incidence and impact of disease. Essentially, the military experience shows more clearly than do civilian data the effect of improvements in health care and health care technology and the military data are more comparable over the decades. The civilian population data on work-loss days show changes not only in technology and health care but also in demand, and the sick leave policies for the civilian work force have changed significantly since 1900. The changes for military personnel, however, were not so extensive. Differences between the military and civilian experiences also exist in the area of hospital services. The increasing income of the population and the increased use of health insurance have increased hospital bed days for civilians since 1900. This does not hold for the military population, because the hospital costs of active service personnel were borne by the government throughout the period. Data on illness in the civilian population, as we have indicated, do not provide continuous historical series prior to 1957.

Admission rate and the noneffective rate per 1,000 of average strength capture the long-term sickness trend. The number of admissions per year, to hospitals or to barracks on sick call, per 1,000 men on active duty is the admissions rate. The noneffective rate measures the average number of men per 1,000 on active duty who are on sick call each day—essentially, patient days per 1,000. These noneffective rates are used here to measure trends in objective sickness rates.

The admissions rate increases during times of war, even when battle-related injuries are excluded; for example, admissions rates for enlisted men in the U.S. Army stationed in the United States rose from 897 per 1,000 in 1897 to 1,929 per 1,000 in 1898. Such changes in admissions rates undoubtedly reflect the effects of harsh wartime conditions on military personnel. The rates remained relatively high for a period after the war, presumably as a result of recurring problems. The rates of admission for 1960, however, were only 27.9 percent of the 1904 admissions rate for the Army. The 1971 rate was 29 percent of the 1904 rate, increased somewhat because of the Vietnam War. The 1960 Navy admissions rate was only 24.4 percent of the 1911 rate (the 1904 rate was not available).

Table 7-3 shows the noneffective rate on account of disease

conditions reported by the Army and the Navy for the years 1904-74. The Army rates dropped to 29 percent of the 1904 level by 1973, and the Navy rates, to 20 percent; the declines, thus, are large. In more recent years, Army data indicate declines through 1960 and small increases since 1960; Navy data show an increase in the aftermath of World War I, but declines throughout the remaining period. These noneffective rates for the armed forces point to marked declines in sickness over the twentieth century.

The data reviewed about height, maturation, and sickness duration as well as the data tabulated by the Army and Navy over a long historical period buttress the mortality statistics. Certainly these data support the finding that the population is healthier now than it was years before.

DETERMINANTS OF SICKNESS LEVELS

The special sensitivity of sickness data to social and economic factors has not gone unnoticed. On the contrary, considerable investigation has been made of the social and economic response of reports on sickness data that help to distinguish between health status and other factors affecting rates of sickness as reported. Indeed, even the health status of one spouse may affect the health status of the other.

The analyses of sickness data, that is, of work-loss days, restricted-activity days, bed days of illness, or percentage of the population with limitations of activity, are reported at some length in a later discussion (Chapter 8). In this section, we review several studies that are particularly relevant.

Silver asked whether work-loss rates are a reliable measure of health status.[37] He hypothesized that work loss reflects differences in economic variables rather than in the "objective" state of health. He assumed that an increase in family income would increase the demand for health, and be reflected in increased work loss including the patient's own time. His regressions, in which income and earnings rates and sex, region, and age were used as independent variables and days lost from work due to illness and injury as the dependent variable, while far from yielding conclusive results, suggest that differences in unadjusted work-loss days may be unreliable measures of variations in health status.

In a study of Medicare by Friedman that addressed the question of impact of services on disability, disability rates were favorably affected by medical care that presumably embodied biomedical advances.[38] Disability rates are represented by restricted-activity days that show a decline for those sixty-five years of age and over for the years from 1959 on, even though deaths have been postponed and income maintenance programs are favorable to withdrawal from work. (At the same time, restricted-activity days are found to be fairly constant for women aged forty-five to sixty-four and increasing for men of the same age who are not covered by Medicare.) Friedman found that by 1969, restricted-activity days for persons sixty-five and over declined 18 percent for men and 11 percent for women.

The change in work ethics as a determinant of growth in claims for disability payments has been researched by the Social Security Administration.[39] Disability for this purpose is defined as the inability "to engage in any substantial gainful activity by reason of a medically determinable physical or mental impairment that has lasted or can be expected to last for at least 12 months or to result in death." Among the factors that lead to increased disability claims, as identified in Social Security Administration studies, are

- changes in economic conditions, especially changes in the labor market
- altered attitudes toward government support
- program and administrative changes[40]

When unemployment is high, the number applying for disability benefits increases. Labor force participation rates of men aged fifty-five to sixty-four have declined in past years. This decline is attributed in part to the response to disability benefits and in part to eligibility for election of old-age benefits even though at a reduced benefit level.

One study by the Urban Institute[41] parcels out the growth in OASDI caseloads for the period 1969-74 among (a) population; (b) prevalence of disability; (c) numbers in insured status; and (d) participation, defined as the number of eligible disabled persons opting to claim benefits. For older men, those aged forty-five to sixty-four, the study found that 20 percent of the growth is due to the increase in the number who opt to retire; for women, the corresponding figure is 50 percent.

In several studies, physical illness is associated with changes in life events that cause changes in mental status.[42,43] Existing data on sickness, whether as the count of work-loss days, restricted-activity days, limitations for work, disability days, removals from the work force due to illness or injury, or institutional populations, are affected by a large variety of factors. Some of these factors have little to do with an objective state of sickness. For example, the existence of diability benefits (or the liberalization of eligibility definitions and amounts of payment) increases the reported number of persons who are disabled. To give another example, work-loss days are responsive to unemployment in the economy or the ability of a spouse to find a job, and they increase even more clearly when sick leave is paid and perhaps when there is favorable general income maintenance support. Differences in perceptions about illness and prevention of sequelae of disease play an important part in determining whether or not illness is reported. Educational status influences those perceptions, as well as the special personal characteristics of those disabled. Two persons with the same physiological or objective condition may have different views about retirement or may respond differently to surveys because of their different economic status, perspectives on illness, and knowledge about consequences of illness and of medical care.

When comparisons are made over time, the differences in each of the major components affecting sickness data are sizable. Some of these differences are suggested when some basic characteristics of the periods are compared.

TRENDS IN SICKNESS DATA

Existing data on the various measures of sickness are often fragmentary. Time loss from work is an example. The time loss from work counts, or the average work days lost per worker when standardized roughly for length of working week, do not uniformly show improvement over the decades. Estimates of the average annual time loss to wage earners due to sickness in the first two decades of the twentieth century are reported elsewhere to be from six to nine days per person, but it is unclear whether the loss is measured in working days or calendar days.[44] While differences between these counts might be expected, Collins's estimates[45] for the civilian population (in contrast to the data on men enlisted in the armed forces) indicate little difference, because limitation of activity is perceived as less on nonwork days. The ten-year record of absences among employees of the Edison Company of Boston for 1914-24 showed an average loss from sickness (exclusive of accidents) of 6.9 calendar days per man and 12.9 calendar days per woman. When accidents (both industrial and nonindustrial) were included, the time loss increased to 8.9 calendar days per man and 14 calendar days per woman.[18]

Boston Edison's experience comes closer in some ways to the

current one, except for its regional bias. That is, the workers were covered by the company's sick leave plan and had fairly liberal coverage. An illness allowance of one day per month was granted for the first twelve months of regular employment and two weeks per calendar year thereafter. For disabilities lasting more than fourteen consecutive days, a disability benefit of full wages was payable up to a maximum of thirteen weeks; after that, the benefit became a proportion of wages.

In 1930, working persons lost an average of 6.1 days due to sickness, but in that year, only a small percentage of lost wages was covered by any sick leave or sick pay plan.[45] (Social Security Administration data go back only to 1948, at which time 16.6 percent of lost work was covered by sick pay.) Today, in contrast, about 40 percent of earnings are compensated and about 60 percent of all employees are covered.

As indicated earlier, a number of studies have pointed to the importance of income maintenance in amount of time away from work. Disability protection, pay levels, existence of multiple employees in households, age of workers, and occupational distributions affect the extent of sick days lost from work. Important, but sometimes overlooked, is the general policy on income maintenance, including welfare and food stamps, that help assure the backstop support often needed in cases of long-term illness.

The granting of sick leave affects the frequency and duration of absences due to illness. An approximate measure of this tendency is provided by the comparison made by Brundage,[18] for the years 1922-24, of the frequency and duration of absences due to disability in a company that paid disability wages with the frequency and duration of this type of absence in a company that did not. The frequency was more than three times as great in the company paying wages as it was in the company without sick leave (Figure 7-2).

Figure 7-3 plots some historical data on the number of cases per 1,000 workers where the workers were sick for eight days or longer.[44] These data were compiled from the records of a number of industrial firms from 1921 to 1952 as a way to assess cash disability benefit loads. The figures indicate little progress over time toward improved health. However, it is obvious that the number of sick days depends on economic variables. The rate of sick days dropped sharply with the onset of the depression and increased rapidly with the tight labor market of World War II. The reported sick days are a joint result of the objective sickness rate and socioeconomic variables.

Apart from work days lost by workers, two other factors in the

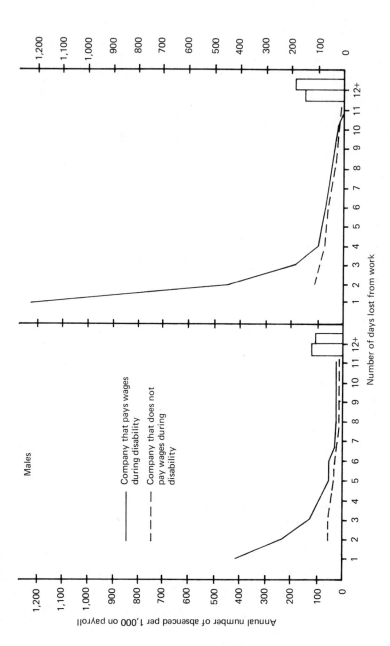

Figure 7-2. Impact of Sick Leave Coverage on Frequency of Work Loss by Duration, 1922-1924

Source: D.K. Brundage: "A 10-Year Record of Absences From Work on Account of Sickness and Accidents." *Public Health Reports*, Vol. 42, No. 8, February 25, 1927, pp. 529-550.

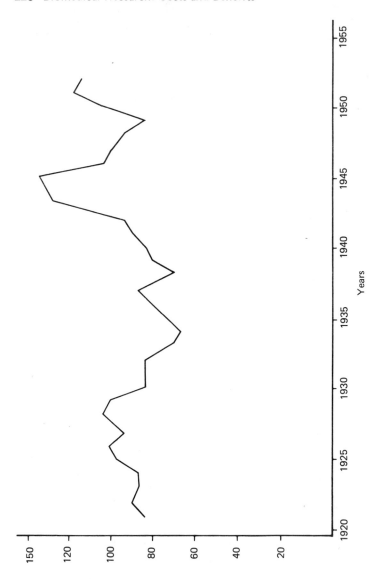

Figure 7-3. Eight Days Sickness, Case Rates per 1,000 Workers

Source: Reference 44.

morbidity that occasions loss in economic productivity are the size of the industrial population and the numbers of persons who have withdrawn from the labor market owing to ill health. The numbers of persons too sick to work are shown in Table 7-5 for selected years. About the turn of the century, approximately 520,000 persons were out of the labor force because of sickness, and about one-third of them were in institutions. By 1930, the numbers of persons out of the work force owing to sickness was almost seven times as large, and some further growth took place in the following forty-five-year period. We project, however, that the number will be below 5.5 million by the year 2000.

Figure 7-4 shows the number not in the labor force during the period 1900-76, and Figure 7-5, the numbers in the institutionalized population.[46] While the number not in the labor force due to disability has remained between 2.25 to 3 million since 1930, the growth in the work force means essentially that the ratio of disabled to total numbers employed has gone down steadily. Figure 7-6 shows the number institutionalized and out of the work force due to illness as a percentage of workers for the years 1957-76. A subsequent drop in this rate is expected by the year 2000. Even in this last, almost twenty-year period shown, the relative numbers of those who withdrew from the labor force due to illness have declined. The decline is far sharper for the institutionalized population. A decline

Table 7-5. Numbers of Persons Unable to Work Due to Sickness (Institutionalized and Noninstitutionalized Populations), Selected Years, 1900-2000 (amounts in thousands)

Year	Total unable to work (institutionalized and non-institutionalized)	Institutional-ized population	Withdrawn from workforce (non-institutionalized)	Total unable to work as percent of numbers employed
1900	520.3	174.6	345.7	1.9%[1]
1930	3,446.4	476.6	2,969.8	7.8
1963	4,059.5	1,461.9	2,597.6	5.9
1975	4.626.2	1,670.2	2,956.0	5.5
2000	5,413.7	1,419.7	3,994.0	4.3

[1] Data reported are clearly understatements of the underlying condition.
Source: Reference 46.

Number of persons
(in thousands)

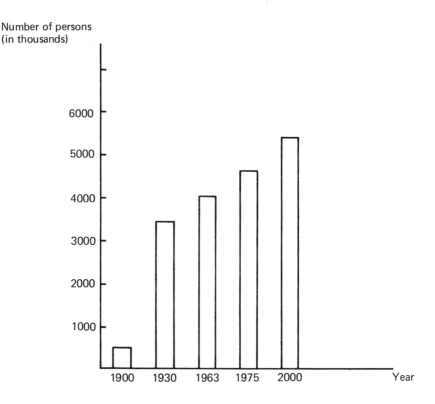

Source: Reference 46.

Figure 7-4. Persons Unable to Work, Institutionalized and Noninstitutionalized, Selected Years, 1900-2000

even in 1 percentage point, however, is of considerable economic importance, as will be discussed in Chapter 9.

THE OBJECTIVE SICKNESS RATE

As indicated earlier (see Figure 7-1), much of the raw morbidity data suggest that the population is sicker now than at the turn of the century or in 1930. Have the declining death rates resulted in more impaired lives in the population and more sickness? Or has the decrease in the death rates been accompanied by corresponding declines in the amount of sickness?

We consider the raw data to be essentially a combination of two components, one the objective sickness rate and the other the socioeconomic-induced rate. Objective sickness is defined as a patho-

Number of persons
(in thousands)

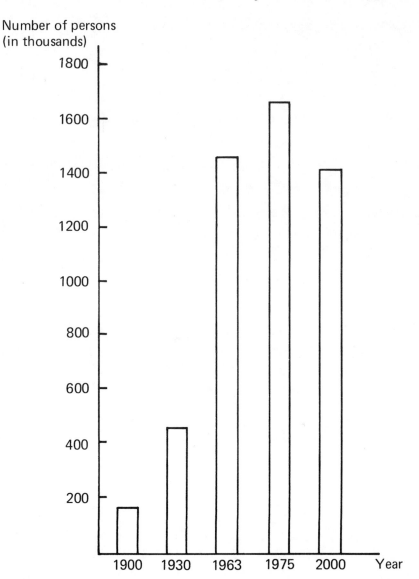

Figure 7-5.   Institutionalized Population, Selected Years, 1900-2000

logical or physiological condition that is more or less uniformly
defined and diagnosed from year to year. The socioeconomic
components of reports of work loss or absence from work due to

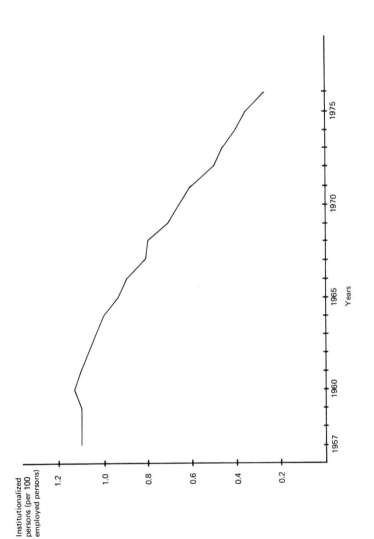

Sources: Computed as a ratio of annual data on the institutional population (average daily census) in mental hospitals, tuberculosis hospitals, and chronic disease hospitals divided by total employment. Employment data are U.S. Labor Department data as published in various issues of *Employment and Earnings*. Institutional data is compiled from Hospital Statistics, American Hospital Association, Chicago, 1977.

Figure 7-6. Institutionalized Population per 100 Employed Persons, Selected Years, 1957-76

sickness change according to such factors as (a) perception of illness; (b) knowledge about illness; and (c) economic capacity to be sick and stay away from work. Earlier reference was made to the historical differences in perceptions about illness. The Fisher report[2][3] enumerated a large number of illnesses that in the first part of the century were "walking" illnesses. However, if persons who would not have considered themselves sick in the early part of the twentieth century were given the perspectives of today, they would tend to be absent from work when illness strikes.

Part of the difference between conduct in the early part of the century extends beyond perception about sickness. It has to do with knowledge about disease, its consequence, and what medical care can achieve. If symptoms of disease are not recognized owing to lack of knowledge about disease, the likelihood of absence from work is reduced. Or, if there is little knowledge about what medical care can do about the symptoms, there is less reaching out for care and less staying at home. (Certainly the capacity of medicine for cures determines the "demand" for care.)

Of special importance in the extent of illness reported or work loss is the economic capacity to stay away from work. In one early report on absences from work because of sickness, it was noted that "many employees are loathe to absent themselves from work when absence involved cessation of pay, even though it may be disagreeable to work when physically indisposed."[18] In fact, a factory physician reported that an employee on a wage basis who was suffering from pneumonia had remained at work until the day his condition became critical.

The economic capacity to stay home from work while sick depends on more than sick leave. It depends on the assets of the family and the income-earning capacity of family members. It rests as well on the whole income maintenance structure that can give support to those who are sick, including the direct cash supports, such as disability benefits, food stamps, and provision for medical care through the medical assistance program. Income maintenance programs of the government are essentially of fairly recent origin, although there were some small efforts in this area before passage of the Social Security Act of 1935. Some medical assistance was provided locally in 1950 under federally aided programs, but Medicaid and Medicare really began after 1965.

What can be learned about the relative importance of objective sickness and socioeconomic reporting of sickness so that adjustments can be made in the data? For the components of the socioeconomic reporting we have identified proxy measures where possible and elasticity coefficients for those proxies drawn from the studies of demand for medical care or of disability. These components and their proxies may be summarized as follows:

Component affecting reporting	*Proxy*
Economic capacity to be sick	Income elasticity of demand for medical care (0.5- to 0.6-percent rise in demand for each 1-percent rise in income supports)
Perception about illness	Percent of mothers in receipt of prenatal care
Knowledge about illness and the potential of medical care	Levels of education: percent high school graduates; percent reaching eighth grade; years of schooling of the population (0.7-percent rise in sickness reported for each 1-percent rise in percent of persons graduating from high school, or 0.2-percent rise in sickness reported for each 1-percent rise in educational level).

An application of this approach is suggested in the next section.

Sickness Rates in 1890 and 1976

In 1890, those who were "sick or disabled as to be unable to pursue their ordinary occupations" were counted in the 1890 census, and the results were compiled for twelve states. If it is assumed, for males aged fifteen and over, that being too sick to work means being bedridden, a comparison can be made with 1976 bed-disability days for males of the same age group. For 1890 the age groupings were slightly different, but close enough for a comparison.

An alternative interpretation of the 1890 census question on being too sick or being disabled is to assume that the relevant comparison is with work-loss days. Today, the average number of men per 1,000 per day that suffer bed disability is substantially higher than the average number per 1,000 employed that suffer a work-loss day on a working day. The only exception is for the over-sixty-five age group; presumably, the very sick in this group retire. Such an interpretation of the 1890 census reduces, but does not eliminate, the reduction in sickness rates between 1890 and 1976.

In addition to the preceding adjustments that simply seek reporting consistency, an adjustment can be made for socioeconomic changes that affect attitude toward sickness or demand for time off from work. A bed-disability day or a day off from work when sick is not a simple objective or technical choice. As indicated earlier, for a certain extent of sickness, economic and social variables will affect whether a person stays in bed or goes to work. As one approximation, we use the income elasticity of demand for health care as a rough guide to the magnitude of this change in demand. We make no pretense that the elasticity coefficient used (0.58) for real income is accurate, but it is, at least, illustrative. It may seem that so large a demand adjustment must be dismissed out of hand. However, the Army and Navy noneffective rates support a finding of a large drop in objective sickness. As stated earlier, the Army and Navy decline in rates should come close to reflecting the decline in the objective sickness rate without being obscured by other changes, such as income and access to care. The characteristics of the Army-Navy data are discussed more fully in Chapter 8. Even though the adjustment we make is not precise by any means, it indicates the nature of the adjustment required to obtain the trend in the underlying sickness rate.

CONCLUSION

The data on sickness for 1890 to 1976 are not fully comparable. In addition, factors other than disease cause survey results to show something other than an objective sickness rate. What seems to be a fairly level sickness rate for the total population from 1890 to 1976 (Table 7-6) is actually an underreported sickness rate for certain age and sex groups (women and children) and the result of staying at home or in bed for less serious illnesses in 1976 than would have been the case in 1890. As can be seen from Table 7-5, when sickness rates for 1890 and 1976 are standardized to a common population base, there is a significant decrease in sickness. On this basis, we estimate that today's underlying sickness rate is somewhere between one-fifth and one-third of what it would have been in 1890 with a population of comparable age. The 20 percent is derived by applying the demand adjustment factor to the 30 per 1,000 adjusted work-loss days in Table 7-7. The one-third is a conservative interpretation of the Army-Navy rates.

Table 7-6.   Males—Bed Disability

	1976 average daily number in bed per 1,000[1]		1890 rate sick per 1,000	
Ages		Ages	On June 1, 1890[2]	With seasonal and regional adjustment[3]
17-24	10.14	15-25	5.33	6.98
25-44	12.88	25-45	11.66	15.27
45-64	21.64	45-65	49.94	65.42
65+	39.18	65+	67.76	88.77
Ages 17+	18.20		23.33	30.56
			(78%)	(60%)
Ages 17+ with 1976 population weights	18.20		28.63	37.50
			(64%)	(49%)

The 1976 daily bed-disability rate per 1,000 as a percent of the 1890 rate for all males seventeen and over is in parentheses for each alternative adjustment.

[1] Source: National Center for Health Statistics: *Current Estimates from the Health Interview Survey, United States–1976*, Series 10, No. 119.

[2] Source: 1890 Census, Vol. 4, Part 1, pp. 474-480. The rate for ages twenty-five to forty-four is a weighted average of the twenty-five to thirty-five and thirty-five to forty-four age group rates.

[3] The seasonal adjustment was made by adjusting acute conditions to annual averages assuming that June 1 levels were equivalent to April-June quarterly levels. This probably underadjusts since April and May have higher disability rates than June (NCHS, Series 10, No. 114). The regional adjustment is simply the ratio of sick per 1,000 for the twelve states reported in the 1890 census divided by the ratio of sick per 1,000 in the three states that were reported by age and sex (Maine, Massachusetts, and Vermont). The seasonal factor was 1.1 and the regional was 1.19. Thus, the adjusted rates were $1.1 \times 1.9 = 1.31$ times the unadjusted rates.

Table 7-7.   Males—Work Loss

		1890 rate sick per 1,000	
Ages	1976 average daily number losing work[1]	On June 1, 1890[1]	With seasonal and regional adjustments[1]
17-24	16.8	5.33	6.98
25-44	20.0	11.66	15.27
45-64	25.2	49.94	65.42
Ages 17+	21.0	19.3	25.3
		(109%)	(83%)
Ages 17+ with 1976 population weight	21.0	22.9	30.0
		(92%)	(70%)

The 1976 daily work-loss rate per 1,000 as a percent of the 1890 rate for all males seventeen to sixty-five is in parentheses for each alternative adjustment.

[1] Sources and adjustments were the same as for Table 7-6.

REFERENCES

1. Fanshel, S., and Bush, J.W.: A health status index and its application to health services outcomes. Operations Research 18:1021-1066, November-December 1970.

2. Chen, M.M., Bush, J.W., Patrick, D.L., and Blischke, W.R.: Linear models of social preferences for constructing a health status index. Paper prepared for meeting of Operations Research Society of America, San Diego, Calif., November 1973.

3. Zeckhauser, R., and Shepard, D.: Where now for saving lives? Law and Contemporary Problems 40:5-45, autumn 1976.

4. Wylie, C.M., and White, B.K.: A measure of disability. Archives of Environmental Health 8:834-839, June 1964.

5. Katz, S., et al.: Studies of illness in the aged: the index of ADL—a standardized measure of biological and psychosocial function. J of the Am Medical Association 185:914-919, September 1963.

6. Mushkin, S.J.: Criteria for program evaluation. Respiratory Disease Task Force on Prevention, Control, and Education. U.S. Department of Health, Education, and Welfare, March 1977.

7. Karnofsky, D.A., and Burchenal, J.H.: The clinical evaluation of chemotherapeutic agents in cancer. *In* Evaluation of chemotherapeutic agents in cancer, edited by R. MacLeod. Columbia University Press, New York, 1949.

8. Gilson, Betty S., Berger, M., Bobbitt, R.A., and Carter, W.B.: The sickness impact profile: development of an outcome measure of health care. Am J of Pub Health 65 (12):1304-1310, December 1975.

9. National Center for Health Statistics: Prevalence of chronic conditions of the genitourinary, nervous, endocrine, metabolic, and blood and blood-forming systems and of the other selected chronic conditions, United States—1973. Vital and Health Statistics, Series 10, No. 109, p. 10, and other publications of Series 10, including Nos. 99, 94, 92, 84, and 83, Rockville, Md.

10. National Center for Health Statistics: Vital and Health Statistics, Series 10, Rockville, Md.

11. U.S. Office of Economic Opportunity: Guide to the documentation and data files of the 1966 and 1967 survey of economic opportunity. Washington, D.C., 1970.

12. Parnes, H.S., et al.: The pre-retirement years: a longitudinal study of the labor market experience of men. Volume I. Manpower Research Monograph No. 15. U.S. Government Printing Office, Washington, D.C., 1970.

13. IMS America Ltd.: National disease and therapeutic index. Ambler, Pa., 1976.

14. National Center for Health Statistics: The national ambulatory medical care survey: 1973 summary, United States, May 1973-April 1974. Vital and Health Statistics, Series 13, No. 21, Rockville, Md.

15. Downes, J., and Collins, S.D.: A Study of illness among families in the eastern health district of Baltimore. Milbank Mem Fund Q, January 1940, p. 14;

and Preas, S., and Phillips, R.: The severity of illness among males and females. Milbank Mem Fund Q, July 1942, p. 233.

16. Sydenstricker, E.: Hagerstown morbidity studies, I-XI. Public Health Rep 41:2069-2088, Sept. 24, 1926; 42:121-131, Jan. 14, 1927; 42:1565-1572, June 10, 1927; 42:1689-1701, June 24, 1927; 42:1939-1957, July 29, 1927; 43:1067-1074, May 4, 1928; 43:1124-1156, May 11, 1928; 43:1259-1276, May 25, 1928; 44:1821-1833, July 26, 1929; 44:2101-2106, Aug. 30, 1929.

17. Stecker, M.L., Frankel, L.K., and Dublin, L.I.: Some recent morbidity data, 1915-1917. Metropolitan Life Insurance Company, New York, 1919.

18. Brundage, D.K.: A ten-year record of absences from work on account of sickness and accidents. Experiences of employees of the Edison Electric Illuminating Company of Boston, 1915 to 1924, inclusive. Public Health Rep 42:529-550, Feb. 25, 1927.

19. The Committee on the Costs of Medical Care: Medical care for the American people. Publication No. 28, final report of the Committee. Arno Press, New York, 1932.

20. Britten, R.H., Collins, S.D., and Fitzgerald, J.F.: National health survey: some general findings. Public Health Rep 55:444, Mar. 15, 1940.

21. U.S. Census Office: Tenth decennial census: 1880. Congressional Series: House Misc. Doc. 42, 47th Congress, 2nd sess., Washington, D.C., June 1, 1880, pp. 1883-1888.

22. U.S. Census Office: Eleventh decennial census: 1890. Congressional Series: House Misc. Doc. 340, 52nd Congress, 1st sess., Washington, D.C', June 1, 1890, pp. 1892-1897.

23. Fisher, I.: National vitality, its wastes and conservation. Report of the National Conservation Commission. Volume III, U.S. Senate Doc. No. 676, 60th Congress, 2nd sess., Washington, D.C., February 1909.

24. Norton, J.P.: Economic advisability of a national department of health. Summary report. Proceedings of the American Association for the Advancement of Science. New York, 1906.

25. Collins, S.D.: Causes of illness in 9,000 families, based on nationwide periodic canvasses, 1928-1931. Public Health Rep 48:283-308, 1933.

26. Koos, E.L.: The health of Regionville. Columbia University Press, New York, 1954.

27. Fisher, I.: The war against the great white plague. Century Magazine 78:627-628, August 1909.

28. Horton, M.: Economic analysis of progress in the medical care of the U.S. Navy and Marine Corps personnel. Including Appendix. PhD thesis, University of Washington, Seattle, 1966; supplemented by data provided by the Surgeon General of the Navy for more recent years.

29. Department of Defense: Annual reports of the Surgeon General, U.S. Army, 1911, 1919, 1938, 1953, 1961, 1973.

30. U.S. Bureau of the Census: Historical statistics of the U.S., colonial times to 1970. Part 1. U.S. Dept. of Commerce, Washington, D.C., September 1975, p. 77, for 1915-70 data; unpublished data from U.S. Center for Disease Control, Atlanta, Ga., for 1975-77.

31. Cited in Mushkin, S.J.: Health as an investment. J of Pol Econ 70:142, October 1962.

32. Goldberger, J.: Pellagra. J of the Am Dietetic Association, Baltimore, IV:221-227, March 1929.

33. Tanner, J.M.: Growth at adolescence. Blackwell Scientific Publications, Oxford, 1962.

34. National Center for Health Statistics: Weight, height, and selected body dimensions of adults, U.S. (1960-62). Vital and Health Statistics, Series 11, No. 8, 1965. Rockville, Md.

35. Klein, R.E., et al.: Is big smart? The relation of growth to cognition. J of Health and Social Behavior 13:219-225, September 1972.

36. Collins, S.D.: Age incidence of specific causes of illness. Public Health Rep 50:1408, 1935. Reprint 1710.

37. Silver, M.: An economic analysis of variations in medical expenses and work-loss rates. *In* Empirical studies in health economics, edited by H.E. Klarman. Johns Hopkins University Press, Baltimore, 1970, pp. 121-144.

38. Friedman, B.: Mortality, disability, and the normative economics of medicare. *In* The role of health insurance in the health services sector, edited by R.N. Rosett. National Bureau of Economic Research, New York, 1976, pp. 365-390.

39. Lando, M.E., and Krute, A.: Disability insurance: program issues and research. Soc Sec Bull 39:3, October 1976.

40. Lando, M.E.: Demographic characteristics of disability applicants: relationship to allowances. Soc Sec Bull 39:15, May 1976.

41. Fletcher, A.E., and Thorpe, Jr., C.O.: Estimates of disabled OASDI beneficiaries (working paper 977-04). Urban Institute, Washington, D.C., April 1976.

42. Rahe, R.H.: Subjects' recent life changes and their near-future illness reports. Annals of Clinical Research 4:250-265, 1972.

43. Holmes, T.H., and Masuda, M.: Life change and illness susceptibility. Paper presented at symposium, Separation and depression: clinical and research aspects. American Association for the Advancement of Science, December 1970.

44. Compiled from a series of reports by Brundage, D., Gafafer, W.M., and Frasier, E.S., appearing in various issues of Public Health Rep. An index of publications in the series from 1920 to 1950 appears in Gafafer, W.M.: Industrial sickness absenteeism among males and females during 1950. Public Health Rep 66 (Part II), Nov. 23, 1951.

45. Collins, S.D.: Cases and days of illness among males and females with special reference to confinement to bed. Public Health Rep 55:54, 1940.

46. Computed from U.S. Bureau of the Census, Decennial Censuses, 1890, 1940, 1960, 1970, supplemented in some instances by estimates prepared by the census for nondecennial years and from U.S. Department of Labor Annual Reports on Employment and Earnings adjusted for historical changes in definition. (The 1930 numbers of workers withdrawn from the labor force are based on the 1940 census but reviewed by comparison with special studies in the 1930s.)

Chapter Eight

Biomedical Research and Disability

What has biomedical research contributed to reducing sickness? Many factors have helped to reduce the heavy toll of childhood diseases and infectious and communicable diseases that once impaired the ability of individuals to work effectively, or to work at all. Over the decades a number of diseases have been attacked so successfully that they are now rare. Pellagra, hookworm, and malaria are examples of diseases that no longer pose a threat to human energy. Similarly, diseases such as dysentery and typhoid that in the early years of the century caused much mortality and morbidity have been controlled by advances in knowledge implemented by public health measures. Diseases for which vaccines have been developed represent still a third class, which includes, measles, whooping cough, diphtheria, tetanus, poliomyelitis, and yellow fever. Recent data indicate the marked progress made in reducing the incidence and suffering from diseases, particularly childhood diseases such as diphtheria and whooping cough. However, although we can compare historical and 1975 rates for diphtheria and whooping cough, the data are not sufficient as tools for analysis. At best, we can say that some part of the change in rates of illness is attributable to biomedical advance.

The linkage is clearer in some instances than in others. For example, the linkage between water supply systems and the reduction in dysentery and typhoid is noted in the early accounts of city health officers and is verified by scientific knowledge.[1] The isolation in sanitoriums of those with tuberculosis is credited with curbing the spread of the disease in the early decades of this century.[1] However, much of what is known is anecdotal. And it is difficult in any instance to determine what share of the gains in control of communicable diseases can be attributed to biomedical science and advances in knowledge.

As the earlier discussion (Chapter 7) on sickness in the population made plain, sickness rates as reported, according to most series, have increased rather than decreased. Even for those series that show a decline, the decline is so small that there is little difference or variation to be explained and parceled out among factors affecting sickness. Tools of assessment that can capture what the "true" impact has been, given the characteristics of the data, are not readily at hand; this is the basic barrier to reaching an understanding of the relation of biomedical advances to sickness.

A MODEL FOR ANALYSIS

It was initially postulated that factors determining sickness rates are similar to, if not the same as, those determining mortality. Accordingly, the market behavioral model formulated for analysis of mortality data was the starting point for analysis of sickness rates.

Familiar demand and supply functions for health and health care are used. Prices and incomes are assumed to determine demand, along with environmental factors and societal characteristics. On the supply side, both the price and characteristics of providers of care and provision of care (represented by knowledge about care) are assumed to be important determinants.

As indicated in Chapter 4, the demand and supply functions can be formally written as follows:

$$Q^d = f \text{ (P, INC, SOC, ENV)}$$

$$Q^s = f \text{ (P, PROV, TECH)}$$

where

Q^d, Q^s = the quantity demanded and the quantity supplied

P = price

INC = a vector of economic variables

SOC = a vector of societal variables

ENV = a vector of environmental variables

PROV = a vector of provider variables

TECH = biomedical research

The equilibrium condition for the market is

$$Q^d = Q^s = Q.$$

However, the definition of Q poses difficult conceptual problems in terms of standard quantification. In Chapter 4, Q is defined to facilitate analysis of mortality rates. In this chapter, Q essentially represents a measure of good health.

The indexes applied for the analysis, however, are not measures of health but of sickness. If, following the conceptual approach of Grossman,[2] we define Q as the number of health days per year, counts of sickness would require transformation. With 365 days per year, the number of sick days per year is, by definition,

$$S = 365 - Q.$$

Similarly, if we substitute Q_1 for Q, and Q_1 is defined as the number of healthy working days per year, work-loss days per year S_1 would be derived as total days of work per year less Q_1:

$$S_1 = TD - Q_1$$

Reduced-form equations with price and work loss as endogenous variables can then be estimated as functions of the exogenous variables. The supply equation is rewritten as

$$P^s = Q\,(S_1, \text{PROV}, \text{TECH}),$$

and substituting into the demand equation for P, the result is

$$S_1 = f\,(\text{INC}, \text{PROV}, \text{ENV}, \text{SOC}, \text{TECH}).$$

Examination of economic studies of disability rate determinants and correlates of utilization of health care points to modification of the model to incorporate additional factors into the equation. While real income per capita as the index used for the variable *INC* may be adequate as a proxy for factors affecting health status such as nutrition, housing, recreation, and capacity to finance medical care, it does not appear to adequately capture the impact of changes in sick leave provision for employees. Sick leave studies suggest that such leave has made a sizable difference in reported sickness.[3]

Not only income levels but also safeguards for income in event of risk are important. Moreover, as suggested earlier, both perception about sickness and knowledge about disease and treatments are determinants of sickness as reported, suggesting inclusion of variables such as mortality as influencing perception, and educational levels as proxies for the public's understanding about diseases.

The model formulated for analysis of mortality required further elaboration. However, this elaboration was hampered by the limited number of observations and the characteristics of sickness data, as indicated in the pages that follow.

Data Limitations

Characteristics of the sickness information that are particular barriers to analysis are (a) the short period over which there are observations; (b) the imprecision of the operational definition of sickness; and (c) the complex relationship between biomedical research and sickness rates.

Information about sickness rates for which uniform definitions were used is available, at most, for twenty years. Data on restricted-activity days and work loss were collected routinely from 1957 on by the National Center for Health Statistics (NCHS). Because 1957-58 was an influenza epidemic year, the representativeness of the statistics for that year was distorted. Furthermore, for two years in the 1970s the survey instrument was modified by the NCHS, thus introducing a further possible bias. The number of observations thus fall short of that needed to test a model that reflects the multiplicity of variables that enter into a complete equation.

To enlarge the number of observations, we turned to the quarterly data reported by NCHS. Analysis of the quarterly data, which incorporated a dummy explanatory variable for seasonality, indicated that the quarterly swings in the data explained almost all of the variations in work-loss days that the analysis was attempting to explain. Thus, still in pursuit of a data base sufficient for a model to explain changes in sickness rates, we adjusted the quarterly observations seasonally to smooth the data points and carried out a new quantification. The findings of this analysis were (a) a sign on the biomedical research variable that was different, from that hypothesized, and (b) coefficients for other variables that were not statistically significant.

Since the quarterly NCHS data did not provide the answer, we looked to the historical studies of sickness and work loss for extension of the number of observations. Examination of the data from the Edison Electric Illuminating Company of Boston's sickness plan inaugurated January 1913,[4] from U.S. Rubber for 1918, 1919, and 1920,[5] and from a series of companies reporting on work absences of eight days or more for the period 1921 to 1952 yielded little.[6] The several early data sources suggest little variance, except as indicated in Chapter 7, in response to economic circumstance. If the historical morbidity data cannot be used, what information can be used?

As we postulated earlier, the population is not sicker today than it was years ago. Sickness rates reported now may be the same or higher than those reported earlier, but the reports are subject to a number of influences that tend to yield misleading results about sickness when objectively defined. Reports of sickness for individuals do not define an individual's objective state of ill health. The reports vary according to the individual's perception about being sick, his or her economic capacity to be sick, the extent of understanding about illness, and the capacity of the medical community to deal with an illness. The last three factors clearly influence the reporting on sickness, while the objective state of sickness is essentially what analysts have in mind when they inquire about the effect of biomedical research on sickness and disability.

Biomedical research tends to reduce objective sickness by advancing knowledge on prevention and disease control. However, it also has had an impact on other factors. Perception about sickness is a function, among other things, of the extent of sickness in the population, particularly in the young population. Advances in knowledge, to the extent that they reduce sickness, raise the level of perception about being sick. Because of its lower incidence, sickness is more likely to be considered a problem. We have already suggested that when the incidence of serious sickness among children is high and many die, the threshold of adults for perceiving illness may tend to be high. Conversely, when death rates are low and serious illness, particularly among children, is rare, adults are more likely to be aware of sickness.

Understanding about illness and the capacity of medicine for cures is also a function of biomedical knowledge. Evidence indicates that the rise in demand for medical services is partially a response to advances in medicine. Moreover, if symptoms are not recognized sickness is likely to be underreported. Also, when medical care is not sought, subclinical symptoms are not detected.

Even the economic capacity to be sick is a function of sickness. Wage and salary payments during periods of illness, financial provision for medical services, and the general level of real income and of income maintenance undoubtedly influence a worker's ability to stay home from work because of illness and to report that illness. Although biomedical advances tend to have less impact on the economic capacity to be sick than on the other socioeconomic factors, the economic capacity to be sick is not entirely independent of advances in biomedical knowledge and the effect of knowledge on productivity and, accordingly, on wage levels.

Other factors that influence reporting of sickness are perhaps not as significant as those identified above, but they warrant some mention. For example, given the definitions now formulated by NCHS, the use of health services itself generates a restricted-activity day. Sickness as reported is increased by utilization rates: the more use, the more sickness. The move toward deinstitutionalization of the population may be presumed to reduce the reported economic days lost from gainful activity due to sickness on the assumption that some persons released from institutions and integrated into the community find jobs. The number of these persons with symptoms may change little, but living in the community may be therapeutic for them. However, days lost from work by those with jobs may be artificially raised by the move to deinstitutionalize the sick population.

Reduced mortality rates among young persons and the postponement of death in general influence the amount of sickness reported. The diabetic whose life has been saved turns up in the count of the sick. Not all cases of postponed death, however, result in impaired lives. On the contrary, the child who is safeguarded against diphtheria also may be spared a long-term heart impairment. The infant whose mother was spared from rubella is less likely to be sick later. The asymptomatic person with hypertension who is receiving medication may not be counted as sick. As Table 8-1 suggests, biomedical research affects each of the factors mirrored in sickness rates, not just the objective state of sickness (or sickness uniformly defined as pathological conditions that are uniformly diagnosed and uniformly reported). In some instances such as disease prevention, the rates go down; in others, such as more identification of disease, they go up. What we wish primarily to know is the extent (or the share) of the biomedical research contribution to the reduction in the objective sickness rate (when the basic figures are adjusted to exclude the "demand" for sickness or socioeconomic variables). The assumption is that biomedical research has reduced the amount of sickness in the population by preventive therapeutic and restorative methods. Few dispute that it has contributed to the dramatic reduction in acute illness. But this reduction has extended life expectancy and has led to more degenerative, chronic diseases.

While the primary emphasis is on the effect of biomedical research

Table 8-1. Impact of Biomedical Research on Sickness Rates
(Plus or Minus), and Factors Influencing Reported Sickness

	Factors affecting reported sickness	*Potential impact of factor on sickness reported*	*Potential impact of research on each factor*
	Objective sickness state	[1]	−
	Acute	[1]	−
	Chronic	[1]	+
	Perception of sickness	+	+
	Understanding of sickness	+	+
	Capacity of Providers		
	Prevention	−	+
Biomedical research	Treatment	−	+
	Identification of illness	+	+
	Use of health services	+	+
	Deinstitutionalization	−	+
	Postponement of deaths	?	+
	With residual condition	+	?
	Without residual condition	−	?
	Economic capacity to be sick	+	+

[1] The objective state of illness reports, but is not influenced by, social, economic, and psychological factors.

on the objective sickness rate, it is important to recognize that biomedical research, in one aspect or other, affects each of the other factors that influence the amount of sickness reported. Biomedical research influences the perception of illness, family understanding about illness, the capacity of physicians to cure, and the use of health services, as suggested in Table 8-1. Advances in knowledge contributed, furthermore, to deinstitutionalization and certainly have affected death rates and length of life expectancy. To the extent to which biomedical research reduces work loss and incapacity to work, it even affects the economic capacity to be sick.

We thus have a set of interactions with biomedical research influencing the range of factors that determine the amount of sickness reported in the population. For example, the capacity of providers to prevent or to cure determines the extent of sickness, and that capacity is determined, in turn, by the state of medical knowledge. As the capacity of providers increases, so do preventive measures and new treatment. Advances in science that identify diseases not diagnosed earlier may make physicians aware of disease conditions that they did not understand earlier; forms of chronic obstructive lung diseases, such as "farmer's lung," are illustrative of this. Family understanding about illness depends on education received outside the medical community, but it is also influenced by earlier contact with public health services and providers of care and their capacity in response to biomedical research. The provision of health services is also a form of health education.

The information now available falls short of permitting us to make a positive statement about the larger number of postponed deaths as a result of research. And it does not give us the basis for even approximating the impact, on balance, of research on reduced death rates of those who have residual conditions and those without such conditions.

Sickness rates that are uniformly defined, uniformly diagnosed, and uniformly reported are the types of information that essentially are sought to yield data on biomedical knowledge as a factor in reducing sickness.

The Objective State

With due recognition of the complex set of forces that operate to influence sickness as reported and the interaction of biomedical research with those forces, we turned to Army and Navy data on sickness, to approach a measure of the concept of the objective state of ill health. Both the Army and the Navy, as indicated in Chapter 7, have information over a series of years on "noneffective" rates. The noneffective rate measures the average number of men per 1,000 on active duty that are on sick call each day. The Navy and Army data reported here exclude injuries. (An Army series that includes non-battle injuries also is used.)

In Chapter 7, we indicated that the Army and Navy data show a substantial downward trend after 1904. But the Army sickness rates moved upward at the time of the Vietnam War, and these rates are not yet down to the mid-1960 levels. The inclusion of war evacuees in the data contributed to the elevated sickness rates. The attitudes of recruits and medical personnel undoubtedly have influenced even these sickness rates.

The longer term trend data are influenced by the increased educational attainment of young persons, by more popular understanding about diseases, and by the improved capacity of providers to treat disease and injury. Although not entirely free of factors that artificially raise sickness rates, the basic characteristics of the military data support their use for assessment of the objective state.

Importantly, the military data are free of the impact on sickness of the immediate economic capacity to be sick. Unlike the civilian sector, income, food, and lodging continue to be furnished by the military without regard to capacity to work; thus, basic necessities do not compel a member of the armed forces to fail to report sickness. Furthermore, the data are fairly uniform in concept across the years. In each case, a medical review established sickness sufficient enough for the patient to be away from effective duty. Although medical knowledge undoubtedly has had some influence on the diagnosis of disease and accordingly this biases the data, no other series of sickness data over a long period has been professionally reviewed for the existence of sickness. The inconsistency in the Army and Navy medical reviews over the years, therefore, is not likely to be of great consequence.

Two questions about the information arise: How representative are the data for the young male population generally? How representative are the data as measures of the objective health condition of the entire population? It is not unreasonable to consider that the trend in sickness as indicated by noneffective rates in the armed forces is representative of the young male population. Of course, each year's noneffective rates are rates for men who have qualified physically for the services. Moreover, the services provide necessary immunizations and other periodic medical care. But the measurement is aimed at the extent to which healthy persons become sick, unless there is reason to think that the proportion of total "healthy" population has changed markedly over the years.

If shifts in the age composition of the armed forces were sizable, they would bias the data in terms of their representativeness for young men in general. The age structure appears, however, to have been fairly stable over the time period. The changes that did occur, namely, an increasing portion of personnel under twenty years of age and over thirty-five (particularly in the Navy) would raise rather than lower more recent sickness rates. The net effect would be to dampen the influence of factors that contribute to reduced sickness.

Perception of sickness, understanding about illness, and attitudes toward the providers of care tend to influence the noneffective rate for the armed forces as they do in civilian life. Attitudes toward society and the extent of alienation probably have a more concentrated impact on noneffective rates in the armed forces than they have in civilian life. On balance, however, these factors tend to have far less impact on armed forces sickness rates as measures of objective conditions than on other data sources.

There is more doubt concerning the second question, about

representativeness of the Army and Navy data for all groups in the population. From one perspective, the information fails to reflect the major gains in reduced sickness among infants and children in the early years of this century. From this perspective the data are biased on the conservative side. At the same time, however, the data do not show the changes in sickness experience of either the female population or the older age groups. Nor do they reflect the impact on sickness rates of mortality improvement in the middle and older age groups that may contribute to more rather than less impairments. The underlying issue is whether the general direction of the trend is accurately portrayed for the population as a whole. We believe it is, as indicated in Chapter 7.

The Army and Navy sickness data as a measure of the objective state of health are applied in a modified way to assess the extent to which biomedical research has contributed to reduced sickness.

A MODEL MODIFIED FOR THE OBJECTIVE CONDITION

Application of an objective sickness concept requires modification of the estimating equation to exclude variables that are not directly relevant. Income as a factor impacting on the general health status (nutrition, housing, and so forth before military service) is included. Sick leave protections that affect the economic capacity to be sick are no longer relevant to an understanding of the variation over time for the military. Two other independent variables are dropped from the model mainly because the proxies used in the analysis of biomedical research and mortality do not appear to capture the characteristics of each of the variables as they determine sickness in the armed forces. The two variables excluded are the environmental measures and the societal measures of stress. They were excluded because the proxies that were applied, namely, unemployment rates and work injuries in civilian jobs, do not relate to the military. However, another variable is included to capture directly the effect of war on sickness rates.

The model as modified is $S_1 = f(\text{INC}, \text{PROV}, \text{TECH}, \text{W})$,

where

S_1 = the noneffective rate for Navy (and Army) personnel

INC   = real income per capita

PROV = the number of Navy (and Army) medical personnel per 1,000

TECH = the number of PhD degrees in biomedical sciences

W = a dummy variable, equal to 1 for war years and 0 for other years

The sickness data and medical personnel data used in the analysis for the Navy were those reported for 1926 to 1962 by Horton in his *Economic Analysis of Progress in the Medical Care of the U.S. Navy and Marine Corps Personnel*,[7] supplemented by data provided by the Department of the Navy for 1963 to 1974. The sickness data used for the Navy represent noneffective rates per 1,000 for disease-related conditions only and exclude injuries. For the Army, two series are analyzed: the noneffective rate due to disease only and the noneffective rate including nonbattle injuries. The data applied relate to two periods, 1930 to 1940 and 1953 to 1973.[8]

A time lag of ten years was applied to the new biomedical PhD's and a distributed lag computation with approximately the same time lag was also carried out. (The reasons for a lag have been set forth in earlier chapters.)

As with the mortality analysis, the high degree of autocorrelation among the variables suggested an adjustment for first-order serial correlation. Again, a variant of the techniques developed by Cochrane and Orcutt[9] was used for the Navy data. Because of the gap in the Army data between 1940 and 1953, there was no simple way to adjust for autocorrelation.

The regression equation used is in double-log form as follows:

$$ln S_1 = \text{Constant} + e_1 \, ln\text{INC} + e_2 \, ln\text{PROV} + e_3 \, ln\text{TECH} + e_4 W$$

where the subscript e's are the estimated coefficients, and the definitions of all variables are those presented above.

The selection of the functional form of the equation is conceptual. It is assumed that over time, a declining marginal physical product accrues to increments in biomedical research. As sickness rates are reduced it becomes more difficult to achieve equal increments of less sickness per unit of medical research input. The assumption is consistent with the hypothesis that biomedical research has been rationally allocated over time; that is, research resources were devoted in a sequence based on extent of the illnesses and ease of attacking the causes. The double-log form approximates this non-linear hypothesis.

FINDINGS ON BIOMEDICAL RESEARCH
AND THE OBJECTIVE CONDITION

The model, when quantified by Navy data, indicates that for each 1-percent added input into biomedical research from 1926 to 1974, objective sickness rates dropped two-tenths of 1 percent. Army data yield much the same result—a two-tenths of 1 percent decline in objective sickness conditions for each 1-percent input into biomedical research for the periods 1930-40 and 1953-73. Since elasticities tend to be higher for a longer time period, the coefficient for the more recent years would be expected to be lower.

The empirical results of the regression for the Navy are summarized in Table 8-2. All estimates are adjusted for autocorrelation and the *t* ratios in parentheses indicate that the figures shown (except the Vietnam War dummy) are statistically significant.

Table 8-3, which shows the regression results for the Armed Forces data, includes noneffective rates due both to disease and to disease plus nonbattle injury rates.

The regression results show a positive sign for providers rather than the expected reduced sickness with more providers. This result is probably reflective of the way in which decisions about recruitment of physician personnel is made by the Army. That is, the personnel are recruited on the basis of defined requirements, which would mean more medical personnel with more sickness.

TECH is measured in the estimates shown by PhD in the biomedical sciences. A uniform ten-year lag is assumed between receipt of degree and the contribution to biomedical research, much in accord with the procedure used in the analysis of biomedical research's contribution to reduced mortality.

The ten-year lag raises methodological concerns. Why ten years rather than another period of time, and in any case, why uniformity over the period? The selection of ten years was explained earlier. However, to answer questions that might be raised about the lag, we computed distributive lags for the TECH variable. The shift in lag markedly affects the findings; generally, it raises the coefficient on TECH and reduces the coefficients for other variables. The estimated coefficients with relatively minor changes in formula become unstable. The distributive lag regressions are shown in Table 8-4 to illustrate the direction of the change. However, it is important to bear in mind that the distributive lag methodology, which may be judged superior to a uniform lag, is not entirely relevant for the purposes of assessing the impact of biomedical research on health

Table 8-2. Regression Findings Applying Navy Data on Sickness Rates
as the Dependent Variable, 1926-74

Variable	No dummy variable for Vietnam War years	Dummy variable for Vietnam War years
Constant	12.0	12.2
INC	−.80	−.83
	(4.78)	(4.89)
TECH	−.20	−.20
	(3.00)	(3.01)
World War II dummy variable	.337	.346
	(3.81)	(3.905)
PROV	−.56	−.545
	(2.32)	(2.25)
Vietnam War dummy	−	.09
		(1.05)
R^2	.79	.80

status. The distributive lag methodology originated in estimating lags
in capital formation; it was subsequently applied in capital analysis,
which has a substantial theoretical base behind quantitative applications. In the present case, the theory is deficient and the application
so manipulates the basic data that coefficients of other important
variables are reduced and become insignificant.

The shift in lag applied to Navy data raised the coefficient on
TECH from −.20 to −.43 and reduced the INC coefficient from
−.80, which is significant, to −0.25, but the −0.25 coefficient is
statistically insignificant.

REDUCTION IN OBJECTIVE SICKNESS
ATTRIBUTED TO BIOMEDICAL RESEARCH

The estimating equation permits a parceling out of the relative shares
of improvement in the objective condition that are attributable to
improved income and living conditions—to more and surer provision
of care—and biomedical advances.

The relative contributions of biomedical research and other factors
to reduction in sickness are estimated from the elasticities derived
from the regression equations coupled with the average annual
growth rates in each variable. The coefficients derived for the
dummy variables for World War II and the Vietnam War have been
ignored in making the estimates because they were transitory
phenomena.

Table 8-3. Regression Findings Applying Army Data on Sickness as the Dependent Variable, 1930-40, 1953-73

Variable	Noneffective rates, disease		Noneffective rates, disease and injury	
	No dummy variable for war years[1]	Dummy variable for war years[1]	No dummy variable for war years[1]	Dummy variable for war years[1]
Constant	6.24	6.18	6.54	6.47
INC	−.44	−.439	−.459	−.45
	(2.51)	(2.97)	(2.53)	(3.36)
TECH	−.167	−.195	−.155	−.190
	(2.15)	(2.99)	(1.95)	(3.20)
War years dummy	−	.19	−	.236
		(3.60)		(4.86)
PROV	+.488	+.579	+.466	+.579
	(3.58)	(4.96)	(3.34)	(5.44)
R^2	.902	.934	.894	.943

[1] The primary war years (1941-52) are not included in the data set but the data for 1940, 1953, and the Vietnam period appear to reflect the impact of war on sickness rates. The dummy variable = 1 was used for 1940 and 1953 and for 1966-72; for other years, the variable = 0.

The following equation is applied in the parceling out of shares:

$$100\% = \sum_{i=1}^{3} e_i \frac{\Delta X_i}{\Delta S_i} + U$$

where the e's signify the elasticities for the three independent variables, Δ is the average annual percentage changes in the dependent and in each of the three independent variables, and U is the unexplained difference.

Based on Navy data for 1926-74, the biomedical PhD variable accounts for 38.5 percent of the reduction in the objective condition of sickness. Income and provider variables account for 54 and 4 percent of the total, respectively (Table 8-5). The Army data yield similar findings; about 39 percent of the reduction in the objective rate of sickness is attributable to biomedical research.[a]

[a]Subsequent to performing the work shown here we were able to obtain data on army noneffective rates for the period 1941-1952 and reestimate the formulation presented above. The results obtained from this amended data set are similar: elasticities of approximately .25 and a relative share of 44 percent for biomedical research.

Table 8-4. Regression Findings Applying Army Data on Sickness as the Dependent Variable and a Distributive Lag for the Variable on Biomedical Research

Variable	Noneffective rates, disease		Noneffective rates, disease and injury	
	No dummy variable	Dummy variable for war years	No dummy variable	Dummy variable for war years
Constant	5.73	4.92	6.27	5.29
INC	−.320	−1.58	−.386	−.191
	(1.13)	(.68)	(1.33)	(.89)
TECH	−.226	−.333	−.191	−.319
	(1.73)	(3.04)	(1.42)	(3.17)
War years dummy	−	.213	−	.256
		(3.93)		(5.15)
PROV	.444	.550	.422	.549
	(3.27)	(4.84)	(3.02)	(5.27)
R^2	.896	.934	.887	.943

The estimated share of reduction in the objective condition of sickness attributable to biomedical research serves as the basis for approximating the share of cost of illness that has been saved as a result of biomedical advances. As indicated in the earlier discussion of the Army and Navy data on noneffective rates as a measure of the objective condition, there are many qualifications in such an approximation.

WORK LOSS AND BIOMEDICAL RESEARCH

In addition to quantifying biomedical research's share of changes in the objective condition, we tried an analysis using unadjusted data on work loss as reported as the dependent variable.

The general model applied was that described at the outset:

$$S_1 = f(\text{PROV, TECH, X}) \text{ with } S_1 = WD - Q_1.$$

The selection of the other variables to be included in the X vector involves difficult choices. The limited number of observations necessarily restricts us to an attempt to capture only the main determinants of changes in sickness over time. Therefore, the factors included must have a substantial effect on sickness rates and also

Table 8-5. Relative Share of Decrease in Objective Sickness Attributable to Biomedical Research, Medical Care, and Income Changes

Variable	Navy data, 1926-74[1]	Army data, 1930-40, 1953-73[2]
Biomedical research (10-year lag)	38.5	39.3
Per capita income	54.0	30.6
Medical personnel per 1,000	4.1	17.4
Unexplained	3.5	12.7
All variables	100.0	100.0
Annual decrease in objective sickness	3.3	3.5

[1] Based on the coefficients in the first equation reported in the text, excluding the Vietnam War dummy.
[2] Based on the second equation in Table 8-3. The percentages are computed on changes from 1930 to 1965 to omit the impact of the Vietnam War. An alternative computation, including the period to 1973 but adjusting the sickness rate downward by the coefficient for the dummy variable for war years, results in a 1.2-percent annual decline in sickness attributable to biomedical research, or a 52.1-percent decline over the period 1930-73.

must have changed considerably over the time period. The components of the X vector were selected from a range of societal and economic variables that are known to affect sickness rates in the population.

The measures of sickness used is work loss, essentially counted here in three ways: (a) the average number of work-loss days per worker (WLD); (b) the percentage of workers who missed time from work due to sickness (%NAWI); and (c) the average duration of a work-loss episode due to acute illness (ACUDUR). Each of these in turn is analyzed in terms of the association with independent variables selected.

The variable PROV is measured by a weighted average of physicians and nurses per capita in the population. TECH is measured again as PHD degrees awarded in the biomedical sciences lagged ten years. The composite societal-economic or X variables pose a special problem in this instance. A large number of societal and economic factors have an impact on sickness rates. These factors include level of earnings, death rates of children, income maintenance payments, education, capacity of providers of care, unemployment, and occupation. Yet the number of years for which data on work loss are available on a continuing and comparable basis is limited. Indeed, there are at most twenty observations for work loss; accordingly, only a small number of variables can be used. Four independent variables in all were considered the practical limit. We therefore chose two variables to be included as proxies for societal-economic influences, namely, real income per capita and a measure of sick leave coverage (the proportion of nonagricultural workers who missed work due to illness but were paid for the time absent) multiplied by an index of the average educational level of the work force as a proxy for understanding about illness.

Table 8-6 shows the regression results for the three dependent work-loss variables, measuring sickness among the work force. These results are estimated from annual data over the 1957-76 period. The elasticity coefficient derived for TECH ranges from a .09-percent decrease to a 0.12-percent decrease in sickness per 1-percent increase in biomedical research. The estimates of average duration have a totally different meaning.

The dependent variable, percentage of employed workers who miss work due to sickness, yields a coefficient of 0.10 per 1 percent change in biomedical activity. The statistics for unadjusted work-loss days show a somewhat higher elasticity estimate, but the figure is not statistically significant. The average duration of a work-loss episode due to acute illness yields a far higher elasticity, but one applicable to a restricted component of the change in sickness; it is a component, however, that has been markedly affected by research and also by early access to care.

The results have many qualifications, but the findings give quantitative support to the contribution of biomedical research to improved health status of the working population.

Income has a mixed effect on sickness rates. Income affects basic family nutrition, housing, and the community environment and the impact of these factors on a person's health status. Availability of income, as we indicated earlier, also determines an individual's economic capacity to be sick. Studies suggest that when sick leave and cash sickness benefits were not available, sickness rates were relatively low. But when those benefits became available, the number of work-loss days rose.

In the regressions, income per capita has a positive coefficient, significantly so in one equation, with reasonably similar magnitudes for each of the dependent variables in terms of income elasticity of work loss. This finding is reasonable because each equation explains alternative measures of disability among the adult labor force.

The other two variables, adjusted sick leave and providers, produce mixed but consistently insignificant results. We have no explanation for the provider variable other than the limited number of observations. To preserve degrees of freedom and reduce multicollinearity, we combined the extent of income compensation for work loss and

Table 8-6.   Determinants of Changes in Work Loss over Time, by Independent and Dependent Variables

Independent variable	Equation number and dependent variable		
	1. Work-loss days (WLD)	*2. Percent of workers who missed work due to illness (%NAWI)*	*3. Average duration of work-loss episode due to acute illness (ACUDUR)*
Intercept	2.059	−7.936	−1.374
Providers	−.622	.203	.588
	(1.058)	(.707)	(.857)
Technology	−.129	−.094	−.419
	(1.534)	(2.288)*	(4.273)*
Income per capita	.308	.468	.457
	(.824)	(2.568)*	(1.048)
Adjusted sick leave	.618	−.224	−.057
	(1.915)	(1.423)	(.151)
N	20	20	20
D-W	2.15	1.61	2.10
R²	.553	.853	.582
F	4.62*	21.75*	5.22*

Note: All variables are measured in logarithms. Coefficients are elasticities with t-statistics reported in parentheses. Equations 1-3 are estimated by ordinary least squares.

*Indicates results significantly different from zero at a .05 level.

Dependent variables

WLD	Work-loss days per year per worker, due to all causes
%NAWI	Percent of employed workers who missed one or more hours of work during the average week due to illness

Independent variables

Providers	A weighted average of the number of physicians and nurses per capita
Technology	The number of new Ph.D.'s awarded in the biomedical sciences lagged ten years
Income	Real income per capita, in 1967 dollars
Adjusted sick leave	Proportion of nonagricultural workers who missed work due to illness but were paid for the time absent, multiplied by an index of the average educational level of the work force

the educational level of the population into a single variable. Since we expected each of the two variables to have a positive coefficient, we combined them by multiplying the extent of income compensation for work-loss days due to illness by an index of the average educational level of the labor force. An alternative specification of this variable, using data on income compensation from the Social Security Administration estimates,[10] resulted in similarly insignificant coefficients. Perhaps the compensation effect, which Paringer found particularly significant for minor illnesses, is partially captured by the income effect over time series data.[11] Another possible interpretation is that the education effect is really of the opposite sign and the two variables counteract each other.

An interesting question that may be answered with such estimates is: What do the elasticity coefficients suggest about work loss if, other things being equal, biomedical research effort did not expand? Table 8-7 presents actual values of the dependent variables, predicted values, and hypothetical values if research effort had remained constant during the period. The estimated impact on work-loss days and percentage of workers not at work due to illness is remarkably similar. Without expansion in research effort, work-loss days would have been 18.7 percent higher than the actual level in 1976 and the percentage not at work due to illness would have been 17 percent higher.

POSTSCRIPT ON EARLIER STUDIES

A review of the literature suggests that little research has been done on the basic question of the contribution of biomedical advances to health status of the population. This dearth of research emphasizes the need for assessment of indicators of advances in biomedical knowledge and the medical and environmental health care in which they are embodied, and assessment of the leads and lags that characterize phases of biomedical research from idea generation to full-scale dissemination.

A review of the earlier analyses of sickness data is presented in

Table 8-7. The Impact of Biomedical Research on Work Loss Due to Sickness, 1957-76

Dependent variable	*Work-loss days*	*Percent of workers who missed work due to illness*
Elasticity estimate	−.129	−.094
1976 value	5.3 days	1.585
Hypothetical 1976 value if research effort had remained constant, 1957-76[1]	6.3 days	1.854
Percent increase from actual 1976 values to hypothetical (difference)	18.7	17.0

[1] Calculated by multiplying the elasticity coefficient by the corresponding values of the independent variable; the 1957 value of the measure of biomedical research was substituted for the 1976 value.

Table 8-8, which is reproduced from a staff memorandum on biomedical research and disability.[12] The summary suggests the types of sickness data that are used in the studies selected, the variety of data sources applied, and the basic findings on determinants.

Two kinds of studies have been made. In one type, disability data are used as dependent variables and an effort is made to explain the changes in disability; in the other, disability is used as one of the independent variables, explanatory of some other factor. Work-loss days is the index used most frequently to reflect work loss due to sickness. These data, however, represent work loss as reported in surveys and do not include work loss representing loss of output as a consequence of sickness of those who have withdrawn from the labor force and are either in the community or institutionalized.

The source of information on work loss is usually the National Center for Health Statistics' Health Interview Survey data.[13] However, the analyses draw from other surveys, including the NBER Thorndike Survey,[14] the National Longitudinal Survey,[15] and the Survey of Economic Opportunity.[16]

Second to work-loss days as a measure of sickness are restricted-activity days, followed by bed-disability days. Again, the main source of data is the National Center for Health Statistics' Health Interview Survey, which does not include the institutionalized population.

Of the studies of disability, the Newhouse study is perhaps the most comprehensive. Newhouse posited a model that divided explanatory factors into four categories: demographic, environmental, medical, and economic.[17] He then tested the model on data aggregated at the standard metropolitan statistical area (SMSA) level. Both linear and log-linear forms of the regression equation were estimated for age-specific work-loss days (age groups seventeen to forty-four and forty-five to sixty-four). He found that poverty is positively related to work-loss days for the older groups, while educational level and number of physician visits are positively related to work-loss days for the younger group. A main conclusion was that determinants of disability are different for different age groups, and failure to consider this may bias the parameter estimates. Earlier studies during the 1920s by Sydenstricker found similar results on variation by age.[18]

Grossman's studies concern the effect of income, education, and sick leave.[2,19] One segment of the model used is an equation specifying the demand curve for the flow of services yielding health capital. The dependent variable is time lost from market and nonmarket activities due to illness and injury. In this study, Grossman found that both work-loss days and restricted-activity days are negatively related to income and positively related to education, family size, and wage rates. Grossman also studied the interaction of health and schooling and found that more schooling leads to better health, although the process by which this occurs is not clear.

A study by Chang and Hu addressed specifically the impact of regulations of the Occupational Safety and Health Administration.[20] They found that occupation is an important variable in explaining sickness, more important than industry classification. The National Health Survey data suggest that persons who are in professional and technical employment have less reported work loss than those in blue collar jobs. In general, Chang and Hu found that workers in chemical manufacturing and transportation jobs have the highest number of disability days, while amusement and recreation employees have the lowest number. Paringer disaggregated disability data by type of illness and found that variables that can explain variation in work loss differ according to the type of illness; minor acute illnesses are most sensitive to economic factors such as sick leave compensation.[11]

General studies have focused on disability as a determinant of labor supply. Scheffler and Iden,[21] Luft,[22] and Parsons[23] found that the labor supply is inversely related to disability. Luft estimated that a man with chronic health problems suffers a 37-percent reduction in yearly earnings, and Parsons estimated that older married men in poor health experience a 61-percent decline in annual hours from a full employment year. It is of some interest that early in the century sickness was found, based on experience, to reduce productivity and earnings by 50 percent.

Few studies have attempted to analyze disability over time, mainly because the data are sparse. Hambor, using unpublished social security program data, built a multiequation recursive model to predict disability applications.[24] He found that disability applications fluctuated with the unemployment rate, but not with changes in labor supply variables. He cautioned readers, however, that the results on the labor supply should not be taken as solid evidence because of problems in data measurement.

Lando and Hopkins[25] also focus on changes in the number of applications for disability benefits under the OASDI program. In the context of a simpler model they confirmed that unemployment rates affect disability application rates, but they also found that the relative benefit level available to disability beneficiaries is significantly related to the number of applicants.

Friedman sought to assess the impact of Medicare by examining

Table 8-8.   Summary of Disability Literature Surveyed

Author	Dependent variables (If regression analysis used)	Data sources	Selected empirical results
		Cross-sectional studies	
Newhouse (1970)	Work-loss days (by age groups)	National Health Survey (SMSAs, July 1963-June 1965)	Poverty is positively related to work-loss days for the older age group (45-64), while education and physician visits are positively related to work-loss days for the younger age group (17-44).
Silver (1970)	Work-loss days	National Health Survey (July 1962-June 1963)	Work-loss days are positively related to family income and inversely related to the earnings rate, suggesting that work-loss days may be an unreliable measure of variations in health status.
Grossman (1972)	The negative of the logarithm of work-loss days (adjusted for weeks worked), and re-stricted days	National Opinion Research Center (1963)	Both dependent variables are negatively related to various measures of income and age, positively related to education, family size, and wage.
Grossman (1976)	Work-loss weeks School-loss weeks	NBER-Thorndike sample (1969 and 1971)	The number of work-loss weeks and school-loss weeks rises as self-rated health status (good, fair, or poor) declines. More schooling appears to cause better health, when other variables are held constant.
Chang and Hu (1978)	Work-loss days Bed-disability days Restricted-activity days	Health Interview Survey (1973)	Income is inversely related to each dependent variable. On average, workers in chemical and allied product manufacturing and transportation have the largest numbers of restricted-activity days, followed by electrical machinery and equipment and medical and health services, while amusement and recreation employees have the smallest number of restricted-activity days.
Paringer (1978)	Work-loss days	Health Interview Survey (1968)	Disaggregation by type of illness and type of occupation is important.
Nagi and Hadley (1972)		Sample of disabled workers (1961-64)	Disability behavior may be affected by economic considerations. More disabled whose family incomes declined sharply exhibited high motivation to return to work.

Davis (1972)		National Longitudinal Survey (1966)	Poor health negatively affects annual weeks worked and earnings for persons at all educational levels.
Burgess and Kingston (1974)		The Service-to-Claimants Project Department of Labor (1969-70)	Persons in good health had significantly shorter durations of unemployment than those in poor health.
Scheffler and Iden (1974)	Labor supply (hours or weeks worked), disability used as an independent variable	Survey of Economic Opportunity (1967)	Disability is inversely related to labor supply.
Lando (1975)		1970 Decennial Census, 5 percent sample	Increased education is associated with lower levels of disability.
Luft (1975)	Labor supply (earnings, weeks worked, etc.). Sets of regressions run on those sick and those healthy	Survey of Economic Opportunity (1967)	The average disabled man suffers a 37 percent reduction in yearly earnings. Disabled blacks are more likely to drop out of the labor force, while disabled whites take cuts in earnings.
Parsons (1977)	Labor supply-hours worked annually Self-rated health status (good, fair, poor) used as independent variables	National Longitudinal Survey (1970)	The decline in annual hours for single men in poor health is 84 percent of a full-employment year, while only 61 percent for married men.
Time-series studies			
Hambor (1975)	Disability applications, awards, allowances	Unpublished social security program data (19631-1972IV)	Unemployment is found to be significant in explaining the level of disability applications and number of disability awards.
Friedman (1976)	Restricted-activity days	Health Interview Survey (1959-71)	The effect of Medicare on disability is estimated to be a reduction in restricted-activity days by 18 percent for men over 65 and 11 percent for women over 65.
Dunlop (1978)	Restricted-activity days, bed-disability days, percent reporting activity limitation	Health Interview Survey (1957-76)	Business cycle proxies, inflation, and unemployment are positively related to disability.

Source: Reference 12.

trends in disability data for those in the forty-five to sixty-four and the sixty-five and over age categories.[26] He attributes to Medicare approximately an 18-percent decline in restricted-activity days for older men and an 11-percent decline for older women. The declines in disability of the older groups is in contrast to the relative stability of restricted-activity days for the forty-five to sixty-four age group.

Another time-series study is currently in process, by Dunlop. He is trying to determine whether a relationship exists between disability and inflation.[27] Tentative results show that both inflation and unemployment are positively related to disability.

Regression analysis is not the only method used to test whether disability is associated with income levels, educational levels, and the like. Nagi and Hadley found, through analysis of sample data, that disability behavior may be affected by economic conditions.[28] Motivation to return to work when disabled appears to be high among those workers who experience sharp declines in their income as a result of the disability. Davis, in still another study, found that poor health negatively affects earnings,[29] while Burgess and Kingston found that unemployed workers experience longer durations of unemployment if they are in poor health.[30] Lando, using census data, showed that increased education is associated with lower levels of disability.[31]

The Social Security Administration's survey of the disabled[32] and the Health Interview Surveys[13] indicate that increased morbidity and disability is associated with older age, being female, nonwhite, and living in the South. These two surveys also show a difference between rural and urban residence. Rural residents are less likely than urban residents to suffer from acute illnesses, but more likely to be disabled. For time-series analysis of the recent past, most of the factors mentioned can safely be ignored because relatively little variation has occurred in, for example, the aggregate age structure of the population. Moreover, the variation that did occur was so steady from year to year that it is difficult to separate from a general time trend. One exception is the female proportion of the labor force. This proportion rose from 32 percent in 1957 to 40 percent in 1976, an increase that suggests the importance of this factor in understanding statistics on sickness. However, female labor force participation is highly correlated with increases in real income from 1957 to 1976 and apparently merely captures the income effect on work-loss days.

These studies are largely econometric in methodology. Another group of studies that mainly assess correlates of medical care use apply the methodology of sociology to achieve an understanding of the various factors that affect sickness in the population.[33]

The groups of studies, both econometric and sociological, while of interest in understanding the phenomenon of "sickness," do not deal with the impact of biomedical research on sickness and accordingly offer little guidance in judging the impact of biomedical research on sickness and reported work loss.

CONTRIBUTION OF
BIOMEDICAL RESEARCH

It seems reasonable, from one perspective, to assume that the share computed as the contribution of biomedical research to reduced mortality is smaller than the contributory share in reduction in work loss. Many of the early gains in knowledge through research concerned diseases that took a toll in human energy and vitality. Debilitating diseases at the turn of the twentieth century had high prevalence rates. For example, eight cases of typhoid were thought to exist for every death at the turn of the century, and each case was reported to result in an average of seventy-five days of incapacity. Death rates for many other debilitating diseases were low, but incapacity was high.

At the time that death rates were dropping most sharply, the application of new knowledge to water supplies, sewerage systems, isolation of patients, and to vaccinations or other disease prevention measures was reducing sickness in the population by what would seem to be an even higher rate. New knowledge, however, has diverse effects on sickness, raising certain diseases from subclinical to clinical levels; contributing to diagnosis of ailments that earlier were obscure; enlarging demand for health services, which tends to increase reports of sickness; increasing the number of impaired lives in the population; and so on. In table 8-1, we attempted to show the multiple impact. However, the multiplicity should not obscure the relation of biomedical research to an objective sickness condition. Even if new medical knowledge has a variety of influences on socioeconomic circumstances and on the reported amount of sickness—and, on balance, helps to raise rates above what they otherwise would be or alternatively keeps them from falling as fast as they otherwise might—it leaves uncertain the relative contribution of biomedical advances to reduction in the objective condition of sickness rates and to lower death rates.

The regression analyses made here, however, on both the objective condition and unadjusted work-loss data indicate that biomedical research has contributed, on balance, to reduced sickness. The information presented to represent the objective condition of sickness is biased by its concentration on young males, and the various work-loss indicators based on national probability samples are available for only a limited number of observations, necessitating a truncating of the model for analysis.

Although the findings must be viewed as tentative and subject to further study, the analyses carried out mark a major step toward understanding the complex links between biomedical research and sickness in the population.

Table 8-9 summarizes the relative shares of sickness reduction attributed to biomedical research. The ranges computed are the basis for approximating the relative reductions in sickness costs that are attributable to biomedical research. This process is discussed in the following chapter.

Table 8-9. Shares of the Reduction in Sickness Attributable to Biomedical Research

Indicator	Percent share
Objective condition of sickness:	
Army data	39.3
Navy data	38.5
Work-loss days, 1957-76	18.7
Percent not at work due to illness (1957-76)	17.0
Mortality reduction attributable to biomedical research	20-30

REFERENCES

1. Report of the National Conservation Commission, vol. III. U.S. Senate Document No. 676, 60th Congress, 2d sess. Washington, D.C., February 1909.

2. Grossman, M.: The demand for health. A theoretical and empirical investigation. National Bureau of Economic Research, New York, 1972.

3. Brundage, D.K.: A 10-year record of absences from work on account of sickness and accidents. Public Health Rep 42:529-550, Feb. 25, 1927.

4. Edison Electric data compiled from a series of reports by Brundage, D.K., Gafafer, W.M., and Frasier, E.S., appearing in various issues of Public Health Rep, from 1914 to the 1940s, three of which are: Gafafer, W.M.: Frequency and duration of disabilities causing absence from work among the employees of a public utility, 1938-42. Public Health Rep 58:1554-1560, Oct. 15, 1943; Gafafer, W.M., and Frasier, E.S.: Titled as above, 1933-37. Public Health Rep 53:1273-1288, July 29, 1938; and Brundage, D.K.: Trend of disabling sickness among employees of a public utility. Public Health Rep 43:1957-1984, July 27, 1928.

5. U.S. Public Health Service Statistical Office: Disabling sickness among employees of a rubber manufacturing establishment in 1918, 1919, and 1920. Some morbidity statistics from the Department of Health of the B.F. Goodrich Co., Akron, Ohio. Public Health Rep 37:3083-3092, Dec. 15, 1922.

6. Compiled from a series of reports by Brundage, D.K., Gafafer, W.M., and Frasier, E.S., appearing in various issues of Public Health Rep. An index of publications in the series from 1920 to 1950 appears in Gafafer, W.M.: Industrial sickness absenteeism among males and females during 1950. Public Health Rep 66:1550-1552, Nov. 23, 1951.

7. Horton, M.: Economic analysis of progress in the medical care of the U.S. Navy and Marine Corps personnel. Doctoral dissertation. University of Washington, Seattle, 1966.

8. Department of Defense: Annual reports of the Surgeon General, U.S. Army, 1911, 1919, 1938, 1953, 1961, 1973.

9. Cochrane, D., and Orcutt, G.H.: Application of least squares regressions to relationships containing autocorrelated error terms. J of the Amer Statistical Association:32-61, 1949.

10. Price, D.: Cash benefits for short-term sickness, 1948-74. Soc Sec Bull 39:22-34, July 1976.

11. Paringer, L.: Determinants of work loss and physician utilization for specific illnesses. Doctoral dissertation. University of Wisconsin, Madison, 1978.

12. Vehorn, C.L., Wagner, D.P., and Landefeld, J.S.: Memorandum on biomedical research and disability. Public Services Laboratory, Georgetown University, Washington, D.C., 1978 (unpublished).

13. National Center for Health Statistics: Health characteristics of persons with chronic activity limitations, United States, 1974. Health Resources Administration, Series 10, No. 112; and other publications of Series 10.

14. Thorndike, R.L., and Hagen, E.: Ten thousand careers. John Wiley and Sons, New York, 1959.

15. Parnes, H.: Longitudinal labor force survey. Ohio State University, Columbus, Ohio, continuing survey (various publications).

16. U.S. Office of Economic Opportunity: Guide to the documentation and data files of the 1966 and 1967 survey of economic opportunity. Washington, D.C., 1970.

17. Newhouse, J.P.: Determinants of days lost from work due to sickness. *In* Empirical studies in health economics, edited by H.E. Klarman. The Johns Hopkins University Press, Baltimore, Md., 1970, pp. 59-70.

18. Sydenstricker, E.: Hagerstown morbidity studies, I-XI. Public Health Rep 41:2069-2088, Sept. 24, 1926; 41:2186-2191, Oct. 8, 1926; 42:121-131, Jan. 14, 1927; 42:1565-1572, June 10, 1927; 42:1689-1701, June 24, 1927; 42:1939-1957, July 29, 1927; 43:1067-1074, May 4, 1928; 43:1124-1156, May 11, 1928; 43:1259-1276, May 25, 1928; 44:1821-1833, July 26, 1929; 44:2101-2106, Aug. 30, 1929.

19. Grossman, M.: The correlation between health and schooling. *In* Household production and consumption, edited by N.E. Terleckji. National Bureau of Economic Research, New York, 1975, pp. 147-211.

20. Chang, C., and Hu, T.: Health status and health services utilization in relation to industry-occupation mix. Pennsylvania State University, University Park, May 31, 1978.

21. Scheffler, R.M., and Iden, G.: The effect of disability on labor supply. Industrial Labor Relations Rev 28:122-132, October 1974.

22. Luft, H.S.: The impact of poor health on earnings. Rev Economics Statistics 57:43-57, February 1975.

23. Parsons, D.O.: Health, family structure, and labor supply. Amer Econ Rev 67:703-712, September 1977.

24. Hambor, J.C.: Unemployment and disability: an econometric analysis with time series data. Social Security Administration, Office of Research and Statistics. Staff paper 20, 1975.

25. Lando, M.E., and Hopkins, T.R.: Modeling applications for disability insurance. Paper presented at the Allied Social Sciences Association meeting, New York City, Dec. 29, 1977.

26. Friedman, B.: Mortality, disability and normative economics of medicare. *In* Theory of health insurance in the health services sector, edited by Richard N. Rosett. National Bureau of Economic Research, New York, 1976.

27. Dunlop, D.: Personal communication, 1978. Study in process at Meharry Medical School, Nashville, Tenn.

28. Nagi, S.Z., and Hadley, L.W.: Disability behavior: income change and motivation to work. Industrial Labor Relations Rev 25:223-233, January 1972.

29. Davis, J.M.: Impact of health on earnings and labor market activity. Monthly Labor Rev 95:46-49, October 1972.

30. Burgess, P.L., and Kingston, J.L.: The effect of health on duration of unemployment. Monthly Labor Rev 97:53-54, April 1974.

31. Lando, M.E.: The effect of unemployment on applications for disability insurance. American Statistical Association Business and Economics Section Proceedings, 1974.

32. Allan, K.H.: First findings of the 1972 survey of the disabled: general characteristics. Soc Sec Bull 10:18-37, October 1976.

33. Aday, L. and Eichhorn, R.: The utilization of health services: indices and correlates: a research bibliography 1972. National Center for Health Services Research and Development. DHEW Publication No. (HSM) 73-3003.

Chapter Nine

Biomedical Research and the Economic Cost of Sickness

What has been the trend in economic cost of sickness? Has biomedical research reduced this cost over the decades?

We turn first to the question of trends in the economic cost of sickness. We use a traditional definition of those economic costs. Cost is defined in terms of the loss to society of economic product, the amount of work time lost due to disability and illness, and the loss in product during those work absences. The loss is incurred because persons are too sick to work—either temporarily, or permanently—and as a result they withdraw from the work force, go into institutions, or are sick at home. To measure the cost, we need to know how many persons are affected, for how long a time during a year, and with what impact on productivity.

Economic cost defined in this way is at best a partial measure of sickness cost. Few would argue that the perspective is sufficiently comprehensive. Sickness affects production in society, but it also has economic, social, and psychological costs for the person who is sick, for his or her family and friends, and for the community as a whole. Some of the costs are immediate or primary costs. There are dollar costs in lost earnings and for health care that fall immediately on the family or on third parties. There are also time costs: the value of time spent in the physician's waiting room, the time spent traveling to a health facility, the time required to visit an ailing relative or friend, and the time spent taking care of the patient at home or being a surrogate for the patient at home. Dollar costs for health care are discussed in a subsequent chapter under the title of health expenditures. Time costs also are approximated (Chapter 13). These time costs, as well as many costs that fall on employers and government as a consequence of illness, are frequently neglected in assessing the burdens of illness. But such costs, including special educational facilities for the handicapped child, special transportation, ramps in streets and subways, and elevator installations in the home, are not inconsequential.

Some costs of sickness continue beyond an immediate period. Those with chronic illnesses, for example, often incur a long-term cost burden both in cash and in time. The costs, again, may be economic in terms of loss in working time and in earnings capacity. They may be social, in that family life is disrupted, tensions accumulate in the home, divorces become more frequent, and normal sex life is impaired. Stress, unsupported, may lead to emotional illness affecting one or more family members.

Some costs, moreover, are intergenerational. Sickness of a parent may impair the health of a child, disrupt educational performance, cause additional school absences, or become a barrier to learning. Sickness of a sibling may have similar long-term effects. The intergenerational impacts are perhaps clearest in the cases of alcoholism of a parent or child abuse, but these impacts are real in other situations as well.

There are gains as well as costs that originate in sickness. Major illness can have a cohesive effect on families, putting the order of things into a perspective and creating mutual support.

The traditional count of the economic cost of sickness omits many of the types of costs mentioned here. Importantly, it also omits the cost of sickness of infants and children, and puts the aged who have retired on an economic waste heap. Those who no longer work have, according to the count, no economic value. The omission from the count of the large burden on families when illness strikes a child particularly conflicts with the basic value structure of society.

In Table 9-1 and supplementary Table 9-2, we outline somewhat more systematically the components of cost. In reviewing these components, certain study results are of special interest. Abt has made a breakthrough in formulating the psychological and social cost of cancer, cost that documents, among other things, family stress and loss of sexual activity.[1] As a rough approximation, Abt sums up the estimated sizes of the different social groups exposed to the psychosocial costs of terminal cancer as follows:

350,000 cancer victims exposed per year
100,000 children of victims exposed per year
175,000 spouses of victims exposed per year

70,000 siblings of victims exposed per year
80,000 parents of victims exposed per year
300,000 friends/co-workers of victims exposed per year
35,000 caregivers of victims exposed per year

One approach to the range of cost is to "correct" the traditional concept by adding cost categories.[2] Methods other than the traditional costing of illness have also been proposed; the most direct of these is to determine what goods and services individual households would be willing to forgo to reduce the risk of sickness. Acton has pioneered in such surveys, but only as they relate to probabilities of survival.[3]

A number of difficult issues are encountered in the survey method of deriving the value to families of good health or absence of sickness. There is no reason to assume that responses are accurate, or even that the hypothetical questions posed are really understood. When eliciting willingness to pay for actual implementation of policies to reduce sickness, there is no way to monitor the truthfulness of response nor to penalize strategic behaviors that may involve misrepresentation of preferences. Validity of the survey instrument, stability of response, and replicability of result are all of technical concern. As of now, the survey technique has not yielded a practical measurement tool that would give us a count of the worth of a reduced risk of sickness for the individual (adult, child, or elderly person), the family, and the community.

The traditional method of costing sickness thus remains, despite criticism, the method most frequently used. We apply this method to estimating the cost of sickness for the selected years being studied— 1900, 1930, 1963, 1975, and 2000. In general, the method, as applied to costing sickness, entails determining the time lost from work due to disease or disability and pricing the output value of that time.

ESTIMATES OF ECONOMIC COST

More specifically, work-loss time is estimated, following Rice,[4] in terms of year equivalents for four categories that in turn are related to data sources: (a) loss of time (derived from the National Center for Health Statistics data on work-loss days per worker by age, sex, and diagnosis converted to work-year equivalents); (b) loss of work time by those not in the work force because of illness who, it is assumed, would have earned wages equal to annual average earnings

Table 9-1. Costs of Illness and Injury: A Classification

- Cost to persons
- Cost to family
- Cost to industry
- Cost to government
- Special cost to providers

I. Primary costs to persons and families

A. Loss in earnings
Loss in enjoyment of consumer goods
Loss in production efficiency

B. Added costs
Medical care costs (providers and public agencies)
Other care costs: patient and family (see supplementary illustration, Figure 9-1, of consumer expenditure impacts of illness)

C. Loss of time
Seeing providers
Visiting sick relatives
Travel to providers
Caring for patients
Serving as proxy in home for patient

D. Primary psychological and social costs to persons and families
Pain
Mental illness, including suicidal behavior, alcoholism, etc.
Family tension, disruption, and divorce
Segregation and isolation
Disfigurement

II. Primary costs to industry

A. Loss in product and work time
B. Material wastage
C. Damage to machinery and plant
D. Delays in production schedules
E. Intergroup conflicts and tensions
F. Increases industrial accidents

III. Secondary (continuing costs of illness)

A. Loss in earnings of patient
B. Loss of product to community
C. Continuing costs of medical care
D. Continuing costs for other services
E. Continuing time costs to patient and family (see Primary costs, item C)

IV. Tertiary (or intergenerational) costs

A. Added costs to children
Increased absences of children from school and impaired performance
Lowered resistance of children to disease
Increased antisocial behavior
B. Exposure to alcoholism, drug addiction, etc.
C. Increase in genetic diseases
D. Reduced long-run productivity

Table 9-2. Consumer Expenditures as a Result of Illness

Consumer Expenditure Survey Categories	*Rationale for Inclusion*
I. Household Help A. Babysitting or other home care for children B. Cleaning, laundering, cooking, or other domestic duties C. Care for invalids (does not include care by nurses)	Need generated by presence of invalid in the home or by hospitalization of family
II. Utilities and Fuels A. Utility or natural gas, electricity, water, garbage/trash collection B. Telephone service	Increased usage due to homebound patient
III. Household Textiles A. Bedroom linens B. Bathroom linens	Increased demand due to confinement of patient to bed
IV. Clothing A. Pajamas, robes, nightgowns, housecoats, house slippers, and other nightwear	
V. Laundry and Dry Cleaning A. Laundry done outside	
VI. In-home Meals	Increased consumption
VII. Nonmedical Rehabilitation A. Weights, vibrators, exercycle	Need occasioned by medical condition
VIII. Household Appliances A. Vaporizer, humidifier, dehumidifier	
IX. Transportation A. Vehicle operating expenses B. Use of public transportation	To and from health care facilities
X. Alterations of and Additions to Owned Property A. Remodeling and additions to rooms	Modifications for invalids

had they not been ill (derived from the earnings and labor force data from the Bureau of the Census and the Department of Labor); (c) loss of work time of those in hospitals and related institutions; and (d) loss of work time over the full year by housewives who are ill (applying data obtained by combining data on bed-disability rates of housewives from the NCHS with census estimates of the number of women who are not in the work force because they are keeping house). Persons who are prevented from working because of illness are assumed to have the same labor force participation as they would have if they were not ill and the same earnings experience as their age and sex counterparts in the population who are well.

As is the case in estimating the cost of premature death, the value of the work-time loss in concept is equal to the marginal product of the workers that is forgone because of their sickness. In the estimates of cost, the work-time loss for each of the selected years was converted to a full-time equivalent basis, and the cost of that work-time loss was calculated by applying a full-time earning estimate to the work-time loss by age. For those who are withdrawn from the labor force due to sickness in 1975 and for the estimates for year 2000, average rather than full-time earnings are used.

If workers with sickness who lost days of work were less productive than other workers, estimates of value of work-time loss are unduly high. However, if those who were out of the labor market or in institutions would, in the absence of illness, have a higher earnings competence, the resulting estimates are understatements.

The use of full-time or average earnings does not capture the social product lost due to inability to engage in household tasks. Imputed earnings were assigned as the output of women who keep house, based on the value of household tasks.

The earnings figures used are single-year earnings, as shown in Table 9-3 for male workers. Special mention is needed, perhaps, of

Table 9-3. Full-time Earnings for Male Workers, by Age, Selected Years, 1900-2000, in Current Dollars

Age	1900	1930	1963	1975	2000
15-19	$ 93	$ 310	$2,582	$ 6,679	$27,330
20-24	223	742	4,435	9,811	40,147
25-29	311	1,034	6,181	13,452	55,046
30-34	387	1,286	7,074	15,948	65,259
35-39	450	1,495	7,555	17,198	70,374
40-44	482	1,599	7,860	18,153	74,282
45-49	480	1,595	7,569	18,397	75,281
50-54	469	1,558	7,179	17,736	72,576
55-59	448	1,487	6,805	17,167	70,247
60-64	421	1,398	6,973	15,813	64,707
65+	240	798	5,532	13,735	56,204

Source: Based on estimates prepared by Public Services Laboratory, Georgetown University, Washington, D.C.

the earnings figures for the year 2000. Those earnings are derived from an economic model of the economy that shows a $9-trillion GNP for the year and assumes productivity to rise 2 percent per annum over the period 1976-2000 and prices as measured by the GNP price deflator to rise 300 percent over the period 1975-2000.

Sickness cost on this basis is a product of many factors. To begin with, each of the segments of sickness cost differ and trends with respect to each vary. These segments are loss of product of those in the work force, loss of work time for those withdrawn from the work force, and illness of housewives. For 1975, the total cost of sickness divided itself by category as follows:

Total	$58 billion[a]
Sickness of those in the work force	21 billion
Sickness of those not in the work force	32 billion
Sickness of housewives	4 billion

[a]Does not add due to rounding.

A major part of sickness cost is attributable to those who have withdrawn from the work force. To suggest the size of this group, we summarize the number of such workers in Table 9-4. The percentages of the aggregate sickness costs that represent the estimated cost of those not in the work force due to illness are as follows: 1930, 60 percent; 1963, 55 percent; 1975, 56 percent; and 2000, 46 percent. The year 1900 sickness cost figures are not comparable because the census reports on those unable to work are not based on the same definitions as those applied later.

Table 9-4. Numbers of Workers Withdrawn from the Labor Force
Due to Illness, Selected Years, 1900-2000
(Disabled workers in thousands)

1900	401.6
1930	3,220.0
1963	3,238.0
1975	3,512.0
2000	*4,666.0*

Source: 1900-75 estimates based on U.S. Census; 2000 estimates prepared by Public Services Laboratory, Georgetown University. The 1930 estimate shown here exceeds the 1939 estimates prepared by I.S. Falk, B.S. Sanders, and D. Federman: "Disability among gainfully occupied persons." Social Security Board, Bureau of Research and Statistics Memorandum No. 61, p. 3, when adjusted for comparability in concept, by about 800,000 persons.

Practices in institutional care of the mentally ill and of employers in hiring handicapped persons or those with diseases have a great deal to do with the distribution of the cost of sickness among work force groups as do other factors that influence decisions about remaining in the work force or withdrawing. One such factor is the extent to which individuals can determine for themselves the amount of work, amount of leisure, and time of work. To the extent that persons work on their own account as self-employed shopkeepers, farmers, or professionals, they can determine their own working hours and adjustments to "not feeling well."

Significant changes have occurred in these economic circumstances. In 1900, the nation was essentially still agricultural and offered much opportunity for impaired persons to reduce their workload or work time during a day rather than withdraw from the work force. Statistics on the importance of self-employment are not readily at hand to document the relative numbers who were able to adjust their work time during periods of illness. However, the Bureau of the Census reports the change in managers, officials, and proprietors, including farmers, as a percentage of the labor force. It matters a good deal whether one of four or less than one of eight workers has flexible control over work time in explaining the behavior about work loss and withdrawal from the work force.

Year	Percent of labor force that were managers, officials, and proprietors
1900	25.7
1930	19.8
1963	14.1
1975	12.4

Source: References 5, 6.

Unemployment rates and retirement practices influence decisions to remain in the work force or to withdraw when illness strikes. High unemployment rates encourage withdrawals from the labor market as part of the phenomenon of the "discouraged worker," and access to retirement benefits even on a reduced-benefit basis further encourage such response. The 1930 figures may reflect the number who withdraw from the labor force due to unemployment and who unduly raised the count of the disabled.

Work patterns of women also influence the distribution of costs of sickness between temporary loss in work time and loss in output attributable to withdrawal from the work force. To some extent, the growth in work-force participation of women has been a compensating factor in the part-time work and early retirement of male workers.

The estimated sickness cost reveals the effect of the concentration of potential work-force participants by age and sex. In 1900, 22 percent of the labor force consisted of males under twenty-five years of age, who had lower earnings than older men; it is expected that by the year 2000, about half this percentage of the labor force will be males sixteen to twenty-four years old (Table 9-5). At the same time, the share of women of all ages in the labor force has moved up sharply from 18 to almost 40 percent since the turn of the century. Since more women are likely participants in the work force when illness strikes, the cost of sickness among women would be larger today than it was years ago despite the dramatic changes that have occurred in how women regard themselves and "female problems."

What are the costs of sickness measured as loss in work time and value of product? The costs are estimated to have risen from $631 million to an amount ninety times that level by 1975, with a further large rise projected for the year 2000 (Table 9-6). Cost of time lost from work increased more than sixfold between 1900 and 1930 in the dollars of each year. In the following thirty-three years, the costs multiplied almost fivefold and more than doubled in the twelve years between 1963 and 1975. For the year 2000, the cost is projected at $366 billion, a sixfold rise compared to 1975.

Again we are confronted with the question: Are illness costs up

Table 9-5. Percentage of Labor Force in Selected Age Groups, Male and Female, 1900-2000

Year	Total	16-24	25-44	45-64	65+
Male					
1900	81.9	22.2	38.2	17.9	3.6
1930	78.1	15.9	36.9	21.5	3.8
1963	66.8	11.9	29.8	22.3	2.9
1975	60.9[1]	14.0	26.4	18.5	2.0
2000	60.6[1]	11.5	27.9	19.2	2.0
Female					
1900	18.1	8.8	6.5	2.4	.5
1930	21.9	8.3	9.3	3.9	.5
1963	33.2	7.0	13.1	11.9	1.2
1975	39.1[1]	10.8	15.8	11.5	1.1
2000	39.4[1]	8.8	17.3	11.9	1.3

[1] Based on unrounded totals.

Sources: Derived from Bureau of Labor Statistics: "Employment and earnings, February 1976." U.S. Department of Labor, Vol. 22, 1976; Bureau of the Census: "Historical statistics of the United States: Colonial times to 1970." U.S. Department of Commerce, 1975; and reference 12.

**Table 9-6.   Total Economic Cost of Sickness (Value of Work-Time Loss),
Selected Years, 1900-2000**

(in millions)

Year	Current dollars	Adjusted to 1975 earnings level
1900	$ 631[1]	$15,030
1930	4,181	30,744
1963	23,745	45,143
1975	57,848	57,848
2000	366,108	89,469

[1] The figures shown here are adjustments of earlier estimates of current dollar costs and are not exactly comparable.

Sources: References 9, 10, 11, and 12 and J.S. Landefeld: "The economic cost of illness, 1963." Public Services Laboratory, Georgetown University, Washington, D.C., 1978.

because there is more sickness (or more reported sickness) in the population, or are other factors responsible for the increases?

Examination of the cost increases suggests that population growth, labor force trends, and price movements mainly account for the rise in sickness costs measured by loss in labor product. Sickness trends alone would have reduced costs if other factors had remained stable. Population growth, in contrast, is one factor that has contributed to the rise. The impact of population growth can best be shown, perhaps, by converting the sickness costs from aggregates to per capita figures, as is done in Table 9-7. On a per capita basis, cost of sickness increased almost fourfold between 1900 and 1930; it more than tripled between 1930 and 1963 and more than doubled in the next twelve-year period.

**Table 9-7.   Total Economic Cost of Sickness (Value of Work-Time Loss)
Per Capita and per Worker, Selected Years, 1900-2000**

Year	Economic cost, current dollars		Economic cost, adjusted to 1975 earnings levels	
	Per capita	*Per worker*	*Per capita*	*Per worker*
1900	$ 8.29	$ 23.41	$197.52	$557.58
1930	33.97	94.63	249.79	695.83
1963	125.98	349.43	239.51	664.32
1975	270.90	695.18	270.90	695.18
2000	1,392.05	2,881.33	340.19	704.14

Source: Computed from Table 9-6 divided by resident population of the United States and number of workers. For past periods, from U.S. Bureau of the Census and U.S. Department of Labor.

Wage increases, perhaps more than any other factor, are responsible for the rise in the economic costs of sickness. Average earnings more than tripled between 1900 and 1930, accounting for 62 percent of the increase in economic costs of sickness. Between 1930 and 1975, average earnings rose even faster—increasing sevenfold—and accounted for 76 percent of the rise over the forty-five-year period.

The rise in earnings over the twentieth century is such that men twenty-five to twenty-nine years old are projected to earn more than $55,000 a year by 2000 in year 2000 inflated dollars, compared to about $13,500 in 1975, more than a fourfold rise in the twenty-five-year period (Table 9-3). The rise in earnings that impacts on counts of sickness cost by providing the basic valuation per day of work loss may be described in these terms: In 1900, the average wage was $1.50 a day; by 1930, wages had risen to $5 a day; and by 1975, to $5 an hour.

Adjustment of the sickness cost estimates for earnings differences greatly reduces the variation from period to period. When cost of sickness is shown on the basis of constant earnings (1975 as a base year), per capita cost and cost per worker for the years 1930, 1963, and 1975 are fairly similar. The year 1900 estimates are lower but, again, this may be due either to an undercount of the numbers who withdrew from the work force because of illness or to the numbers of farmers and shopkeepers who adjusted their work day and week due to illness without withdrawing from the work force. The higher per capita estimate for year 2000 reflects the relatively larger number of workers than dependent age groups projected by year 2000. On a per worker basis, there is really little growth in sickness cost.

The real question arises: Why is there any growth in the estimates when the basic data underlying sickness cost (work-loss days either for those temporarily out of the work force or those who have withdrawn due to illness) trend downward? We have already suggested the biases in data that affect the estimates somewhat for 1900 and 1930; in the way of an undercount for 1900 and a possible overcount for 1930. If the total work force, in place of persons working, is used as the denominator, the decrease in sickness begins to show.

The distribution of work-loss days by age and sex and the difference in earnings of these groups also affect the estimates. Adjustment to a uniform average earnings basis from one period to another does not take account of the differences in causes of illness, or of the age distribution of those afflicted and the characteristic differences in their earnings level. The basic sickness cost data are derived based on work loss by disease, age, and sex that is valued in terms of earnings by age and sex.

On an aggregate rather than a per capita or per worker basis, sickness cost was 6.6 times as high in 1930 as in 1900; corrected for earnings level to a 1975 base, the cost was twice as high in 1930 as in 1900 (Table 9-8). Sickness costs were 1.5 times their 1930 level by 1963 at 1975 average earnings, and 1.3 times the 1963 level by 1975. The explanation for the upward movement in sickness costs lies, as indicated earlier, in the distribution of work loss by disease and by age, sex, and earnings.

The Basic Work-loss Data

Since 1930, even without correction to reflect objective sickness rates or to exclude the impact of socioeconomic conditions on reported sickness, the trend in the reported work-loss days is down, as shown in Table 9-9. As indicated earlier, the 1900 figure is an approximate one; there are no reported data on days lost from work due to sickness for that year. Census data yield information, however, on numbers in institutions and those not in the work force due to illness, but the data are essentially not comparable with current census and Department of Labor data.

One study for the year 1906 places days of average illness per annum at nine with an economic burden computed at $1.4 billion, of which one-half is reckoned to represent the wage loss at $1 a day, and the other half, illness expenses.[7] Anecdotal information reported elsewhere about the same year cites an average loss of five days a year from work on account of headaches, toothaches, colds, and similar minor ailments, leaving still to be resolved the average number of days of work loss due to more serious illnesses.[8] Assuming that the total days are about double those five days, a total of 10 days of work loss would not seem unreasonable for the first part of the century. Fisher used an average of 13 days per annum in his report to

Table 9-8. Ratio of Economic Cost of Sickness from Start of Period to End of Period (Vaiue of Work-Time Loss), Selected Years, 1900-2000

Year	*Current dollars*	*Adjusted to 1975 earnings level*
1900-30	6.6	2.0
1930-63	5.7	1.5
1963-75	2.5	1.3
1975-2000	6.3	1.6

Source: Computed from Table 9-6.

Table 9-9. Trend in Market Sector Work Loss, 1900-2000, Work-Loss
Days per Worker

Year	Temporary work-loss days	Total work-loss days (Includes those who have withdrawn from the work force)
1900	12.0[1]	16.2–32.4[4]
1930	6.1[2]	26.5[1]
1963	5.9[3]	17.6[1]
1975	5.2[3]	15.5[1]
2000	4.8[1]	13.8[1]

[1] Derived from references 9 and 12.
[2] S. Collins: "Cases and Days of Illness Among Males and Females with Special Reference to Confinement in Bed." *Public Health Reports,* January 12, 1940, p. 17.
[3] National Center for Health Statistics: *Current Estimates from the Health Interview Survey: United States, 1962-63 and 1975,* Series 10.
[4] Institutionalized and unable to work population losses based on assumption that 1900 rates of disability were equal to 1930 rates.

the president of 1908 and went on to cite returns gathered from 79 benefit societies in Scotland, which showed the average duration of sickness for each member under seventy years of age as 10 days per year, 2 of which were assumed to be bedfast, 5 days, of walking sickness, and 3 days, of permanent sickness. Our own computation uses a figure of 12 days, which, among other things, assumes 280 work days in 1900 as compared to 245 used for other years to reflect the longer work week in 1900 compared to now and, at least partially, the longer hours per day.[9]

The data as reported, however, do not reflect the full change in sickness. For the full change we turn again to the Army-Navy noneffective rates to correct the reported days of work-time loss. Applying the average Army-Navy data as an index (1973=100), we compute the approximate temporary work-loss days and total work-time loss in days as shown in Table 9-10. The number of days of sickness per year, while large, seems entirely consistent with the Fisher description of the condition of health in 1908. Many workers labeled minor certain illnesses that today would fall in the serious class and many persons went to work sick because there were no income protections against illness. The adjusted numbers show a far larger drop in sickness than do the actual statistical reports.

Sickness Cost, By Disease

We have already indicated that part of the explanation of the trends in sickness cost is attributable to the changing patterns of

Table 9-10.   Estimated Objective Sickness Rates per Worker, 1900-75

Year	Temporary work-loss days	Total work-loss days per worker, including those withdrawn from the work force
1900	49.0	66.1–132.3[1]
1930	18.0	78.0
1963	6.9	20.7
1975	5.2	15.5

[1] Institutionalized and unable to work population losses based on assumption that 1900 rates of disability were equal to 1930 rates.

illness. These patterns are suggested by the cost estimates. Clearly, there has been a decline in sickness cost for infective and parasitic disease, for complications of pregnancy and childbirth, and for diseases of the blood. By 1975, the cost of infective and parasitic disease, for example, was less than half of what it was estimated to be in 1900 and approximately one-quarter of what the cost was in 1930 at constant earnings levels. It is again useful to restate the basis for the sickness estimate and to note that it does not take account of the important decline in infective and parasitic sickness of children between 1900 and 1930.

The dramatic reduction in infective and parasitic diseases to which medical science has contributed is shown by the large decline in the relative cost of these diseases. They accounted for one-quarter of total cost of sickness in 1900 even though the sickness estimate is confined to cost of those of working age. By 1975, less than 3 percent of sickness cost was attributable to infective and parasitic diseases.

For 1975, more than 70 percent of the costs attributable to sickness fall into five categories of illness or injury: mental disorders; diseases of the circulatory system; diseases of the respiratory system; diseases of the musculoskeletal system; and accidents, poisonings, and violence. The cost of sickness is differently arrayed than is the cost of death. Neoplasms that rank second as a cause of death account for less than 2 percent of sickness costs in 1975. Mental disorders that have a low mortality rank have a high rank as a cost of sickness. In most of the years over the past seventy-five-year period, mental disorders ranked high as a cause of illness, and in 1975, mental disorders and circulatory diseases each accounted for 15.1 percent of sickness costs. The cost of accidents, poisonings, and violence rose sharply between 1900 and 1930 but in recent years seems to have declined in relative importance as a share of costs. The cost of diseases of the respiratory system declined markedly in relative importance between 1900 and 1930 but has held almost the same relative cost rank in subsequent years. Far more representative of changing patterns are the diseases of the circulatory system; in 1975, they claimed 15 percent of the costs of work loss, in contrast to about 4 percent of the total in 1900. Differences in diagnosis, as well as the overall aging of the working population owing to the larger number of older women working, have much to do with this shift.

Table 9-11 shows the total sickness cost for the major diseases and injury at 1975 earnings levels. Between 1900 and 1930, the cost of work loss attributable to sickness doubled. The rate of increases in sickness cost has slowed down, and further decline in the rate of increase is projected. The larger participation of women in the work force who earn smaller amounts than men and the shift in age distribution largely account for these changes. The distribution of cost among disease and injury categories are shown in Table 9-12 and Figure 9-1.

We find, once again, that economic and demographic conditions and the diseases that afflict the population, rather than the overall sickness rates among the work force, account for the changing cost of sickness.

Table 9-11. Sickness Costs for Major Disease and Injury Categories, Selected Years, 1900-2000, at 1975 Earnings Level[1]
(in millions)

Disease and injury category	1900	1930	1975	2000
Total	$15,030.0	$30,744.0	$57,848.0	$89,469.0
Mental disorders	1,767.1	3,596.3	8,751.2	11,636.9
Diseases of the circulatory system	574.2	2,556.6	8,743.6	11,800.3
Diseases of the respiratory system	4,066.1	4,569.9	8,542.1	14,129.3
Diseases of the musculoskeletal system and connective tissue	1,125.7	1,952.2	7,351.4	11,371.9
Accidents, poisonings, and violence	675.8	4,365.4	5,669.2	9,867.5
Infective and parasitic diseases	3,356.3	5,211.8	1,559.0	2,932.1
Neoplasms	56.0	354.4	1,105.0	1,854.8
Other	3,408.8	8,137.5	16,126.0	25,876.2

Source: Computed from references 9-12 to adjust for average earnings differences, with 1975 used as the base year.

Table 9-12. Distribution of Sickness Costs among Disease and Injury Categories, Selected Years, 1900-2000

Disease and injury category (ranked by relative cost) 1975	Percentage of sickness cost			
	1900	*1930*	*1975*	*2000*
Total	100.0	100.0	100.0	100.0
Mental disorders	11.8	11.7	15.1	*13.0*
Diseases of the circulatory system	3.8	8.3	15.1	*13.2*
Diseases of the respiratory system	27.1	14.9	14.8	*15.8*
Diseases of the musculoskeletal system	7.5	6.4	12.7	*12.7*
Accidents, poisonings, and violence	4.5	14.2	9.8	*11.0*
Infective and parasitic diseases	22.3	17.0	2.7	*3.3*
Neoplasms	.4	1.2	1.9	*2.1*
Other	22.7	26.5	27.9	*28.9*

Computed from Table 9-11.

SICKNESS COST AND BIOMEDICAL RESEARCH

The assessment of sickness cost tells us little of what biomedical research has achieved by way of reducing the cost of sickness. The exceptions are the saving in infectious and parasitic diseases, in diseases connected with childbearing, and in blood diseases. Has biomedical research, then, made little, if any, additional contribution?

In the traditional analyses of how biomedical advances affect sickness cost, it is assumed that the disease is wiped out as a result of the research. There are diseases, as we have indicated, for which just this has happened historically. The appropriate measure of gain from biomedical research in these instances may be the total historic cost of the sickness. If, however, biomedical research should succeed in reducing the incidence of a disease by providing cures or prevention for some persons, but not others, as is the case in antismoking campaigns, the cost saved by the preventive or curative steps falls short of the full-scale amount. Thus, the gains from the research that resulted in the antismoking campaign of the Public Health Service would be less than the full cost of disease. But the product of the biomedical research may not reduce incidence. It may reduce severity or it may increase incidence of one disease as a feedback

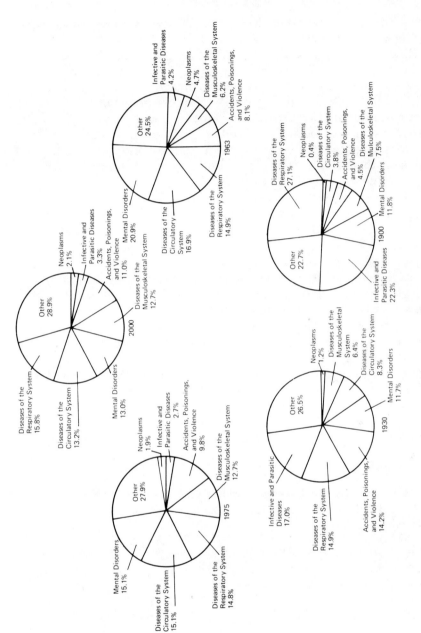

Figure 9-1. Percentage of Sickness Cost, by Diseases and Injury Category

effect of reducing another. Reduction in heart disease, for example, is increasing the cancer rate.

How then do we assess the overall dollar impact of biomedical research on sickness over the decades of the twentieth century? We first estimate the saving based on the objective sickness rate, or the adjusted estimates of average work-time loss priced at the per diem earnings rate of 1975 for the employed population of 1975. The difference in cost between periods in sickness cost valued at 1975 earnings essentially represents the total reduction in the cost of sickness that has taken place. Some part of that reduction is attributable to biomedical advances.

What was the actual objective sickness rate per worker for each of the selected years? Assuming the work-loss days per worker for each of the periods is sufficiently adequate as a measure of the extent of sickness in those years, it is then reasonable to adjust those work-loss days to reflect the differences between the socioeconomic reporting of sickness (constrained by economic capacity, perception, and knowledge) and the objective sickness rate (see Table 9-13). Given these adjusted rates, we then value each day at 1975 levels for the employed population of 1975. The difference from one period to another is the saving due to reduced work-loss time (corrected for underreporting).

Estimates based on objective sickness rates may be compared with the raw unadjusted work-time loss numbers, setting a lower bound on the total saving in sickness cost.

Only a share of the reduction in cost is attributable to biomedical research. That share is derived from the analysis presented in Chapter

Table 9-13. Estimated Saving in Sickness Cost, in Billions, over Selected Periods, 1900-75, at Standard Earnings and Labor Market Participation Rates

Estimate 1. Saving in cost of sickness at objective sickness rates (billions of 1975 dollars)

Selected periods	Saving in temporary work loss	Saving in total work loss
1900-30	$129.0	—
1930-63	46.2	$238.4
1930-75	53.3	260.1
1900-75	182.2	210.5

Estimate 2. Simulated 1975 saving in sickness cost, taking account of the difference between 1930 sickness rates by disease for each age and sex group and 1975 rates (at 1975 earnings and work-force participation)

Unadjusted saving	$21 billion
Adjusted for objective sickness rate	$63 billion

8. We have estimated the percentage of the reduction in the objective sickness rate attributable to biomedical sciences at 39 percent.

Another approach to assessing the effect of biomedical research is to estimate the change in sickness cost, taking account of differences in sickness rates by disease and also the change in the distribution of the work force by age and sex and of earnings by age and sex. In the first computation, allowance is made only for period-to-period differences in average earnings without taking account of the disease patterns or the composition of the work force.

SIMULATED COST, BY DISEASE

The 1930 work-loss costs were simulated for 1975 population and work-force characteristics and these costs, in turn, were compared with the actual 1975 experience. The estimates, which initially were prepared using the unadjusted illness data, need to be adjusted for the average difference between the objective sickness rate and the actual reported rates.

We first applied 1930 sickness rates to the 1975 population, taking account of the work-force characteristics of 1975. The result is an estimated 1975 cost under 1930 illness experience. At 1930 unadjusted rates, we find that sickness would have cost $79 billion, a figure about $21 billion, or about 37 percent, above the 1975 actual cost. Accordingly, the $21 billion represents essentially an estimate of the saving in sickness cost due to the reduction in work loss, but it does not take account of the marked differences between 1930 and 1975 in income protections against sickness, capacity of medicine to treat, educational levels of the population, and perception about disease.

The simulation was carried out for each of the categories of time lost from work, namely, work absences of workers, those not in the work force due to illness (including those in institutions and those in the noninstitutionalized population), and loss of working time by housewives. The simulated costs are as follows (in billions):

Work loss time by:	1975 costs at 1930 illness rates	1975 costs at 1975 illness rates
Total	$79.1	$57.8
Those in the work force	27.5	21.3
Those not in the work force	46.1	32.2
Housewives	5.5	4.4

About $14 billion, or two-thirds, of the $21 billion saving in cost is attributable to the reduction in the numbers who would have withdrawn from the labor force under 1930 conditions. While the estimates are incomplete as measures of "saving," they provide a perspective on the changes in disease problems that are significant in understanding the impact of biomedical advances.

As indicated earlier, in 1930 the three most costly categories were infective and parasitic diseases; diseases of the respiratory system; and accidents, poisonings, and violence. If these three most costly categories and the others that affected workers in 1930 were experienced in 1975 by the 1975 population at 1975 work experience and earnings rates, sickness costs would have been higher in 1975 than they in fact were. The largest percentage differences would be in complications of pregnancy and childbearing, infective and parasitic diseases, and diseases of the blood and bloodforming organs (Table 9-14). Under 1975 economic conditions, more salaried women would be affected by the complications of pregnancy that characterized childbearing of 1930, and thus, by the almost

Table 9-14.   Ratio of 1975 Simulated Costs (If 1930 Illness Prevailed) of Morbidity to Actual 1975 Costs

Disease and injury category	*Ratio of cost of illness at 1930 to actual 1975*
Total[1]	1.37
Infective and parasitic diseases	8.18
Neoplasms	.86
Endocrine, nutritional, and metabolic diseases	.64
Diseases of the blood and blood-forming organs	4.75
Mental disorders	1.09
Diseases of the nervous system and sense organs	.83
Eye diseases[2]	(.57)
Diseases of the circulatory system	.76
Diseases of the respiratory system	1.39
Diseases of the digestive system	2.12
Diseases of the oral cavity, salivary glands, and jaws[2]	(.17)
Diseases of the genitourinary system	1.73
Complications of pregnancy, childbirth, and puerperium	11.84
Diseases of the skin and subcutaneous tissue	2.53
Diseases of the musculoskeletal system and connective tissue	.67
Congenital anomalies	—
Certain causes of perinatal morbidity and mortality	—
Symptoms and ill-defined conditions	.48
Accidents, poisonings, and violence	1.94

[1] Total may not add due to rounding.
[2] Included in previous total.

Source: A. Berk and L. Paringer: "Economic costs of illness, 1930-1975." Public Services Laboratory, Georgetown University, Washington, D.C., 1977.

twelvefold rise in cost. Similarly, infective and parasitic disease costs would be far greater today—eight times as large if 1930 sickness conditions prevailed. Infective and parasitic diseases, which represented 17 percent of all morbidity costs in 1930 and totaled $709 million in 1930, would have been $12.8 billion, given 1930 sickness rates under 1975 economic conditions. Actual 1975 economic costs for these illnesses totaled only $1.6 billion. The figures also indicate substantial reductions in the economic cost of infective diseases and diseases connected with childbearing when we adjust for earnings levels and economic conditions. Biomedical research has probably had its most important impact on the incidence of these illnesses. Primary prevention measures have succeeded in wiping out the dangers of contracting contagious diseases, and prenatal care, along with antibiotics to fight infections, have reduced the high costs of maternity deaths and maternal illnesses and of respiratory infections.

Diseases of the blood and blood-forming organs also show a very interesting change over time. In 1975, the cost of blood diseases was $281 billion. If we estimated the costs of these illnesses in 1930 under 1975 conditions, this cost would be $1.3 billion. Anemia is a major illness in this category. Changes in diagnoses of illnesses may account for part of the change in costs. To the extent that leukemia and other blood cancers may have been diagnosed as diseases of the blood and blood-forming organs, rather than neoplasms, this may cause some noncomparability among the estimates of this category of illness costs. However, the antibiotics have undoubtedly played a large role in changing the cost of blood diseases. Other causes of morbidity for which greater costs are simulated are accidents, poisonings, and violence; mental disorders; and diseases of the respiratory system, of the digestive system, and of the genitourinary system.

The reduction in the work accident rates over the period may partly account for the cost saving in accidents, poisonings, and violence. It is of some note that the injury category is less costly today than it would have been under earlier circumstances; the seemingly violent mood of the current times would have suggested higher costs rather than cost saving.

Efforts at deinstitutionalizing the mentally ill may be responsible for reducing the costs of institutionalization of persons with mental disorders, but at the same time, a sizable rise in cost is estimated for those who are employed. Some formerly institutionalized persons are now functioning in society but are not yet members of the labor force. All told, the saving in costs of mental disorders appears small.

Reductions in the incidence of influenza and pneumonia and improved treatment techniques, which have reduced illness severity, have been largely responsible for the reduction in the impact of respiratory illnesses on the economic cost. Under 1930 illness conditions, the costs of respiratory illness would have been about $11.9 billion or $3.3 billion greater than they actually were in 1975.

Diseases of the digestive system also showed a reduction in economic costs between 1930 and 1975. The simulated 1975 costs were $7.3 billion, two times as great as the actual costs. Again, the largest reductions in costs were among those who reported being unable to work. In 1930, illnesses, such as ulcers, appendicitis, and hernias, caused bed duration of more than forty-five days far more frequently than they do today. Improved treatment methods have made it possible for more people with these conditions to carry on normal work activities.

Diseases of the genitourinary system have also witnessed a decrease in economic cost since 1930. The 1975 costs would have been over one-and-a-half times greater than they actually were if 1930 illness conditions had existed. In 1930, diseases of the genitourinary system were comprised of such illnesses as nephritis, cystitis, salpingitis, menstrual disorders, and complications of circumcision. Antibiotics and changes in general medical care (for example, circumcisions are now routinely done at birth) have contributed to the reduction in morbidity. It is also possible that psychological changes surrounding health problems, such as menstrual disorders, have led to a decrease in the reporting of such illnesses.

Costs for several disease categories would have been lower in 1975 if 1930 sickness rates prevailed but economic and population characteristics were the same as 1975. Among the categories for which costs would have been less in 1975 under 1930 conditions are neoplasms; endocrine, nutritional, and metabolic diseases; diseases of the nervous system, circulatory system, and musculoskeletal system and connective tissue. Indeed, at 1930 rates the cost of work time lost due to cancer morbidity would be low, relative to that of other major diseases. This is in sharp contrast to the cost of premature cancer deaths.

At least part of the increase in cancer costs may be due to improved diagnostic methods and an increased willingness by its victims to report the disease. However, increased smoking and environmental health hazards are contributing to an increase in the disease prevalence. For circulatory illnesses, an increase in the cost of sickness could be a consequence of a reduction in the death rate.

Heart attacks and stroke may not be as likely to result in death as they were in 1930. However, the results of such illnesses could incapacitate the individuals affected for extended periods so that, while there is a reduction in the cost of mortality, there apparently is also an increase in the cost of sickness.

Endocrine, nutritional, and metabolic diseases have also increased in economic importance, as have diseases of the nervous system and sense organs. Some illnesses such as diabetes, no longer result in high death rates, and thus morbidity measures have become increasingly important. The age-adjusted death rate from diabetes in 1975, for example, was about half the rate of 1930. A similar influence may also be occurring with respect to some diseases of the nervous system and sense organs; for example, because eye and ear diseases are now being treated more frequently and more effectively, we might expect an increase in the economic cost.

A final category for which increases, rather than savings, in economic cost is indicated is the group of diseases of the musculo-skeletal system and connective tissue. Arthritis and rheumatism are two major illnesses in this disease category. One possible reason for the growth in economic cost of these illnesses is that, as mortality rates have declined and life expectancy has increased, the population has become older and more susceptible to these degenerative diseases.

In summary, then, while the cost of sickness on the whole would have been higher in 1975, at 1930 rates, this has not been the case for all illnesses. Certain illnesses, such as infective and parasitic diseases and diseases of childbirth, have experienced rather dramatic reductions in relative costs, while others, such as heart disease, cancer, and metabolic diseases, have experienced cost increases.

Table 9-15 displays the cost savings and increases, with the disease and injury categories arrayed in the order of cost saving. The saving in the three major categories is estimated at $20.5 billion. This saving is offset in part by the higher cost diseases. The ratio of simulated costs to actual 1975 costs is shown in Table 9-14.

The saving in cost is not entirely attributable to biomedical advances. Many factors have played a part, including greater access to medical care, higher incomes, improved income maintenance, better education, and changes in perception about sickness. But the saving estimate is little more than a partial estimate of the change in sickness experience over the forty-five-year period.

An additional bit of political arithmetic is suggested by the difference between the actual reported data and the objective sickness rates. The objective sickness rates between 1930 and 1975

Table 9-15.   Total Sickness Cost Saving, 1930-75, Based on Simulation, by Disease and Injury Categories
(in billions)

Category arrayed by cost saving	Cost in billions
Total (net saving)	$21.3
Infective and parasitic diseases	11.2
Accidents, poisonings, and violence	5.4
Diseases of the digestive system	3.9
Diseases of the respiratory system	3.3
Complications of pregnancy, childbirth, and puerperium	2.1
Diseases of the genitourinary system	1.3
Diseases of the blood and bloodforming organs	1.1
Mental disorders	.8
Diseases of the skin and subcutaneous tissue	.6
Neoplasms	−.2
Endocrine, nutritional, and metabolic diseases	−.6
Symptoms and ill-defined conditions	−.7
Diseases of the nervous system and sense organs	−1.0
Diseases of the circulatory system	−2.1
Diseases of the musculoskeletal system and connective tissue	−2.4

increase threefold over the actual unadjusted rates. If, as a rough approximation, we apply that difference to the cost derived by the simulation, we would increase the aggregate saving in cost from $21 billion to three times that amount, or $63 billion. Again, the share of the saving in the objective rate of sickness may be taken at 39 percent of the total, resulting in a saving of $25 billion attributable to biomedical research.

SUMMARY

The approaches to an estimate of the saving in sickness cost attributable to biomedical research are summarized in Table 9-16. The estimates are far from precise but they do begin to set some bounds and limits on the complex question of the effect of biomedical research on sickness costs. Perhaps the best justification for the estimates summarized here is that they are sufficiently provocative to initiate a questioning process that may yield a far better set of estimates in the years ahead.

Table 9-16. Two Estimates of Saving in Sickness Attributable to Biomedical Advances over Designated Periods, in Billions of 1975 Dollars

Selected periods	Temporary wage loss	Total wage loss
Estimate 1		
1900-30	$50.3	—
1930-63	18.0	$ 93.0
1930-75	20.8	101.4
1900-75	71.1	82.1
Estimate 2		
1930-75 simulation		
Unadjusted sickness rates	—	$ 8
Adjusted sickness rates	—	25

Computed at 39 percent of the total saving in sickness cost based on Table 9-13.

REFERENCES

1. Abt, C.: The social costs of cancer. Social Indicators Research 2:175-190, 1975.

2. Mushkin, S., and Landefeld, J.S.: Non-health sector costs of disease and injury. Submitted to Medical Care, 1979.

3. Acton, J.: Measuring the social impact of heart and circulatory disease programs: Preliminary framework and estimates. Rand Corporation, Santa Monica, Calif., April 1975.

4. Rice, D.: Estimating the cost of illness. Health Economics, Series No. 6. U.S. Public Health Services, Washington, D.C., 1966.

5. U.S. Bureau of the Census: Historical statistics of the United States, colonial times to 1970. Bicentennial ed. U.S. Government Printing Office, Washington, D.C., 1975.

6. U.S. Department of Labor: Employment and training: report to the President, 1963 and 1975. Washington, D.C., 1963, 1975.

7. Norton, J.P.: Economic advisability of a national department of health. Proceedings of the American Association for the Advancement of Science, Ithaca, N.Y., published 1907.

8. Fisher, I.: Report of the National Conservation Commission. Report on national vitality: its wastes and conservation. Bulletin of One Hundred on National Health, Washington, D.C., No. 30, 1909, p. 656.

9. Berk, A., and Paringer, L.C.: Cost of illness and disease, 1900. Public Services Laboratory, Georgetown University, Washington, D.C., 1977 (revised 1979).

10. Berk, A., and Paringer, L.C.: Cost of illness and disease, 1930. Public Services Laboratory, Georgetown University, Washington, D.C., 1977.

11. Paringer, L.C., and Berk, A.: Costs of illness and disease, fiscal year 1975. Public Services Laboratory, Georgetown University, Washington, D.C., 1977.

12. Mushkin, S.J., et al.: Cost of disease and illness in the United States in the year 2000. Public Health Rep 93:493-588, September-October 1978.

Chapter Ten

The Cost of Debility

Assessment of biomedical research funds, in terms of cost of disease, is likely to fall short of its mark unless the cost of debility is counted, that is, the cost of loss in output or increase in production cost per unit of output due to sickness. Debility cost, with successful attacks on disease problems, could be wiped out. Indeed, as is indicated later, progress toward this end has been made.

In the traditional accounting of the economic cost of sickness, only the time lost from work is included. But an additional cost is incurred when workers who have a headache, backache, cold, toothache, and the like come to work. These costs are not ordinarily included in the calculations, partly because the data base for determining the cost of debility is most inadequate. At best, only a rough approximation can be achieved at this time.

Neglect of the cost of debility in sickness cost studies does not originate in the notion that such costs are unimportant. It is widely recognized that minor ailments afflict millions in the population. Indeed, gains in productivity due to reduction in debility from diseases now virtually eradicated have been vital in the economic growth of the United States. But there continues to be a disease load that impairs the output of workers while at work. The common cold, for example, remains costly in terms of economic output of the affected workers. Each year, millions of persons suffer with colds and similar minor diseases that are not severe enough to keep them from work. What are the economic costs of these diseases, or, stated differently, what would be the gains in productivity if the sickness that evidences itself in debility were eliminated?

The formulation of debility as loss in worker efficiency due to illness while at work has been measured crudely in the past to identify need for public action on disease control. Several yardsticks of the effect of debility on worker efficiency have been used. Several others have been discussed. These include

1. Output in a plant with recorded information on number of machines in operation before and after disease control measures are taken
2. Wages earned on a piece-rate basis by those with a disease compared to those free of the disease
3. Wages of workers in an area with a high disease prevalence compared to wages of similar workers in areas free of the disease
4. Output on a farm in which a disease problem is controlled, measured against output of a control group of workers
5. Laboratory tests of work energy of groups of workers afflicted with a disease, measured against work capacity of a normal control group

There are some historic records of studies of increased worker output after disease control is instituted.[1] The control-group type of experiment has been discussed, and an effort has been made toward such experimentation. Demands from the control groups for treatment in an area with a high rate of endemic disease have been met, but no experiment, as far as we know, has been carried through to definitive findings. A laboratory approach to the problem of work energy is another method of assessing health and productivity.

The alternative to these case studies is to compile mass data on output and on disease prevalence among workers and to analyze the data to find the effects of pertinent variables, including the extent of the disease.

All of these yardsticks address one facet of the measurement problem, namely, what is the loss in output due to sickness or what is the gain in output with cure? Still another unknown remains– the numbers of workers who on an average day, week, or year are afflicted. Total debility costs comprise two components: the effect on output per workday and the number of workdays on which workers at work are not well. Data are not readily at hand for either of these components.

In this chapter, we identify the several types of debility and present estimates of those components of debility that can be measured at least on an approximate basis (together with their qualifications).

TYPES OF DEBILITY

Debility extends beyond the common cold to other sicknesses that impair performance on the job. Three types of debility may be distinguished:

1. Temporary and acute sickness or not feeling well, exemplified by the cold, toothache, or headache, which, while impairing performance for a short time, does not have a continuing effect on productivity.
2. Physical or mental impairment that follows a major illness and that lowers vitality or alters attitudes toward work in ways that can impair job performance. Examples are the work performances of persons who return to their jobs after recovering from a heart attack or from major surgery.
3. Impairment of those with static disabilities or stabilized chronic conditions if such impairment reduces output while on the job. In this category fall, for example, the paraplegics, the deaf, and the nonsighted.

Individual differences among persons' responses to illness or impairment, differences in severity of illness, variation in the symptoms of each illness, and the diverse nature of the employments and of the requirements placed on jobholders, result in lack of uniformity in effect of illness on job performance. Thus, there are uneven distributions in the impact on output among individuals for each class of sickness or disability and among sicknesses.

The full impact on productivity is essentially a composite number that, on the one hand, reflects the high output of impaired persons who, given an opportunity to work, have a special work ethic and, on the other, reflects the reduction in output per worker (or increased cost per unit of output) that may result from impairments.

We estimate separately the cost of each type of debility identified because of the separate data sources available, to approximate numbers in the population at risk and loss in output.

TEMPORARY ACUTE SICKNESS

The number of people with temporary sickness perhaps poses the largest data problem. Despite the frequent references to the common cold as a costly disease that warrants more research attention, or to the common toothache, the statistics gathered do not provide a clear picture of the extent of these ailments.

Data Collection Problems

The basic statistics gathered by the National Center for Health Statistics (NCHS) do not provide the information needed. The NCHS collects information, for example, on work-loss and bed-disability days. Data on less serious restricted-activity days are also collected, but these are presented in a format that precludes segregation of such days into minor acute conditions occurring on working days and on other days. Excluded from restricted-activity days by definition, moreover, are minor acute conditions that do not involve a substantial reduction in normal activities for the whole day or require medical attention.

Despite the orientation of the Health Interview Survey toward relatively serious disabling acute conditions, NCHS data suggest a higher than average prevalence of less serious conditions and the aftereffects of acute episodes. For example, in fiscal year 1975, of the 5 total restricted-activity days per acute condition, only 2.2 involved bed disability.[2] Another bit of data on the extent of minor acute illness over and above work-loss and bed-disability days comes from the information on the incidence of acute conditions by measures of the impact of illness. As Table 10-1 points out, nearly 18 percent of acute illness cases are medically attended but do not involve a restriction of activity.[3] Some medically attended cases may have a debilitating effect but do not involve restricted activity as defined. In other words, the splitting headache that takes a worker to the health room for an aspirin in the morning and is gone in the afternoon would not be counted among restricted-activity days, despite its possible impact on work performance. Nor would the industrial accident be counted that required care only at the workplace for a cut or bruise.

As Table 10-1 shows, about 408 million new cases are estimated as the annual number of acute conditions. Of these, 181 million, or 44.4 percent, restrict activity. The Health Interview Survey defines a restricted-activity day rather strictly:

A day of restricted activity is one on which a person *substantially* reduces his normal activity for the *whole* day because of illness or injury. Restricted activity does not imply complete inactivity, but it does imply only the minimum of usual activities. A special nap for an hour after lunch does not constitute cutting down on usual activities, nor does the elimination of a heavy chore such as cleaning ashes out of the furnace or hanging out the wash. If a farmer or housewife carries on only the minimum of the day's chores, however, this is a day of restricted activity.[4]

By definition, the day of restricted activity provides little guidance on the full count of the extent of debility attributable to temporary sickness or injury. The incidence data of NCHS, moreover, exclude minor acute conditions that do not result in restricted activity or require medical attention.

How large, then, is the extent of minor ailments—numbers afflicted and length of illness—that can impair performance on the job? Some pieces of information suggest that the number of cases exceeds that of the annual 408 million conditions.

At an early phase of the NCHS data collection, the health interview schedule included the question, "Were you sick at any time last week or the week before?" An intern at NCHS tabulated the results of this question for 1973-74 and reported that those who responded affirmatively to the question exceeded by 30 percent the number with restricted activity.

Years back, some data were collected about the incidence of colds. Collins, in analyzing the Committee on the Costs of Medical Care (CCMC) data, noted as a characteristic of the information reported on sickness conditions the understatement of colds. "If all of the

Table 10-1. Number and Percentage Distribution of Incidence of Acute Conditions, by Measures of Impact of Illness, According to Condition Group: United States, July 1974-June 1975

	Incidence of acute conditions (number in thousands)	Percent distribution		
Condition group		percent	Medically attended only	Medically attended and activity restricting	Activity restricting
All acute conditions	407,831	100.0	17.8	37.8	44.4
Infective and parasitic diseases	42,114	100.0	11.2	44.1	37.8
Respiratory conditions	219,958	100.0	9.4	31.8	58.8
Upper respiratory conditions	108,312	100.0	14.9	27.6	57.5
Influenza	102,231	100.0	2.8	32.6	64.6
Other respiratory conditions	9,415	100.0	16.7	72.4	10.9
Digestive system conditions	18,737	100.0	16.2	33.2	50.6
Injuries	71,342	100.0	36.6	47.8	15.6
All other acute conditions	55,681	100.0	32.3	45.3	22.4

Source: Reference 3.

many trivial colds had been recorded, as in a few special respiratory studies, the rates for such affections would have been about 10 times those recorded in these studies. The cases here included (CCMC) are probably those of more than average severity."[5] One of those special respiratory studies referred to, that by van Volkenburgh and Frost, found that "the mean number of colds per person during the year 1929-1930 was 3.07, and the mean duration of symptoms was 15.9 days, the average time during which symptoms were present being 49 days."[6]

In the NCHS data, selected acute conditions that generate debility costs seem to be greatly underreported. The underreporting is probably a consequence of the definitions established to capture by statistics major illnesses and to omit minor, temporary sickness. Nevertheless, the NCHS data on incidence of acute disease per person clearly omit many cases. According to NCHS, on the average, each person has less than half a cold during a year; influenza occurs about as frequently as colds. Digestive conditions fare even more poorly than colds in the statistics; only one person in ten is shown to have a stomach upset during a year. Headaches, according to the statistics, occur far less frequently. Table 10-2 gives the number of acute conditions per person per year for selected condition groups, according to NCHS data.

Another way to show these data is to derive from the incidence numbers per person per year a figure on the number of years that would elapse, on the average, between cases in each of the condition groups at the incidence rates shown. These figures are shown in the second column of Table 10-2. (The years elapsing between cases is simply the reciprocal of the incidence per year figure shown in the first column.)

The NCHS data as reported indicate that only 2 percent of the

Table 10-2. Incidence of Selected Acute Conditions: Per Person and by Number of Years Elapsing between Cases

| | Number of acute conditions per person | |
Condition group	Incidence per year	Years elapsing between cases
Common cold	.45	2
Influenza	.47	2
Digestive system conditions	.10	10
Diseases of the ear	.07	14
Headaches	.02	50

Source: Computed from data shown in reference 3.

population will have a headache during a year and 10 percent, a stomach upset. Stated differently, each person is shown to have a headache once every fifty years and a stomach upset, every ten.

In an attempt to obtain some notion of the extent of acute temporary illness, when defined less restrictively than incidence is defined by NCHS, we conducted a simple survey of workers. The results are not intended to be regarded as scientific, but rather as merely suggestive of a more complete account of minor acute illness.

In the District of Columbia, fifty-three office workers were asked about the incidence and duration of acute illness, where incidence was defined in terms of the presence of the condition rather than in terms of whether the condition exceeded a prescribed level of severity. Individuals were asked if they had any of the following acute conditions in the past year:

- Infective and parasitic
- Respiratory conditions: upper respiratory (common cold); influenza (with or without digestive manifestations); other respiratory illnesses (pneumonia, bronchitis)
- Digestive system conditions: as a result of dental or gastrointestinal problems
- Injuries: fractures, dislocations, sprains, cuts
- Other acute conditions: diseases of the ear; headaches; diseases of the skin

If they answered "yes" to any of these conditions, they were asked how many times they had the condition and the average duration of the illness. To clarify what constituted "having" the condition, they were told to base their responses on the severity of the symptoms that signified presence of the condition.

The average number of acute full-time equivalent illness days per person obtained from the survey was 52.3 days for all conditions. In contrast, the 1975 Health Interview Survey (HIS) reported an average of 9.6 restricted-activity days per person associated with acute conditions of the total 17.9 restricted-activity days—both acute and chronic—for the entire population. If we assume that restricted-activity days of the working population (12 days) are divided between acute and chronic, roughly in the same proportion, about 6.4 days would account for acute conditions. The disparity between 52.3 and 6.4 is so large that even a figure one-half as large would indicate a prevalence of illness significantly higher than that reported under NCHS definitions.

Table 10-3 displays NCHS incidence figures and our informal survey results. Although our survey findings are only suggestive, they indicate a substantially higher incidence rate when the measure of illness is presence of sickness rather than severity of disease. The largest differences are for minor conditions such as common colds, digestive problems, earaches, and headaches. (It is interesting that the informal survey incidence was 2.7 colds a year, a figure very close to the 3 colds a year reported by van Volkenburgh and Frost in 1930;[6] also, for office workers, 25 headaches a year or 1 every two weeks seems more reasonable than 1 every fifty years, as reported by NCHS data.) For more disabling conditions, such as influenza, the differences are small.

We had made various efforts to obtain data from other sources before we undertook the crude survey. We had contacted several agencies and firms to ask staff in personnel offices for information on workers who came to work sick, and we asked nurses in the health rooms what data they kept on workers who came to them for assistance. We also sought records from the Public Health Service to determine the volume of services provided. Unfortunately, record-keeping of the kind that would yield information on the extent of debility was not at hand. Earlier, Fuchs had reviewed the literature only to find that the emphasis of company health plans was on turnover rates, accident rates, absenteeism, and workmen's compensation premiums rather than on output per hour. Little seemed to be known about output.[7]

Loss in Output

The loss in output or added costs per unit of output per day as a consequence of temporary sickness poses an equally difficult, if not greater, data problem.

Table 10-3. Alternative Measures of the Incidence of Selected Acute Conditions

	Acute conditions per person per year	
Condition	*Findings among 53 office workers*	*NCHS data on medical attention and/or restriction of activity*
Common cold	2.70	0.45
Influenza	0.38	0.42[1]
Digestive system conditions	2.19	0.09[1]
Diseases of the ear	0.68	0.07
Headaches	25.82	0.02

[1] Rates for working-age persons seventeen and over; similar data not available in 1975 for other conditions.

Again, we ask: What is known about the output of sick persons who come to work?

Earlier in this chapter, different measures of the extent of loss in output were enumerated. Some studies of the enumerated measures support the finding that worker efficiency is reduced by about 30 percent or more as a consequence of sickness for the days of sickness. Stated differently, if selected diseases were conquered, productivity of the workers now affected with these diseases would rise by perhaps 30 percent per workday.

In the United States, results of studies of malaria control during the first part of the century point to such a finding.[1] Textile mill output per worker, assessed in terms of the number of machines in operation before and after a malaria control program was initiated, indicated such a product difference. The introduction of an anti-malaria program in the Philippines resulted in not only a reduction in absenteeism but also an increase in productivity per worker of approximately one-third.[8]

At least seven studies were done on the effect of schistosomiasis on worker productivity. Four of the studies found declines in worker productivity of approximately one-third, while a fifth study in Egypt estimated that the productivity loss was between 4 and 20 percent.[9] Two studies found no significant reduction in productivity, although one of these reported a bias in sample selection, which included only new workers in the group afflicted with schistosomiasis,[10] while the other study appeared to have problems with model misspecification.[11]

To our knowledge, the only recent study in the United States related to debility was a survey of Equitable Life Insurance employees. This study found that simple stress-related disorders, including anxiety, tension, or migraine headaches, cause significant reductions in productivity. Employees estimated that the "average hourly interference effect" was approximately 25 percent, a figure surprisingly close to the estimated impact of debility due to malaria years ago in the United States and in less developed countries.[12]

Essentially, by combining the earlier information on days of sickness with selected acute conditions and output loss per day, we can approximate the total dollar loss attributable to debility associated with temporary acute conditions.

We estimate the cost of temporary debility at $34.5 to $41.5 billion for those in the work force.

In making this approximation, we allowed for the sickness days already reported by NCHS and included in the cost of sickness set forth in Chapter 9. The estimates represent the net difference between the survey results for selected conditions and NCHS data on restricted-activity days from acute conditions. To the extent conditions other than those included in the survey are underreported, this accounting of debility is an underestimate.

If we assume, alternatively, losses in output of 25 percent and 30 percent due to sickness, the per diem cost (on a full-time equivalent basis) would be alternatively $12.66 to $15.19, with these amounts computed on an average daily earnings level for 1975 of $50.64 for the employed population of 83.2 million.

The earlier computation suggested an average of 45.9 unreported days during the work year when workers were not up to par. If five-sevenths of these were working days, the average worker experienced 32.8 debility days a year. On those days, workers who were on the job had colds, toothaches, headaches, or other temporary conditions.

Cost of debility that is caused by temporary acute conditions may be calculated as follows: Assuming as many as 32.8 full-time equilvalent sickness days during periods of work, additional to that reported in the NCHS morbidity data, the costs could be $34.5 to $41.5 billion.

PHYSICAL OR MENTAL IMPAIRMENT
FOLLOWING A MAJOR ILLNESS

A second type of debility is attributable to the slowdown that often accompanies patients' concern about themselves as an aftermath of a major illness, such as a heart attack or major surgery.

For some patients, the earlier bouts with major illness may require job changes. For some, the job requirements are such that the diminution of physical or mental vigor may not necessitate job changes, even though work capacity may be impaired. On the other hand, for some there may be a focusing of energy or a sharpening of purpose that contrasts with earlier performance and increases rather than diminishes output.

Of 1.9 million workers whose activities are limited because of heart disease or major surgery, about 400,000 of these represent workers who have had a first bout with heart disease during the year. These 400,000 are among the 1.3 million new cases of heart disease each year.[13]

We estimate that of the 17.9 million surgical operations performed in 1975 on patients fifteen years of age and older in short-stay hospitals, the work capacity of at least 1.5 million workers is diminished for a period following surgery. The kinds of surgery included in this count and the estimated number of workers affected are shown in Table 10-4. Heart surgery is excluded to avoid double counting.[14]

The numbers are clearly crude. Individual differences in response to illness, the variations in severity of that illness, and job task requirements have a good deal to do with the numbers of workers whose output is diminished as a result of a diseased condition.

The 1970 Census reported that 5.9 percent of the age group eighteen to forty-four years had a partial work disability. For the age group forty-five to sixty-four, the corresponding percentage was twice as high (11.8 percent). With today's population, this would mean that upward of 5.5 million would respond affirmatively to the following census inquiry: "Does this person have a health or physical condition which limits the kind or amount of work he can do at a job?"

We assume that individual responses to this type of question would vary greatly, particularly for those who are adjusting to a major illness or surgery. While the inquiry about limitations extends beyond the scope of the type of debility being considered here to permanent or long-term impairments, it also does not include cases of special concern here because of the likelihood that some of those affected would deny a limitation. To illustrate, we draw on the reports to NCHS on limitation of activity reported by persons with severe vision limitations.[15] Severe limitation is defined as inability to read ordinary newspaper print with glasses, and impairment indicates no useful vision in either eye. More than 1.3 million persons are reported to have severe vision impairment, yet 811,000 of these

Table 10-4. Estimated Number of Workers with Temporary Debilitating Effects Following Major Surgery

Surgical category	Number of workers (in thousands)
Total	1,539
Neurosurgery	198
Operations on thyroid, parathyroid, thymus, and adrenals	60
Cholecystectomy	272
Resection of small intestine or colon	93
Dilation of urethra	124
Prostatectomy	208
Mastectomy	155
Hysterectomy	336
Excision of bone	93

Source: Reference 14.

persons indicated that the lack of sight did not cause limitations of activity. However, only 123,000 reported that they were usually working.

The factual base to draw on for establishing the numbers at risk in this category of debility is far from adequate. At best, these numbers must be pieced together from the existing health statistics and medical care data. But even more inadequate is information about the loss in productivity. Nor is this information likely to come easily, because of offsetting factors at work. Most likely, productivity would be impaired more if continued employment were not provided for those who suffer a heart attack or undergo major surgery. Society would lose much experience and the enhanced output that comes with years of learning on the job. And the well-being of the individual affected would be greatly impaired. Continued employment is indeed part of long-term therapy, a factor that generates much concern about job discrimination against the cancer patient and others.

Given the uncertainty about output impacts, we used alternative measures. We started with the 25- to 30-percent loss in output that has been attributed to acute illnesses and adjusted for various shares of a work year that would be affected on the average before a fuller adjustment to the illness, as follows:

Period of disability	Percent	Loss Dollars (in millions)
2 months	25-30%	$ 884-1,105
3 months	25-30	1,443-1,803
6 months	25-30	2,839-3,548

If we assume alternative days of debility at the 25-percent loss in output level, the losses would range from $884 million to $2,839 million. At the 30-percent loss in output level, the corresponding losses would total $1,105 million to $3,548 million.

The uncertainty about the estimates poses a question: Why try the accounting? The answer is that, despite the many dollars spent for research on health services, little has been done to assess and quantify debility costs. The identification of the issue may stir others to take on research directed to a better understanding of the problem. Quantification, on an approximate basis, should encourage researchers to quarrel with the numbers and achieve through the challenge a better set of estimates.

STATIC OR STABILIZED
DISABILITY IMPAIRMENTS

An additional type of debility is attributable to loss of output that develops out of long-term impairments, such as loss of limbs or hearing and stabilized or controlled chronic impairments.

To approximate the total numbers involved, we summed up the numbers of persons with selected impairments who were usually working, limiting the summary as far as the data permit to severe conditions. To these approximations we added arthritis, rheumatism, and diabetes as major conditions affecting work output of those with the long-term conditions who hold jobs.[16] Table 10-5 shows the figures compiled by disease category.

To approach a conservative estimate we excluded many long-term conditions. Persons with speech defects and those with loss of fingers are not included, for example, despite the output impact of such impairments. The reported prevalence of arthritis was scaled down to include only the percentage with arthritis who reported that the condition bothered them a great deal.

Table 10-5. Static or Stabilized Impairments, Latest Year Circa 1975, of Persons Usually Working

Impairments	Numbers at risk (in millions)
Selected impairments	4.4
Severe visual impairment	.1
Severe hearing impairment	.3
Paralysis	.3
Absence of major extremity	.1
Orthopedic impairment:	
Back or spine	1.3
Upper extremities and shoulders	1.2
Lower extremity and hip	.6
Other and multiple	.5
Selected chronic diseases	5.7
Asthma	1.8
Arthritis	2.0
Rheumatism	.5
Diabetes	1.4

Source: Estimated from data of the National Center for Health Statistics, DHEW. In some instances, the number has been reduced to include only those bothered a great deal or "some" by the disease. For those with hearing impairments, only those with deafness in both ears and deaf mutes are included.

What, on balance, is the yearly output loss attributable to such conditions?

In some studies, estimates were made of the earnings differentials between groups with certain types of disabilities and a similar demographic population that is "well."[1 7] These differentials, however, do not provide the yardstick needed to assess the costs of debility, since the lower earnings of the "sick" group is an aggregation of losses due to (*a*) days of lost work due to illness; (*b*) incremental unemployability among the disabled; and (*c*) reductions in hourly earnings for actual hours and weeks worked among the disabled. The last category appears useful for approximating the output loss associated with sickness and impairment. Although most studies of the impact of disability do not separate the several effects, the study by Luft, "The Impact of Poor Health on Earnings,"[1 7] specifically breaks down the losses in earnings of those with long-term disabilities into the reductions in labor force participation, weeks worked per year, hours worked per week, and earnings per hour. Using labor market models, Luft estimated the differentials for each of these variables between a "well" and a "sick" population (Table 10-6). The sick population was composed of individuals who had chronic activity limitations in their major activity. In deriving the differences in earnings variables between the well and the sick groups, Luft adjusted for the differences in the characteristics of the two populations—age, education, family type, and so on.

Using Luft's adjusted differences in earnings components between the well and sick, it is possible to estimate the earnings or production losses for disabled workers due to debility alone. What is needed is an estimate of the reduction in earnings while at work. Luft shows about a 10-percent loss in earnings per hour as a measure of output differences between the well and the sick. For those with static impairments, 4.4 million persons, we assume a loss in output of one-half this 10 percent or a total loss of 5 percent. We did not allow for the improved productivity that characterizes many impaired workers' performances or the reduced output of those with stabilized chronic diseases. The estimated loss in output is $2.7 billion on this basis. Clearly, if losses attributable to chronic diseases were taken into account, the amount would be higher.

So far, little account has been taken of chronic mental illness. The National Institute of Mental Health points out that mental disabilities are substantially underreported in the Health Interview Survey: "The number of those shown by the NCHS data as unable to carry on their major activity due to mental illness is estimated to be one-fourth of the actual number in the population. . . ."[1 8]

Table 10-6. Mean Values of Components of Earnings for "Well" Persons and the Gross and Adjusted Differences between "Well" and "Sick" Persons

	Labor force participation	Unemployment rate	Weeks worked	Hourly wage	Hours worked[1]	Weekly earnings	Earnings per year[2]
White men							
Well	.9533	.0236	46.31	3.29	43.30	139.79	6,633
Gross difference[3]	.1679	−.0217	3.98	.59	1.69	25.75	1,875
Adjusted difference[4]	.1775	−.0165	4.39	.38	1.58	18.26	1,416
Black men							
Well	.9342	.0640	44.69	2.32	40.35	93.64	4,148
Gross difference[3]	.2545	−.0320	6.45	.41	4.62	19.89	1,305
Adjusted difference[4]	.2692	−.0321	7.15	.24	4.45	12.89	1,010
White women							
Well	.5960	.0303	37.78	2.14	35.93	76.43	2,654
Gross difference[3]	.1897	−.0106	5.57	.32	2.89	16.70	951
Adjusted difference[4]	.1797	−.0096	8.16	.21	3.52	13.51	951
Black women							
Well	.7062	.0644	36.77	1.59	35.19	59.12	1,917
Gross difference[3]	.1974	−.0214	6.37	.23	7.01	18.75	877
Adjusted difference[4]	.2171	−.0221	7.73	−.06	5.46	15.96	481

[1] Estimated values for hourly wage are used in the computation of the adjusted figures for hours worked in place of the actual wage rate.

[2] Estimated values for weeks worked are used in the computation of the adjusted figures for earnings per year in place of the actual number of weeks worked.

[3] Gross difference is equal to the value for the "well" population minus the observed value for the "sick" population.

[4] Adjusted difference is equal to the value for the "well" population minus the estimated behavior for the "sick" population as computed from the regressions on the "well" population and the economic characteristics of the "sick" population.

Source: Reproduced from reference 17.

Conley, Conwell, and Willner, in "The Cost of Mental Illness, 1968," estimated that $1.9 billion was lost to the economy due to less productive employment among workers with mental illness than among other workers.[19] The increase in hourly earnings between 1968 and 1975 inflates this loss to an estimated $2.8 billion. Although this loss is not directly comparable to the productivity losses derived from Luft's estimates, they are not too dissimilar, because Conley and associates estimated the costs of excessive absenteeism and excessive unemployment among the mentally ill separately from the loss of less productive employment among mentally ill workers.

All told, the losses in output in the third category of debility (stabilized or controlled chronic impairments), conservatively estimated, are $2.7 billion for those with selected impairments and $2.8 billion for those with chronic mental illness, or a total of $5.5 billion.

We attempted still another computation to determine the order of magnitude of debility losses attributable to all chronic illnesses. Luft's analysis permits an assessment of the product loss attributable to each of the following factors: labor force participation, unemployment, hours worked per week, and hourly earnings. Assuming the labor force participation rates of disabled persons, by sex and race, used in Luft's study, we estimate a total number of disabled at 7.6 million, as indicated in Table 10-7. Their losses in product would be represented by the differences in wages per hour between well and sick workers for actual hours worked per week and number of weeks worked per year by the sick (actual time at work with impaired work capacity). In combination, these factors yield a difference between sick and well of 10 percent. The estimated debility losses of the chronically disabled are also shown in Table 10-7.

IMPACT OF DEBILITY ON OTHER COSTS OF PRODUCTION

We have thus far discussed the cost of debility in terms of the workers who are ill or disabled. These workers produce less because they are sick or raise the costs of production by their performance. Production costs are affected in a variety of ways:

- Materials are wasted
- Machinery and buildings are damaged
- Production lines are delayed
- Industrial accidents are increased
- Intergroup relations are impaired

Table 10-7. Estimated Debility Losses of the Chronically Disabled, 1975

Sex	Annual productivity losses (per person)	Number of disabled workers (thousands)	Debility losses (millions)
Males	$1,282	4,814.3	$6,173.1
Females	312	2,752.6	859.3
Total		7,566.9	7,032.4

In the pages that follow we present a summary of an analysis by Landefeld that represents an initial effort to measure the impact of illness on costs of production, using specifically industrial accidents as indicative of the costs that the sick worker imposes.[20]

Acute illness is an irritant that, among other things, diverts the worker's attention and slows his or her reflexes, thereby increasing the likelihood of an accident. As a consequence, workers other than those who are sick are also affected and industry bears additional costs.

Relevant literature on industrial safety indicates that existing models of the work injuries (Smith,[21] Chelius,[22] and Oi[23]) do not include a variable for the effects of sickness. Statistical evidence thus did not exist to confirm an inverse relationship between debility and work injuries.

As a test of the hypothesis that sickness among the workers at work causes work accidents, a regression was run on work injury rates using influenza data as the proxy for all sickness. The other explanatory variables were the relative cost of labor, the rate at which new inexperienced employees are hired, and a dummy variable for the introduction of the Occupational Safety and Health Administration in 1970. The relative cost of labor is included on the hypothesis that as the rate of labor relative to other inputs rises, the employer will presumably have a higher investment in the worker and will make investments in durable safety equipment to protect the worker.

New hire rates are used as a proxy for both inexperienced accident-prone workers and the level of business activity, since high levels of demand should be accompanied by a tight labor market and an increase in the new hire rate. The dummy variable for the introduction of OSHA was employed on the assumption that increased attention to safety would lead to greater awareness and increased reporting of accidents.

Three regressions were run (Table 10-8). The first regression uses only the three independent variables—new hires, influenza incidence,

Table 10-8. Determinants of Work Injury Rates: Fiscal Years 1961-75

1 INJ =   1.92 +   .276 NH +   .095 DIDRE +   .145 DOSH
            (11.93)   (5.53)   (2.17)   (7.93)

   R^2 = .93   DW = 2.23

2 INJ =   1.92 +   .255 NH +   .097 DIDRE +   .211 RLC1 +   .159 DOSH
            (11.64)   (4.00)   (2.14)   (0.54)   (4.96)

   R^2 = .93   DW = 2.27

3 INJ =   1.98 +   .266 NH +   .085 DIDRE +   .219 RLC2 +   .12 DOSH
            (9.20)   (4.68)   (1.69)   (0.43)   (2.82)

   R^2 = .93 DW   DW = 2.10

NOTE: These equations were estimated in a double-log linear functional form.

Variable List

INJ = Occupational injury and illness rate, per one hundred full-time employees. FY 1961-70 from Bureau of Labor Statistics data published in *Historial Statistics of the United States,* Volume 2; FY 1971-75 from Bureau of Labor Statistics data published in the *Statistical Abstract of the United States, 1976.*

NH = New hires rate per one hundred employees per month. U.S. Bureau of Labor Statistics, *Employment and Earnings,* monthly.

DIDRE = Influenza debility rate. Derived from average influenza debility data reported in *Annual Report, Division of Federal Employer Health, FY 1971-73,* and influenza incidence rates for employed persons reported by the Health Interview Survey in *Acute Conditions Incidence and Associated Disability, U.S., FY 1961-75.*

DOSH = Introduction of OSHA.

RLC1 = Relative labor cost 1. This is real wage rate divided by price index for fixed investment in durable equipment. From *Economic Report of the President,* 1977.

RLC2 = Relative labor cost 2. This is unit labor cost divided by price index for fixed investment in durable equipment.

and the introduction of OSHA as a dummy variable. New hires are used to proxy all the labor market effects, while the influenza debility rate is a proxy for the cyclical accident risk associated with minor acute illness. The other two regressions report a more complete model with two alternative specifications of the relative cost of labor, real wage rates divided by the price index for fixed investment in durable equipment (RLC1) and unit labor cost divided by the price index for fixed investment in durable equipment (RLC2).

All three regressions report similar coefficients for the effect of influenza. All of the coefficients are significant at the 80-percent level for a two-tailed hypothesis test, and two are significant at the

95-percent level. Admittedly, the data set is small and the results must be interpreted with caution, but they do seem to indicate support for the hypothesis that in years of increased sickness, there are more industrial accidents.

The magnitude of the effect of sickness may be estimated by noting that the coefficient estimates imply that debility in 1975 accounted for between 11.8 and 13.4 percent of total accident costs in that year. These percentages provide the basis for estimating the costs involved when combined with the National Safety Council estimates of the total cost of work accidents (in 1975, $16 billion). More than half of the total cost of work accidents ($10.9 billion) is represented by fire losses, insurance administration, and indirect work loss by noninjured workers. According to the National Safety Council, the cost indirectly related to work accidents "represents the money value of time lost by workers other than the injured worker. It includes the time lost in investigating accidents, writing reports, retraining workers to replace lost personnel, and disruptions of production schedules."[24, 25] The council estimates other indirect costs of work accidents in terms of time costs to other workers. These time losses were approximately equal to the costs directly related to the injuries (wage loss of injured workers, medical expenses, and insurance administration costs). As the council points out, the use of a one-to-one relationship between costs directly related to work injuries and costs indirectly related probably errs on the conservative side, since estimates by other investigators have placed the ratio as high as one to four or one to five. Also, other than fire losses associated with work injuries, no estimate is made for property damages associated with work injuries and accidents.

Of the total 1975 estimated cost of work injuries, only $5.1 billion, or that portion attributable to work-loss days of primary workers and their medical expenses, would be included in conventional estimates of the cost of illness. Yet, according to our estimates, 12 or 13 percent of the remaining $10.9 billion of insurance, fire, and production losses of other workers are attributable to the impaired functioning capacity of employees at work suffering from minor debilitating illness. In other words, $1,286 to $1,461 million of the costs of work accidents should be added to the cost of debilitating illness (Table 10-9).

SUMMARY OF DEBILITY COSTS

For the three classes of debility of primary workers, the estimates presented here total $40.9 to $50.5 billion, as indicated in Table 10-10. The figures, to recapitulate, are most approximate. The basic

Table 10-9.   Estimated Accident Costs, in Millions, Attributable to Debility, 1975

Type of cost	Estimate I (11.8 percent of total accident costs)	Estimate II (13.4 percent of total accident costs)
Total costs attributable to debility	$1,888.0	$2,144.0
Wage loss	401.2	455.6
Medical expense	200.6	227.8
Insurance administration	224.2	254.6
Fire loss	236.0	268.0
Wastage of materials and other damages	n.a.	n.a.
Other production losses (indirect)	826.0	938.0
LESS: Costs counted in conventional estimates of the cost of illness (wage loss and medical expenses)	601.8	683.4
EQUALS: Extra costs of debility	1,286.2	1,460.6

Source: Computed from National Safety Council cost data.

information needed to approximate more accurately the loss in productivity of those workers who are at work but who are sick requires data on the number of workers who are at risk and the extent of loss of their product. Additionally, there are other costs in loss of product due to debility and industrial accidents. We estimate these additional costs minimally at $1.3 to 1.5 billion.

We have tried to approach the debility loss count conservatively, aware of the extent to which the figures are judgmentally, rather than statistically, determined. In doing so, we may have greatly understated the losses—even in a nation such as the United States. In less developed nations where schistosomiasis and other infective and

Table 10-10.   Approximate Cost of Debility, by Type of Cost

Type of debility cost	Cost (in billions)
Total	$42.2-52.0
Losses of output of primary workers	40.9-50.5
Acute temporary conditions	34.5-41.5
Impairments following a major illness	0.9-3.5
Static impairments	5.5
Other losses in industrial accidents	1.3-1.5

parasitic diseases continue to be widespread, the loss in productivity due to debility is a far more serious barrier to economic development than it is in this nation.

However, in the United States, the common cold and the headache account for losses in product as large or even larger than do the several types of cancers at the various cancer sites. Debility losses due to headaches and the common cold accounted for an estimated $24 to $30 billion in production losses in 1975, while absenteeism and premature death accounted for $23 billion.

REFERENCES

1. von Ezdorf, R.H.: Demonstrations of malaria control (1916). Public Health Rep 31:614-629, 1916.

2. National Center for Health Statistics: Acute conditions: incidence and associated disability, United States, July 1974-June 1975. Vital and Health Statistics, Series 10, No. 114, 1977.

3. National Center for Health Statistics: Acute conditions: incidence and associated disability, United States, July 1974-June 1975. Vital and Health Statistics, Series 10, No. 114, 1977.

4. National Center for Health Statistics: Current estimates from the health interview survey, United States, 1975. Vital and Health Statistics, Series 10, No. 115, pp. 50-51.

5. Collins, S.D.: Age incidence of specific causes of illness. Public Health Rep 50:4, 1935.

6. van Volkenburgh, V.A., and Frost, W.H.: Acute minor respiratory diseases prevailing in a group of families residing in Baltimore, Maryland, 1928-1930. American Journal of Hygiene, January 1933.

7. Fuchs, V.R.: The contribution of health services to the American economy. *In* Essays in the economics of health and medical care, edited by V.R. Fuchs. National Bureau of Economic Research, New York, 1972.

8. Winslow, C.: The cost of sickness and the price of health. World Health Organization, Geneva, 1951.

9. For a review of the effects of schistosomiasis, see Sorkin, A.L.: Health and economic development. D.C. Heath and Company, Lexington, Mass., 1977.

10. Collins, K.J., et al.: Physiological performance and work capacity of Sudanese cane cutters with schistosoma mansoni infection. The American Journal of Tropical Medicine and Hygiene 27:410-421, 1976.

11. Weisbrod, B.A., et al.: Disease and economic development: the impact of parasitic diseases in St. Lucia. University of Wisconsin Press, Madison, 1973, pp. 81-82.

12. Reported in Task Panel Reports submitted to the President's Commission on Mental Health, Vol. II, Appendix, Washington, D.C., 1978, p. 511.

13. National Center for Health Statistics: Prevalence of chronic circulatory conditions, United States, 1972. Vital and Health Statistics, Series 10, No. 94, pp. 12, 20.

14. National Center for Health Statistics: Utilization of short-stay hospitals: annual summary for the United States, 1975. Vital and Health Statistics, Series 13, No. 31, p. 54.

15. National Center for Health Statistics: Prevalence of selected impairments, United States, 1971. Vital and Health Statistics, Series 10, No. 99; Characteristics of persons with corrective lenses, United States, 1971. Vital and Health Statistics, Series 10, No. 93.

16. National Center for Health Statistics: Selected data from Vital and Health Statistics on chronic disease from Series 10, including Nos. 112, 101, 99, 96, 94, and 92.

17. For a brief survey of this literature, see Luft, H.S.: The impact of poor health on earnings. Review of Economics 57:46, February 1975.

18. Levine, D.S., and Levine, D.R.: The cost of mental illness, 1971. National Institute for Mental Health, Series B, No. 7, Washington, D.C., 1975, p. 42.

19. Conley, R.W., Conwell, M., and Willner, S.G.: The cost of mental illness, 1968. National Institute for Mental Health, Statistical Note 30, Rockville, Md., 1970.

20. Landefeld, J.S.: Control of debility: an approach to accident prevention with benefits to industry and worker safety. Public Services Laboratory, Georgetown University, September 1978.

21. Smith, R.S.: The occupational safety and health act. American Enterprise Institute, Washington, D.C., 1976, pp. 87-104.

22. Chelius, J.R.: The control of industrial accidents: economic theory and empirical evidence. Law and Contemporary Problems 38, summer/autumn 1974.

23. Oi, W.Y.: On the economics of industrial safety. Law and Contemporary Problems 38, summer/autumn 1974.

24. National Safety Council: Accident facts. National Safety Council, Chicago, 1976.

25. National Safety Council: Estimating procedure for the annual cost of accidents. National Safety Council, Chicago, 1974, 1977.

Chapter Eleven

Trends in Health Expenditures

The concept that biomedical advances prevent disease and illness in a primary sense and accordingly reduce the costs of care stems from the results of early research. Indeed, the traditional studies of illness and of individual disease costs basically assume that the disease will be wiped out by the advances in medical sciences. Studies by Weisbrod, Mushkin, Fein, Klarman, and Rice, [1-5] among others, essentially make such an assumption. Only the medical care required to give reality to the advances in medicine is seen as an offsetting factor to the cost saving.

When the major focus of research was on the infectious and communicable diseases, this method of considering medical treatment and related expenditures seemed to be in accord with what was actually being achieved. But as the focus shifted to the chronic impairments and the development of half-way technologies, health expenditures often were enlarged rather than reduced. Indeed, research itself has come to be challenged as a contributor to the ever-advancing pace of growth in health expenditures.

The Administration's concern with cost containment has focused attention on the cost-generating impact of new medical technology. The estimated $163 billion spent for health care in 1977—and the rapid rise in that outlay—underscores the high costs of care and emphasizes the need to scrutinize the factors responsible for the growth. Some are questioning the unchecked application of new technology and are proposing action to consider the potential health cost impacts of proposed biomedical research designs.

In fact, some are urging a new review process that would mark a departure from past research policies, in that it would allow the federal government to direct the way in which biomedical research develops. The research grant, instead of being a stimulus and a support to unfettered scientific progress, would become a means of harnessing research in the interest of containing health care costs. Direction of biomedical research would be but one step among many in the reluctant but persistent move toward regulating health care to check cost increases.

The Administration is attempting in its health policies to stem the tide of mounting medical care costs in several ways. It is encouraging new delivery systems for health care, such as health maintenance organizations (HMOs); reviews of health care services provided under federal programs by Professional Standards Review Organizations (PSROs); certificates of need are being applied more rigorously to new construction or modification of health facilities; and more extensive and larger cost sharing is being proposed for third-party payment plans. A lid on hospital revenue increases is being urged to control the costs of hospital care.

Cost increases have been particularly large in hospitals where third-party payments have relaxed the financial constraints on the institution and created, as Fuchs[6] states, "an unprecedented opportunity for physicians and hospital administrators to . . . improve the quality of care as they see it. This means more equipment, more personnel, more tests, more X-rays and so on." He asks: "Are physicians and hospitals merely fulfilling their own 'technological imperative'?"

It is far from an easy task to discern the impact of research on spending for health. Earlier, we described briefly the complex interaction of sickness, utilization of health services, and mortality. We identified changes that increase sickness and those that reduce sickness in the population, bearing in mind that most uses of medical care and health expenditures, although a declining share, originate in sickness.

In this chapter and Chapter 12, we attempt to examine the factors that have contributed to increased spending for health care. Many uncertainties make this examination far from definitive. However, we conclude that health expenditures have not been increased in any major way by new medical findings and other health research from 1930 to 1975 (Figure 11-1). The capacity of health care through new research to treat and prevent deaths may have contributed somewhat to the growth in outlays in the thirty years from 1900 to 1930, but the data base is far from adequate for definitive findings. While for the more recent period research appears to have added to the rise in

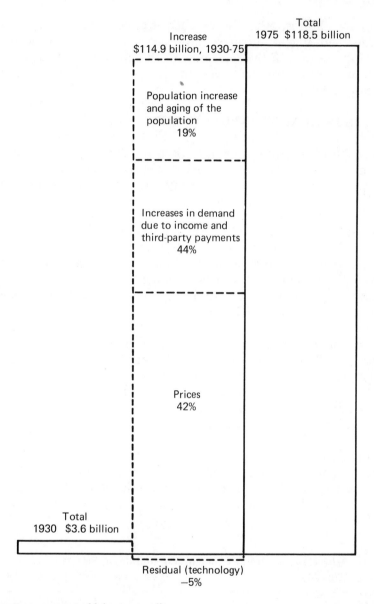

Figure 11-1. Direct Health Expenditures, 1930-75, and Factors Accounting for the Increase

Percentages may not add due to rounding.

Source: S.J. Mushkin, L.C. Paringer, and M.M. Chen: "Returns to Biomedical Research, 1900-1975: An Initial Assessment of Impacts on Health Expenditures," in R.H. Egdahl and P.M. Gertman (eds.), *Technology and the Quality of Health Care*, Aspen Systems Corp., Germantown, Md., pp. 105-120, 1978.

health expenditures, other factors such as price increases, third-party coverage, and higher incomes have been far more significant in explaining the rise. In the remainder of this chapter, we examine the growth in spending for health care in the aggregate and for categories of disease and illness.

GROWTH IN HEALTH EXPENDITURES

National health expenditures have risen rapidly since the advent of Medicare and Medicaid. Broadened third-party payments markedly influenced access to care for many low- and moderate-income families. Removal of the constraints on use that a pay-as-you-go system of health care required increased use of services. The absences of a price limitation at time of use altered demand relative to other family budget needs. While other costs, such as the pain of diagnostic and treatment methods and the loss of personal control that characterizes a patient's life in a "horizontal" position, may deter excessive use of services, growth has been characteristic of national spending for health (Table 11-1).

Demand for care, however, has been on the rise for many decades. This rise can be attributed, in part, to improved living conditions, greater availability of services, and the expanded capacity of the medical profession for diagnosis and cure.

Among the forces at work influencing expenditures for care are the health status of the population, its demographic composition, income status, inflationary trends, and environmental characteristics.

Health Status of the Population

While a part of health expenditures represents preventive health care, research, building of capacity for health services, and the like, in the main, health expenditures are made for diagnostic, therapeutic,

Table 11-1.   National Health Expenditures, in Billions, Selected Years, 1900-2000

Fiscal year	In current dollars	In constant 1975 dollars[1]
1900	$ .5	$ 5.3
1930	3.6	15.6
1963	34.3	64.2
1975	118.5	118.5
2000	1,013.6	416.4

[1] Deflated by the medical care price index.

Sources: References 36-40.

rehabilitative, and restorative health services. The amount of such health care sought reflects the health status of the population, the rates of sickness among population groups, and the basic factors of nutrition, living arrangements, neighborhood, and environment that impact on mortality and morbidity.

Health expenditures were low at the turn of the century, even when sickness rates were high. Many in the population had little access to medical care; rural communities, for example, lacked physical facilities and health personnel. Economic barriers to care were high, while substandard living conditions heightened the incidence of critical conditions and infectious diseases.

Age and Demand for Health Care

Around the averages of demand for care are wide variations by age and sex, as well as by education and other characteristics. Older persons use 2.5 to 3 times as much physician and hospital care as others in the population. Infants and young children also are relatively high users of care. Two sets of figures are summarized here—the 1930 use rates by age and sex from the Committee on Cost of Medical Care study [7, 8] and the 1975 data from the National Center for Health Statistics (Table 11-2).[9] Comparison of these data indicates the following:

- Use rates for health services have risen over the period
- The rise in use of physician services has gone up more than use of hospital care
- Rates of males has gone up more than that of females
- Younger persons used less hospital care in 1975 than in 1930 but more physician services

Income Elasticity

The shift in access to health care by family income has markedly influenced the growth in health expenditures. In 1975, physician visits per person per year were greater for the lower income families than for those with higher incomes. Access to medical care is now more evenly divided than it was before the establishment of Medicaid, Medicare, and other third-party payments. At each age group, those with family incomes of $15,000 or more in 1975 made the same or lower use of services than those with incomes of less than $5,000.

The percentage of income devoted to medical care rose as average income rose from 1900 to 1930, suggesting an income elasticity of medical care expenditures that is greater than 1 (Figure 11-2). This

Table 11-2.   Use Rates for Selected Health Services by Age and Sex,
1930, 1975

	Hospital days per 1,000 persons		Physician visits per 1,000 persons	
Age group	1930	1975	1930	1975
Total	886[1]	1,031	2,949[1]	5,052
Males	795	934	2,410	4,315
Under 17	601[2]	370	2,120[2]	4,475
17-44	668[2]	625	2,072[2]	3,527
45-64	894[2]	1,605	2,895[2]	4,727
65+	2,895	2,803	4,325	6,369
Females	950	1,121	3,423	5,738
Under 17	507[2]	311	2,059[2]	4,014
17-44	1,188[2]	1,068	3,478[2]	6,282
45-64	833[2]	1,471	4,025[2]	6,452
65+	1,155	2,642	6,185	6,775

[1] These totals are adjusted.
[2] Data for age groups as shown were not available for 1930. The numbers for 1930 are
simple averages of the following categories:

<5		15-19		45-54	
5-9	<17	20-24	17-44	55-64	45-64
10-14		25-34			
15-19		35-44			

Sources: Derived from references 7 and 8; National Center for Health Statistics: "Current
estimates from the health interview survey, United States–1975." *Vital and Health
Statistics,* Series 10, No. 115, pp. 23, 29.

result is not borne out, however, in looking at the cross-sectional
income elasticity displayed by families in the 1930 CCMC study.[10]
Estimation of the arc elasticity between the $1,600 and $7,500
income range gives us a figure of 0.9 (.89). Thus, as income increases
1 percent, expenditures by families for health care rise 0.9 percent.

The CCMC study reported average charges for medical services by
income group and distributions of charges for medical care by size.
From 1928 to 1931, average charges for all income groups combined
were $108.14. As a percentage of $108.14, the charges by income
class were as follows:

All communities, by income level	Amount	Percent average charge
All incomes	$108.14	100.0
Under $1,200	49.17	45.5
$1,200-2,000	66.81	61.8
$2,000-3,000	94.84	87.7
$3,000-5,000	137.92	127.5
$5,000-10,000	249.35	230.6
$10,000 and over	503.19	465.3

Source: Reference 10.

Characteristically, the major burden of costs of health care fall on those who incur illness. For 1930, families incurring out-of-pocket costs of $200 or more or of more than 8 percent of average income were as follows:

Income level	Percent of average income
All income groups	13.6
Under $1,200	4.8
$1,200 to 2,000	7.1
$2,000 to 3,000	12.6
$3,000 to 5,000	19.1
$5,000 to 10,000	35.9
$10,000 and over	58.1

Source: Reference 11, p. 289.

Chapin, in 1909, found similar variations in medical care spending by income group.[1][2] Of the 318 families in his study, only 5 families, in New York City, reported spending more than $100 which, when price is adjusted, is the equivalent of more than $200 in 1930.

Chapin also collected some data on health expenditures by income class, which is summarized as follows:

Family income	Annual medical care expenditures, per family
$600-699	$13.78
$700-799	14.02
$800-899	22.19
$900-999	23.30

Source: Reference 12.

The income elasticity of medical care expenditures between $650 and $950 is 1.37, suggesting that in 1909, the percentage of income devoted to health expenditures rose as income rose. The relatively small number of observations in this study makes these figures far less reliable than those in the CCMC study.

Considerable research has focused attention on estimating the income elasticity of demand for medical care. The National Center for Health Statistics presents data on health expenditures per family per year by income as follows:

Family income	Out-of-pocket expenses for family members Including health insurance premiums	Excluding health insurance premiums
Less than $5,000	$437	$329
$5,000-9,999	568	422
$10,000-14,999	706	530
$15,000 or more	911	688

Source: Reference 13.

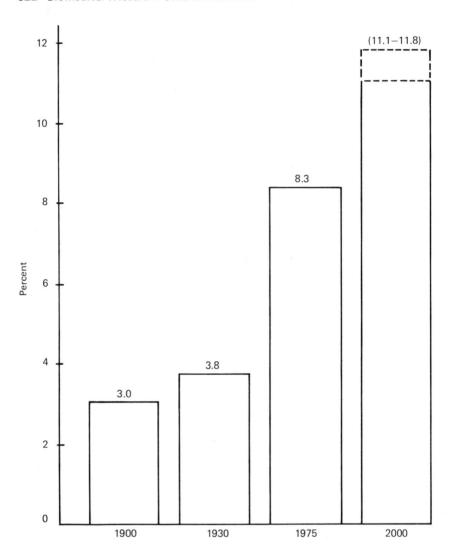

Sources: References 36, 37, 39, and 40.

Figure 11-2. Direct Costs of Illness as a Percentage of the GNP for Selected Years

The income elasticity of medical care expenditures, including health insurance premiums from $7,500 to $12,500 income, is 0.43. Even when we exclude health insurance, the elasticity is 0.45, again a figure that is considerably less than 1. Over time, access to medical care and expenditures for care have tended to depend less on high income and wealth and more on public programs.

In all of these budget studies, the income variable used is current income that includes transitory components. Andersen and Benham attempted to estimate the income elasticity of demand by using permanent income. They found that, when other factors were not controlled (price, quality, demographic variables, and preventive care), the elasticity of demand was indeed greater with the use of permanent rather than current income.[14] They also found that when they controlled for the level of illness, the permanent income elasticities tended to increase. The Benham and Andersen study restricted its focus to expenditures on physicians and dentists; however, it does suggest that one might expect to find a higher income elasticity in a time series than in a cross-sectional study. The elasticity of physicians' service expenditure with respect to income was less than unity in the analysis of changes in spending in relation to permanent income; dental care expenditures, however, were found to be highly income elastic.

From 1900 to 1930, per capita real income rose 51 percent and from 1930 to 1975, 121 percent. If we assume a unit elasticity, health expenditures would have grown 51 percent over the initial thirty years and 121 percent in the next forty-five years. If the elasticity is about half unity, the growth per capita would have been more than 25 percent from 1900 to 1936 and 60 percent in the next forty-five-year period. Clearly, the growth was greater than these elasticities would suggest (Table 11-3).

Inflationary Forces

Price increases have boosted the level of health expenditures so that the real resources used have increased by less than the aggregate numbers suggest. For all commodities, the cost of living was about one-seventh as high in 1900 as in 1977 and twice as high in 1930 as in 1900. Even modest assumptions about the future place price increases in the economy in the years ahead to the year 2000 at 3.3 to 3.6 percent per annum.

The more rapid advance of medical care prices than of prices for other goods and services has come to be a familiar characteristic. Medical care prices rose at 1.4 percentage points above the cost of living during the period 1950-65; and 1 percentage point above the cost of living since 1965. In contrast, the period of 1930 to 1950 witnessed a growth in medical prices somewhat below that of the cost of living generally. Much uncertainty surrounds any determination of comparative price changes for the first thirty years of

Table 11-3. National Health Expenditures Per Capita, Selected Years, 1900-2000

Fiscal year	In current dollars	In constant 1975 dollars[1]
1900	$ 7	$ 70
1930	30	127
1963	181	339
1975	557	557
2000	3,854	1,583

[1] Deflated by the medical care price index.

Sources: Derived from references 36-40.

the twentieth century. Data were not collected on a comprehensive basis in the first part of the century, and what is available is fragmentary. A special study for the Bureau of Labor Statistics places the overall cost of living index at 25 for 1900, compared to 50 for 1930.[15] We have estimated the rise in the medical care price index at about 127 percent over the period 1900-30 from an index of 16.5 in 1900 to 37.5 in 1930, but this figure is most approximate. Several different approaches were taken in estimating the 1900 and 1930 figures, including comparing combinations of the estimates of cost of hospital care per annum, nurses, wages, and selected drug items (see Chapter 12) and applying an estimate of physician fees developed by Ethel Hoover and CCMC data.

Price increases alone are not responsible for the increase as the adjusted-for-price figures indicate. Even at a constant price basis, national health expenditures rose from $5.3 billion in 1900 to nearly three times that, $15.6 billion, by 1930. Between 1930 and 1963, national health expenditures at 1975 prices increased more than fourfold. Even in the twelve-year period 1963-75, expenditures moved from $64.2 billion to $118.5 billion (Table 11-1).

Per capita expenditures for health care on a constant price basis testify to the magnitude of the historical change. Expenditures that even in 1975 dollars amount to only $70 per capita in 1900 nearly doubled per capita by 1930, and increased nearly five times the 1900 level by 1963. In the twenty-five years from 1975 to 2000, a further, almost threefold rise is expected, bringing to $1,583 per capita outlays for health care and related services (Table 11-3).

An unknowable factor influencing health and the cost of health care is the changing characteristics of the environment. Despite large government expenditures to guard against environmental health hazards, the crisis in energy supply and the possible relaxation of pollution standards with the possible threat of increases in carcinogenic materials in work and living environments may create new health care cost problems.

The growth in health expenditures also has claimed a rising share of the nation's economic resources, as shown in Figure 11-2; the share clearly reflects the reduction of price constraints on use of health care by American families and the shift of funding to Medicare, Medicaid, and other third-party arrangements.

ADVANCES IN KNOWLEDGE AND THE EXPENDITURE GROWTH

Have advances in knowledge about disease and about diagnosis, treatment, and prevention contributed to the mounting health care bill? What type of answer is supported by analysis of the data and studies available?

Variation in Expenditure
Growth, by Disease

The expectations of traditional studies that biomedical research would achieve cures and disease prevention is certainly suggested by the historical record for certain diseases. A number of diseases have indeed been eliminated or drastically reduced. In the aggregate, per capita real expenditures in 1975 medical care dollars for infective and parasitic diseases and certain causes of perinatal disease dropped between 1930 and 1975; the decrease was about 20 percent. But in most of the disease categories, expenditures per capita in real terms have grown, and in some the growth has been four and five times above the average. The disease categories with the largest percentage increase are diseases of the circulatory system and neoplasms (Table 11-4). The rise in spending for these diseases mirrors the shift in mortality over the decades toward the degenerative diseases.

In some cases, the reduction in health expenditures for diagnosis and treatment of a disease came after sizable public investments in water supplies and sanitation facilities and private investment in milk supplies. These costs are not reflected in the national health expenditures, but they had much to do with reduction in number of patients and health care for those with dysentery, typhoid, and malaria. For other diseases—poliomyelitis and rubella, for example—great strides have been made toward primary prevention by development of vaccines. The development of polio vaccine marked a dramatic episode in the history of medicine, along with the earlier work on whooping cough, diphtheria, and smallpox. Polio vaccine has greatly reduced the costs of the disease; the long period of chronic

Table 11-4. Real Per Capita Health Expenditures, 1975=100, by Disease Category, Selected Years, 1900-1975

Selected diseases arrayed by size of per capita expenditures, 1975	*Expenditures per capita*		
	1975	*1930*	*1900*
Total[1]	$467.09	$109.36	$67.67
Diseases of the circulatory system	75.29	3.72	6.60
Diseases of the digestive system	68.46	24.83	11.07
Mental disorders	44.24	6.28	2.91
Diseases of the respiratory system	35.59	20.38	11.75
Diseases of the nervous system and sense organs	35.06	8.97	2.82
Accidents, poisonings, and violence	32.18	8.16	4.47
Neoplasms	24.81	1.41	1.55
Diseases of the musculoskeletal system	24.03	4.36	7.09

[1] Deflated by the medical care price index.
Sources: References 37, 39, and 40.

impairment following costly hospitalization has been checked, and the number of cases has dropped markedly, although there is concern about the percentage of children who are now unvaccinated.

Rubella, which can lead to congenital defects in children, including deaf-mutism, eye and heart disease, and possibly mental retardation if the mother contracts the disease during the early stages of pregnancy, can now be prevented. Less than a decade ago, the first of the vaccine was tested.

Secondary prevention or disease control also has been furthered by research. In some ways, the control measures that do not prevent disease but provide a treatment or lessen the deterioration or part of it are far more significant now than they were earlier, largely because of the progress already made on primary prevention of many infectious and parasitic diseases. Antibiotics are an example of a treatment that originated in medical research but tended to lower cost of illness. However, in some cases, the health care cost has been raised by new procedures and new equipment.

Cost of Disease, Per Patient

Another approach focuses on medical care costs per patient by diagnosis. Scitovsky and McCall re-analyzed data on the cost of care in the Palo Alto Medical Clinic for selected illnesses for the years 1951, 1967, and 1971 to document the change in real inputs (after price adjustment) for those illnesses.[16] Data were analyzed on treatments for otitis media, acute appendicitis, maternity care, breast cancer, forearm fractures, pneumonia, duodenal ulcer, and myocardial infarction.

Scitovsky and McCall's findings permit comparisons for selected disease categories of average costs of treatment, with prices held constant, to arrive at a measure of changes in quantity, quality, or scope of services. The mean averages of 1964 treatment costs, in 1971 prices, are shown in Table 11-5.

The Scitovsky-McCall data show reductions in cost for maternity care, cancer of the breast, and nonhospital care for pneumonia and duodenal ulcer. The reductions in maternity care costs are attributed to reductions in hospital stays, from an average 3.8 days per case in 1964 to 2.8 days in 1971, and the rise in the percentage of deliveries without a general anesthetic. For cancer of the breast, reduced hospital stay again was a factor, as well as partial substitution of modified mastectomies for radical mastectomies, at a somewhat lower surgical fee. For the pneumonias and duodenal ulcers, physician visits were reported to decline, and a small reduction in X rays was reported, along with somewhat less expensive laboratory tests.

The major increases are shown for treatment of myocardial infarction and fractures treated by closed reduction with no general anesthetic. In the latter instance, the authors suggest advances in treatment that permitted a larger share of patients to be treated as outpatients (in and out of the hospital in one day), with considerable cost saving. Intensive care of cardiac patients, however, has spread considerably since 1964, with an attendant rise in laboratory tests,

Table 11-5. Mean Averages of Treatment Costs, in 1971 Prices

	Treatment methods		
	1964	*1971*	*Percentage change per annum, 1964-71*
Disease category	*(1971 prices)*		
Otitis media (children)	$ 24	$ 25	0.6
Appendicitis			
Simple	1,040	1,063	0.3
Perforated	1,812	2,062	1.9
Maternity care	881	807	−1.2
Cancer of the breast	2,582	2,557	−0.7
Forearm fractures			
Cast only	94	97	0.4
Closed reduction, no general anesthetic	199	246	3.0
Myocardial infarction	2,461	3,780	4.2
Pneumonia (nonhospital care)	99	85	−2.1
Duodonal ulcer (nonhospital care)	212	187	−1.8

Source: Reference 13.

electrocardiograms, intravenous feedings, X rays, and inhalation therapies.

Generally, use of drugs and laboratory tests rose, while the number of days of hospital care declined. These data pose an important question: To what extent do reduced days of hospital care result from improved surgical techniques and the biomedical advances that these techniques reflect? Similarly, the query arises as to the effectiveness of the increased X ray and laboratory tests and the use of intravenous solutions, electrocardiograms, and inhalation therapies—factors that have raised costs of care.

The use of 1971 prices for each item of treatment does not free the data entirely from the effect of medical advances, because 1971 prices for any class of treatment—a day of hospital care, a physician's office visit, a chest X ray, a particular laboratory test—already reflect the impact of medical advances on those prices. The percentage change per year attributable to medical advances between 1964 and 1971 is thus somewhat understated.

To broaden the consideration, we show the following average charges in 1930 by diagnostic group for classes of diagnoses for which there is some, even though approximate, similarity between the CCMC data[7] and the Scitovsky-McCall data.

Diagnostic category	1971 (1971 prices)	1930 (priced at 1971 BLS prices)
Maternity care	$ 807	$394
Diseases of the ear and mastoid	25	82
Cancer	2,557	870
Pneumonia	85	218

The data are suggestive rather than truly comparable. The comparisons essentially point to a need for far more analysis of the net impact of technological advances on the cost of illness to obtain more accurate data about the relation between such advances and health care costs.

In one of our Public Services Laboratory (PSL) studies (still in process), data for 1930, from the work of Lee and Jones[17] on use of physicians, hospitals, drugs, and other medical services for the diagnosis and treatment of selected diseases under high 1930 standards of quality of care, is being compared to estimates of use of services in a similar 1970 study by Schonfeld and others at Yale University.[18] The incompleteness of the 1970 materials requires great caution in their use without extensive supplementation.

A first cut on findings, however, supports the Scitovsky analysis that the changes over time in real resource use vary by disease or illness. However, unlike the Scitovsky findings that emphasize increases, the PSL findings indicate only that changes in real costs, on balance, depend on the diseases assessed. The 1930/1970 comparisons show that a large number of diseases with high prevalence in 1930 are similar to pneumonia and maternity care in the Scitovsky study, and resources declined rather than increased over the period. Differences in general findings are probably a function of the shift in base year of comparison. In 1930, many infectious and communicable diseases required substantial hospitalization and physician services; preventive measures and drug-specific therapies have reduced costs considerably for those diseases.

Table 11-6 shows the most expensive causes of illness in 1930 and the percent of all charges represented by those diseases. Comparable figures for 1975 are not available. The multiplicity of funding sources has made it difficult to compile data on costs of medical care by type of illness. An approximation of comparative ranking for 1930 and 1975 is that presented below, drawing on Tables 11-6 and 11-8. We have identified diseases for which the categories may be reasonably similar.

	Percent of total charges 1930	*Percent of total health expenditures*	
		1930	*1975*
Cancer	1.7	1.3	5.3
Pregnancy and perinatal morbidity	9.2	5.8	3.5
Diseases of the genitourinary system	3.3 (female only)	4.4	5.6
Diseases of the circulatory system	2.5	3.4	16.1
Diseases of the oral cavity	20.4	15.8	7.8
Diseases of the respiratory system	8.9 (minor plus pneumonia only)	18.6	7.6

The comparisons suggest reductions in health care and in the cost of pregnancy, respiratory diseases, and dental diseases. Increases are suggested for cancer, diseases of the genitourinary system, and diseases of the circulatory system. Again, the improvement in health care for the acute diseases and shifts to chronic diseases that afflict the population today are indicated.

Table 11-6.   Medical Care for the Most Expensive Cause of Illness, 1930

Illness	Average charge per case	Percent of total charges
Total		
Cancer	$342	1.7
Appendicitis	168	5.8
Hernia and intestinal obstruction	132	1.4
Confinement, abortion, and miscarriage	95	9.2
Diseases of the gall bladder	80	1.8
Nonvenereal diseases of female genitourinary system	63	3.3
Pneumonia	59	1.7
Diseases of the heart and arteries	50	2.5
Rheumatism	31	1.3
Diseases of the ear and mastoid process	30	2.3
Care of teeth	19	20.4
Minor respiratory	6	7.2
Health and checkup examination	3	1.1

Source: Reference 10, p. 105.

Capital Cost Growth

Still other methods are used to assess the issue, namely, the growth in capital costs associated with medical care. Examples of high-cost capital equipment, such as CAT scanners or cardiac intensive care units in hospitals, emphasize the role of capital equipment as a factor in the rise of health care costs.[19]

Are capital costs the villain in the skyrocketing of medical care costs? Against the backdrop of testimony before the President's Biomedical Research Panel, which claimed that "at least half of the increase in hospital expenditures (between 1965 and 1975) is related to more intensive use of real resources" rather than price,[20] a review was undertaken of what is known about technology's impact on costs.

According to the review by Rycroft and Vehorn, discussions of technology seem to be restricted to capital-intensive equipment.[21] However, sometimes any factor "not otherwise accounted for" is labeled technology. Indeed, any change in process is included in that category from one perspective: technology is not consistently defined in the literature. A technological change is used, at times, to refer to any change in resources used—ranging from additional laboratory tests (including more frequent use of the same kind of test) to fully equipped intensive care units. New drug therapies, new surgical instruments, new hearing aids, and prosthetic devices are included.

Technology defined as a change in resources used is not synonymous with knowledge advances of biomedical research findings. Repeated use of the same laboratory test for a patient, for example, does not necessarily come about as a result of either better understanding about disease or some research finding. Rather, repeated use of a test may be a safeguard against malpractice suits, or it may result from the greater weight given to "science" in medicine and the tendency of residents in hospitals and other providers to read test results as "objective" measures of the condition of the patient. Medical education and depersonalized medical care, aided by third-party coverage, may be responsible for more medical services.

As Davis emphasized several years ago,[22] given the cost pass-through of reimbursement for hospital care, there is little incentive to adopt innovations that reduce costs. With third-party payments, demand responds more or less automatically to technological change, in the way of new products or more repetitive application of diagnostic or therapeutic methods.

Earlier studies have been hampered, in determining the impact of new technology, by the difficulties of measuring changes in output (or patient outcomes) and by lack of yardsticks or measures of technology.

Most of the major studies of technology and medical care costs, including some of the more recent studies, deal with hospital costs only. While hospital costs are a substantial part of health care costs, these hospital costs omit sixty cents out of each dollar of health expenditures. Studies by a number of experts are confined to hospital care, for example, the study by Lave and Lave,[23] Feldstein,[24] Anderson and May,[25] Salkever,[26] Davis,[27] and Worthington.[28] Both the analysis by Feldstein and Taylor for the Council on Wage and Price Stability[29] and the Congressional Budget Office analysis[30] are also confined to hospital costs. The study by Fuchs and Kramer[31] however, deals with physician services, and that of Worthington[28] includes physician services as well as hospital care.

To illustrate the findings, the regression analysis by Davis[27] shows that demand variables (insurance, real income per capita, population density, and other demographic characteristics, and physicians and hospitals per capita) accounted for 45 percent of the rise in hospital expenses; case-mix variables, for 7 percent; wages (payroll expenses per full-time employee), for 10 percent; and technology, for 38 percent. Technology in this analysis is a time-trend variable for the period 1962-68. Feldstein and Taylor[29] found that technology, measured by nonpayroll costs deflated by price, added 7.2 percent to the annual growth rate of hospital costs. (Hospital labor costs rose 9 percent per year and nonlabor costs, 11 percent, of which 3.6 percent was price and the remainder, technology.)

Economic incentives under insurance plans drive all costs up in the delivery of covered health services. The incentive structure is such that it leads to cost-raising rather than cost-saving innovation. In this regard, insurance in health care is similar to procurement in the Department of Defense. Incentives to continuously change the product are induced by insurance that allows both physician and patient to demand the "best possible care" with little regard to costs.

The basic analysis in several of these studies is based on the relationship of payroll to nonpayroll costs. If nonpayroll costs rise faster than payroll costs, capital outlays are a primary cause of cost inflation.

"Nonpayroll expenses" (as reported by the American Hospital Association), the basic data in a number of the studies, are defined, however, to include intern and resident pay, payroll supplements, interest charges, food expenditures, and so forth. Intern and resident pay represents a real labor factor cost. Payroll supplements similarly are a labor factor cost. Changes in interest over time are influenced by the shift in sources of funds for capital outlays of hospitals from grants to loans and do not reflect a change in real capital use. To the extent that food and laundry are provided under contract, payroll costs associated with food preparation and laundry may be included in nonpayroll costs. Until comparable data over time are applied in analysis, the results with respect to technology and health costs will remain unclear.

Health care, however, over the historical period, has not been an exception to the characteristic growing capital intensity nor is it an exception to the requirements for more complex personnel skills for the more complex machines. The striking contrast between yesterday's physician carrying his "little black bag" on visits to ailing patients and the present-day hospital clinic or physician's office makes clear that health care has become more capital intensive. Far larger sums are invested in facilities and equipment, and the professional and related skills have broadened, with respect to numbers of occupations and amount and scope of training required.

For most of the occupational groups engaged in the provision of health care, there is more equipment today per professional person. But pharmacists possibly have less capital equipment now than in 1900 because of the change in method of compounding drugs, and private duty nurses generally may work with only slightly more equipment.

More capital intensity does not mean upward pressures on costs of care. For industry in general, capital intensity tends to be indicative of possible economies of scale. And R&D in industry is often intended to lower costs of production. Research in the health sciences also has a cost-reducing aspect for second-, third-, and fourth-generation equipment. X-ray machines today, for example, are less complex and costly than the early models. New devices in some instances reduce the cost of care and enhance quality at the same time. Dental drilling equipment illustrates a change of this type, and microblood specimens and mutagenesis testing for carcinogens in industry are still further examples.

PATTERNS OF HEALTH CARE

The technological and institutional structure of health care has changed markedly over the years. The early part of this century witnessed implementation of basic public health measures; reform of medical education to improve medical research and clinical teaching; the development of special hospitals for mental illness, tuberculosis, and contagious diseases; and the gradual emergence of the medical center.

The shift in relative importance of hospital and physicians' services represents one aspect of medical technology that gives far greater importance to the medical center as the hub of patient care, research, and physician education. Physician and hospital care services accounted for almost sixty cents of each dollar spent for health care in 1975. However, when physician care is represented as an index using 100 as the unit and other health expenditures are represented as a fraction of that unit, it becomes plain that hospital care expenditures in 1975 were more than twice those for physician care; in 1930, they were lower (Figure 11-3).

Between 1900 and 1930, expenditures for hospital care changed very little, compared to physicians' services. When computed as a share of total health expenditures, hospital care was 18 percent of the total in both 1900 and 1930 (Table 11-7). By 1975, hospital care accounted for almost 40 percent of national health expenditures, roughly a doubling of the share of outlays since 1930. Hospital use indeed was in a stage of transition in 1930. As Carpenter pointed out in his review for the Committee on Costs of Medical Care, "Not many years ago the problem of the hospitalization of patients of moderate means scarcely existed . . . there were few patients of moderate means in hospitals. . . . Today this situation has been radically altered. . . . Patients of all social groups, the moderately well-to-do no less than the rich and the poor, are seeking hospital care in ever increasing numbers."[32] By 1940, hospital expenditures climbed above spending for physicians' services. Writing about these changing trends, Falk and associates noted: "Just as office practice has largely moved from the physician's home to a retail business district, so has the care of many bed patients been transferred from the patient's home to the hospital."[10] Both of these trends have opened possibilities, the authors continue, "for the development of more efficient technical procedures, as well as for the conservation of the time and resources of a busy practitioner." In the 1930s also, Lewinski-Cowin noted that

> the complicated techniques of modern medicine and modern surgery require elaborate apparatus and laboratory services for diagnostic and therapeutic purposes; as techniques have developed, the costs of hospital maintenance have mounted steadily. In the United States, the average daily cost of maintaining a patient, exclusive of interest on capital investment and depreciation charges, is about $5.00 in a hospital for acute conditions and about $3.00 in a hospital for the care of patients afflicted with chronic maladies.[33]

In 1900, per diem costs of short-term hospital care were half the 1930 level of around $2.25 to $2.50, varying by region and hospital. In 1975, these daily costs were $151.

The position of dentists' services has altered relative to physicians' services in the past seventy-five years, moving from 27 percent of expenditures for physicians' services in 1900 to 34 percent in 1975. However, by looking at the entire span of time, we miss the fact that in 1930, expenditures for dentists' services had risen to almost half of those for physicians' services. (Table 11-6 illustrates the importance of dental care to total charges in 1930.)

One observer, commenting on the development of dentistry between 1900 and 1930, wrote: "If we should compare the patients waiting in a dentists' office, about the year 1900, with such patients at the present time, we would find that the swollen faces and miserable countenances of the earlier years have largely disappeared. . . . With the passing of time, the importance of dentistry and oral hygiene to general health has come to be recognized."[34]

As indicated earlier, between 1930 and 1975, dental expenditures declined relative to those for physicians' services. This decline may be explained at least in part by the fact that dentistry remained, throughout the period, a component of health care for which use was constrained by price and differences in income. These two factors contributed to the wide variations in patients' use. In contrast, hospital and physicians' services were increasingly covered by third-

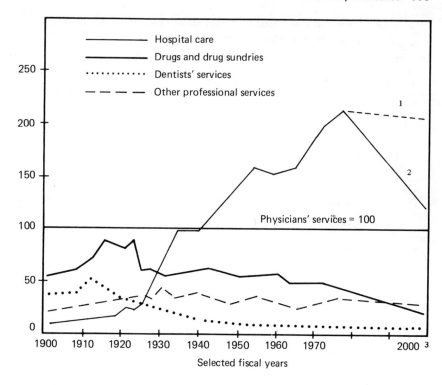

Figure 11-3. Expenditures for Health Care Relative to the Cost of Physicians' Services, 1900-2000

[1] Dotted line assumes hospital prices rise 3 percent more per year than general prices.
[2] Dashed line assumes 1.2 percent faster.
[3] Year 2000 estimates are made assuming enactment of national health insurance.
Source: Reference 36.

party payments. As a share of total health expenditures, dental expenditures went from 10.4 percent in 1900 to 13.2 percent in 1930 and back down to 6.3 percent in 1975.

Still another major shift in relative importance occurred in drug expenditures. Drug outlays have declined as a proportion of total health expenditures; more drugs are being sold by prescriptions, and a larger share of those are prepared by the drug manufacturers. In 1975, drugs and drug sundries accounted for 8.9 percent of total national health expenditures; in 1930, they were 16.6 percent; and in 1900, still a higher share, 21.2 percent. Relative to expenditures for physicians' services, drug expenditures have not changed as much, moving from 54 percent of physician expenditures in 1900 to 60 percent in 1930 and back down to 48 percent in 1975. Increased use

Table 11-7. Percent Allocation of Direct Health Expenditures, by Class of Expenditures, 1900, 1930, 1975

Class of expenditure	Percent allocation of expenditures		
	1900	1930	1975
Total	100.0	100.0	100.0
Hospital care	18.1	18.2	39.3
Physicians' services	39.2	27.6	18.6
Dentists' services	10.4	13.2	6.3
Other professional services	5.8	6.9	1.8
Drugs and drug sundries	21.2	16.6	8.9
Eyeglasses and appliances	2.0	3.7	1.9
Nursing home care	—	—	7.6
Expenses for prepayment and administration	—	3.0	3.9
Government public health activities	3.3	2.6	2.9
Other health services	—	2.5	2.5
Research	—	—	2.3
Construction	—	5.7	3.8
Public			1.1
Private			2.7

Sources: References 37, 39, and 40.

of hospitals for care and the use of drugs in hospitals may account for the recent period's small decline.

More dramatic than the change in relative expenditures for drugs is the shift in type of drug outlays. In 1975, three-quarters of all drug expenditures were for prescribed drugs and the remaining one-quarter, nonprescribed drugs. In 1930, the proportions were reversed; about three-quarters of drug purchases represented home remedies and over-the-counter purchases. For 1900, the estimated division was 70 percent, nonprescribed drugs, 30 percent, prescribed drugs. "The usual expenditure for medicine, when there is no long illness in the family, is about $5 for household remedies, such as salts, magnesia, and cough medicine," wrote More in her study of Wage-Earners' Budgets, initiated in November 1903.[35] Some 200 families were surveyed, 50 of whom kept accounts on behalf of the inquiry. In 1930, the expenditures, as reflected in charges for medicine, amounted to $14.33 per family buying medicines. By 1975, family purchases of drugs reached $149 per family.

The share of outlays for nursing services, included among other professional services, has declined over the years. The aggregate share for professional services has dropped, despite the large number of professions represented. The share for private-duty nursing has declined even more. Private-duty nursing accounted for almost half the amount spent for physician care at the turn of the century, but by 1977 it had dropped to a small fraction of costs.

EXPENDITURES, BY DISEASE CATEGORY

Spending by cause of illness has changed over the years, as have incidence, diagnosis, and therapies. Table 11-8 presents estimates of aggregate health expenditures by disease category in 1900, 1930, and 1975; Table 11-9 details the percentage distribution of those expenditures; and Table 11-10 shows the per capita expenditures by category in current dollars.

Expenditures for diseases and other cause-of-illness categories have changed as therapies have changed and as the mix of health services used in the diagnosis and treatment of disease has been modified. Not only have treatments changed, but also diagnosis of disease and classification of diseases as revisions have been made in the International Classification of Diseases.

Does spending for health care mirror the sickness in the population? In general, expenditure patterns do reflect illnesses, and changes in relative expenditures tend to mirror the differences in mortality and morbidity.

The order of rankings of expenditures changed markedly by 1975. On the one hand, expenditures for complications of pregnancy declined in relative importance as did outlays for infective and parasitic diseases. On the other hand, a far larger share of outlays was attributable to diseases of the circulatory system and to mental disorders. In 1975, respiratory diseases claimed less than half the share of expenditures that they had in 1930. Neoplasms that by 1975 represented the second largest cause of death ranked eighth in order of expenditures.

How, we ask, have direct expenditures for health care changed by causes of illness during the years of great biomedical advances? By 1975, health expenditures were less concentrated in a few disease categories than they had been earlier. While diseases of the digestive system continued to be important in terms of expenditures, accounting for 14.7 percent of all health expenditures, diseases of the respiratory system had fallen considerably in relative importance. By 1975, only 7.6 percent of health expenditures were made for respiratory ailments compared to 18.6 percent in 1930 and 17.3 percent in 1900. Expenditures for infective and parasitic diseases showed the greatest decline in relative importance by 1975, moving from 15 percent of total expenditures in 1900 to only 2 percent in 1975. A notable change from 1900 and 1930 to 1975 was the

Table 11-8. Direct Health Expenditures, in Millions, by Disease Category, 1900, 1930, 1975

Disease category	Health expenditures (allocated amounts only)		
	1900	*1930*	*1975*
Total[1]	$526	$3,132	$99,374
Infective and parasitic diseases	80	340	2,027
Neoplasms	12	40	5,279
Endocrine, nutritional, and metabolic diseases	1	55	3,337
Diseases of the blood and blood-forming organs	1	15	676
Mental disorders	23	180	9,411
Diseases of the nervous system and sense organs	22	257	7,459
Eye diseases[2]	(−)	(156)	(4,648)
Diseases of the circulatory system	51	107	16,017
Cerebrovascular diseases[2]	(19)	(9)	(2,633)
Diseases of the respiratory system	91	583	7,571
Diseases of the digestive system	86	711	14,564
Diseases of the oral cavity, salivary glands, and jaws[2]	(−)	(494)	(7,777)
Diseases of the genitourinary system	23	138	5,575
Complications of pregnancy, childbirth, and puerperium	37	169	3,387
Diseases of the skin and subcutaneous tissue	4	77	2,120
Diseases of the musculoskeletal system and connective tissue	55	125	5,113
Congenital anomalies	1	11	432
Certain causes of perinatal morbidity and mortality	−	11	64
Symptoms and ill-defined conditions	4	45	3,180
Accidents, poisonings, and violence	35	233	6,846
Other	−	35	6,316

[1] Totals may not add due to rounding.
[2] Included in previous total.
Sources: References 37, 39, and 40.

increase in importance of diseases of the circulatory system, which account for the largest share of health expenditures today.

Table 11-9 shows the percentage distribution estimated for direct health expenditures for each of the years 1900, 1930, and 1975. The total expenditures per capita by illness category are shown in Table 11-10.

Little change occurred between 1900 and 1930 in the diseases which claimed a major share of expenditures. However, in 1930, digestive diseases ranked ahead of respiratory diseases, perhaps owing to the greater use of dental services in 1930 than in 1900.

Diseases of the respiratory system ranked second in 1930 but claimed first place in expenditures for 1900. Relative expenditures

Table 11-9. Distribution of Direct Health Expenditures, by Disease Category, 1900, 1930, 1975

Disease	Percent distribution		
	1900	*1930*	*1975*
Total[1]	100.0	100.0	100.0
Infective and parasitic diseases	15.2	10.9	2.0
Neoplasms	2.3	1.3	5.3
Endocrine, nutritional, and metabolic diseases	.2	1.8	3.4
Diseases of the blood and blood-forming organs	.2	0.5	0.7
Mental disorders	4.4	5.7	9.5
Diseases of the nervous system and sense organs	4.2	8.2	7.5
Eye diseases[2]	(−)	(5.0)	(4.7)
Diseases of the circulatory system	9.7	3.4	16.1
Cerebrovascular diseases[2]	(3.6)	(0.3)	(2.6)
Diseases of the respiratory system	17.3	18.6	7.6
Diseases of the digestive system	16.3	22.7	14.7
Diseases of the oral cavity, salivary glands, and jaws[2]	(−)	(15.8)	(7.8)
Diseases of the genitourinary system	4.4	4.4	5.6
Complications of pregnancy, childbirth, and puerperium	7.0	5.4	3.4
Diseases of the skin and subcutaneous tissue	.8	2.5	2.1
Diseases of the musculoskeletal system and connective tissue	10.5	4.0	5.1
Congenital anomalies	−	0.4	0.4
Certain causes of perinatal morbidity and mortality	.2	0.4	0.1
Symptoms and ill-defined conditions	.8	1.4	3.2
Accidents, poisonings, and violence	6.7	7.4	6.9
Other	−	1.1	6.4

[1] Totals may not add due to rounding.
[2] Included in previous total.
Sources: References 37, 39, and 40.

for complications of pregnancy and childbirth dropped off somewhat between 1900 and 1930. Expenditures for mental disorders were among the highest in 1930 but not in 1900; in contrast, diseases of the musculoskeletal system and connective tissue were among the top 80 percent in 1900 but not in 1930.

In 1930, as in 1900, diseases of the respiratory system, the digestive system, and infective and parasitic diseases continued to be important in terms of the share of direct expenditures devoted to them. In 1900, these three groups of diseases accounted for 48.8

Table 11-10. Per Capita Health Expenditures, by Disease Category, 1900, 1930, 1975

Disease category	Per capita health expenditures (allocated amounts only)		
	1900	1930	1975
Total[1]	$6.97	$25.59	$467.09
Infective and parasitic diseases	1.06	2.77	9.53
Neoplasms	.16	.33	24.81
Endocrine, nutritional, and metabolic diseases	.01	.45	15.69
Diseases of the blood and blood-forming organs	.01	.12	3.18
Mental disorders	.30	1.47	44.24
Diseases of the nervous system and sense organs	.29	2.10	35.06
Eye diseases	(−)	(1.27)	21.85
Diseases of the circulatory system	.68	.87	75.29
Cerebrovascular diseases[2]	(.25)	(.08)	(12.38)
Diseases of the respiratory system	1.21	4.77	35.59
Diseases of the digestive system	1.14	5.81	68.46
Diseases of the oral cavity, salivary glands, and jaws[2]	(−)	(4.03)	(36.55)
Diseases of the genitourinary system	.30	1.13	26.20
Complications of pregnancy, childbirth, and puerperium	.49	1.38	15.92
Diseases of the skin and subcutaneous tissue	.05	.63	9.96
Diseases of the musculoskeletal system and connective tissue	.73	1.02	24.03
Congenital anomalies	.01	.09	2.03
Certain causes of perinatal morbidity and mortality	−	.09	.30
Symptoms and ill-defined conditions	.05	.37	14.95
Accidents, poisonings, and violence	.46	1.91	32.18
Other	−	.29	29.69

[1] Totals may not add due to rounding.
[2] Included in previous total.
Sources: Derived from references 37, 39, and 40.

percent of direct health expenditures, and in 1930, they represented 52.2 percent of direct health expenditures.

The level of expenditure for each time period is, of course, considerably different. The per capita health outlay of $467 in 1975 contrasts sharply with the less than $7 per capita in 1900. By disease class, the variation among the years is more diverse. About $1 per capita was spent on each of the categories that were so important in the mortality and morbidity of 1900 (infective and parasitic diseases, respiratory diseases, and digestive diseases); those sums had grown to

$36 per capita for respiratory disease care in 1975 and $68 for digestive diseases. Even infective and parasitic diseases, despite the marked decline in incidence, totaled almost $10 per capita. Diseases of the circulatory system for which spending averaged about 68 cents in 1900 grew to $75 for 1975. Neoplasms, which claimed 16 cents per capita in 1900, grew to almost $25 per capita by 1975.

As shown in Figure 11-4, projections for the year 2000 show that 45 percent of the total outlay is expected to go for the five major disease categories, in this order of importance: circulatory, digestive, mental, respiratory, and neoplasms.[36]

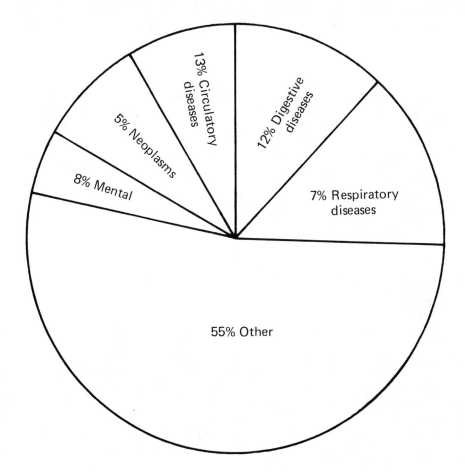

Figure 11-4. Direct Costs of Health Care, Year 2000

REFERENCES

1. Weisbrod, B.A.: Costs and benefits of medical research: a case study of poliomyelitis. J of Pol Econ 79: 527-544, May-June 1971.
2. Mushkin, S.J.: Health as an investment. J of Pol Econ 70: 129-157, October 1962.
3. Fein, R.: The economics of mental illness. Basic Books, New York, 1959.
4. Klarman, H.E.: Syphilis control programs in measuring benefits of public investments. *In* Measuring benefits of government expenditures, edited by R. Dorfman. Brookings Institution, Washington, D.C., 1965, pp. 367-414.
5. Rice, D.P.: Economic costs of cardiovascular diseases and cancer, 1962. *In* Report to the President, A national program to conquer heart disease, cancer and stroke, vol. 2. U.S. Government Printing Office, Washington, D.C., February 1965, pp. 439-630.
6. Fuchs, V.R.: Who shall live? Health, economics and social choice. Basic Books, New York, 1974, pp. 94-95.
7. Collins, S.: Hospital care for specific diseases. Reprint No. 2405, Public Health Rep 57: 1399-1428, Sept. 18, 1942, and 1439-1460, Sept. 25, 1942.
8. _____. Frequency and volume of doctors' calls among males and females in 9,000 families based on nationwide periodic canvasses, 1928-31. Reprint No. 2205. Public Health Rep 55: 1977-2020, Nov. 1, 1940.
9. National Center for Health Statistics: Current estimates from the health interview survey, United States 1974. Vital and Health Statistics, Series 10, No. 100.
10. Falk, I.S., Rorem, R., and Ring, M.: The costs of medical care: a summary of investigations on the economic aspects of the prevention and care of illness. University of Chicago Press, Committee on the Costs of Medical Care Publication No. 27, January 1933.
11. Falk, I.S., Klem, M.C., Sinai, N.: The incidence of illness and the receipt and costs of medical care among representative family groups. University of Chicago Press, Committee on the Costs of Medical Care Publication No. 26, January 1933.
12. Chapin, R.C.: The standard of living among workingmen's families in New York City. Charities Publication Committee, New York, 1909, p. 186.
13. National Center for Health Statistics: Family out-of-pocket health expenses, United States, 1970. Vital and Health Statistics Series 10, No. 103, p. 10.
14. Andersen, R., and Benham, L.: Factors affecting the relationship between family income and medical care consumption. *In* Empirical studies in health economics, edited by H.E. Klarman. The Johns Hopkins Press, Baltimore, Md., 1976.
15. U.S. Bureau of the Census: Historical statistics of the United States: colonial times to 1970. Bicentennial ed. Part 1. Washington, D.C., September 1975, p. 211.
16. Scitovsky, A.A., and McCall, N.: Changes in the costs of treatment of selected illness, 1951-1964-1971. NCHSR, Research Digest Series, DHEW Publication No. (HRH)77-3161, July 1976.

17. Lee, R.I., Jones, L.W., and Jones, B.: The fundamentals of good medical care. University of Chicago Press, Committee on the Costs of Medical Care, Chicago, 1933.

18. Schonfeld, H.K., Heston, J.F., and Falk, I.S.: Standards for good medical care: based on the opinions of clinicians associated with the Yale-New Haven Medical Center with respect to 242 diseases. Volume I-IV. DHEW Publication No. (SSA) 75-11926, February 1975.

19. Hearings on HR 6575, March 3-7, 1977. Proposed legislation concerning containment of hospital costs.

20. Gaus, C.R.: Biomedical research and health care costs. Testimony of the Social Security Administration before the President's Biomedical Research Panel, September 1975, p. 3.

21. Rycroft, R.S., and Vehorn, C.L.: Medical cost and medical technology: a review of selected literature. Public Services Laboratory staff report, Georgetown University, Washington, D.C., August 1977.

22. Davis, K.: The role of technology demand and labor markets in the determination of hospital costs. *In* The economics of health and medical care, edited by M. Perlman. John Wiley & Sons, New York, 1974, pp. 283-301.

23. Lave, J., and Lave, L.: Hospital cost functions. Am Econ Rev 60: 379-395, June 1970.

24. Feldstein, M.: The rising cost of hospital care. Information Resources Press, Washington, D.C., 1971.

25. Anderson, R., and May, J.J.: Factors associated with the increasing cost of hospital care. The Annals. The American Academy of Political Science, 1972.

26. Salkever, D.: A micro-economic study of hospital cost inflation. J of Pol Econ 80: 1144-66, November-December 1972.

27. Davis, K.: Theories of hospital inflation: some empirical evidence. Journal of Human Resources 8: 181-201, Spring 1973.

28. Worthington, N.L.: Expenditures for hospital care and physicians' services: factors affecting annual changes. Soc Sec Bull, 3-15, November 1975.

29. Feldstein, M., and Taylor, A.: The rapid rise of hospital costs. Executive Office of the President, Council on Wage and Price Stability, Staff report, January 1977.

30. Congressional Budget Office: Expenditures for health care: federal programs and their effects. Washington, D.C., August 1977.

31. Fuchs, V.R., and Kramer, M.J.: Determinants of expenditures for physicians' services in the United States, 1948-1968. National Center for Health Services Research and Development, December 1972.

32. Carpenter, N.: Hospital services for patients of moderate means: a study of certain American hospitals. University of Chicago Press, Committee on Costs of Medical Care Publication No. 4, April 1930.

33. Lewinski-Cowin, E.H.: Hospitals. Encyclopedia of the social sciences. The Macmillan Company, New York, 1937 edition.

34. Allen, P.: Medical facilities in the United States. Committee on Costs of Medical Care Publication No. 3, Washington, D.C., 1929, p. 29.

35. More, L.B.: Wage earners' budgets: a study of standards and cost of living

in New York City. Greenwich House Series of Social Studies, No. 1. Henry Hott and Company, New York, 1907.

36. Mushkin, S.J., et al.: Cost of illness and disease in the United States in the year 2000. Public Health Rep 93: 493-588, September-October 1978.

37. Paringer, L.C., and Berk, A.: Costs of illness and disease, fiscal year 1975. Public Services Laboratory, Georgetown University, Washington, D.C., 1977.

38. Rice, D.: Estimating the cost of illness. U.S. Public Health Service, Health Economics Series No. 6, 1966.

39. Berk, A., and Paringer, L.C.: Cost of illness and disease, 1930. Public Services Laboratory, Georgetown University, Washington, D.C., 1977.

40. Berk, A., and Paringer, L.C.: Cost of illness and disease, 1900. Public Services Laboratory, Georgetown University, Washington, D.C., 1977 (revised 1979).

Chapter Twelve

Health Expenditures and Biomedical Research

Despite the major controversy about technology and health expenditures, most studies that address the issue do not differentiate technological change from biomedical research, and they define technological change broadly to mean any change in the production process (or production function) for health care. Biomedical research itself is not measured as a determinant of expenditures, although numerous studies have been made of expenditure growth, for example, those of Lave and Lave,[1] Salkever,[2] Davis,[3] and Klarman.[4]

The questions still remain: What impact has biomedical research had on health expenditures? Has this research as embodied in public health or medical practices added, on balance, to cost of care or has it reduced the cost of care? Are there differences in the experience for different disease categories? We took two approaches in examining the questions. We first looked to a residual analysis of the expenditures for health care in terms of the several factors contributing to growth of outlays. Second, we applied the market model used throughout the study to health expenditures as a dependent variable.

RESIDUAL FACTOR ANALYSIS

In the residual factor analysis, a model is formulated that essentially explains the total percentage rise in direct health expenditures. The expenditure growth is assumed to equal the product of the percentage rise in expenditures adjusted for the effect of aging of the population, price rises, the percentage change in demand attributable to the rise in income and third-party payments, and the unexplained residual. This analysis is presented in "Returns to Biomedical Research, 1900-75: An Initial Assessment of Impacts on Health Expenditures."[5] The discussion presented here draws on that analysis.

ANALYSIS OF 1930-75 CHANGES

The approach involves identifying the determinants of medical expenditure increases and measuring technological change as the residual. This residual can be either positive or negative. A number of studies have been made of the growth of health expenditures and their determinants. Among those who have analyzed the causes of growth are Feldstein,[6] Klarman and associates,[4] and Fuchs.[7] From these studies, it is assumed that the total percentage rise in direct health expenditures is equal to the product of the percentage rise in population, adjusted for the effect of aging of the population, rises in prices, the percentage change in demand attributable to the rise in income and third-party payments, and the unexplained residual.

Contrary to the current conventional views about technological change and its impacts on health expenditures, we find, based on our analysis, that from 1930 to 1975 expenditures were reduced rather than increased by the advances in medicine. Of the total rise—some 3,150 percent in health outlays over the 45-year period—the net consequence of biomedical advances as reflected in the residual is small when compared to the effect of other factors such as price, income, third-party payments, and population.

Table 12-1 shows the aggregate rise in health expenditures, the increase in each of the factors over the period, and the share of the change attributable to each.

The formulation used for estimating the impact of each of the five variables and the residual factor on health expenditures was the following:

$$(1 + \% \ \Delta H) = (1 + \% \ \Delta PoEpo)(1 + \% \ \Delta PrEpr)(1 + \% \ \Delta YEy)$$
$$(1 + \% \ \Delta AEa)(1 + \% \ \Delta TPEtp)(1 + \% \ \Delta X)$$

where

$\% \ \Delta H, \% \ \Delta Po, \% \ \Delta Pr, \% \ \Delta Y, \% \ \Delta A,$[a] $\% \ \Delta TP$

---

[a]The effect of the age distribution was determined by using 1974 per capita health expenditures by age and comparing the average per capita expenditure using the 1975 and 1930 age distributions of the population as follows:

are equal, respectively, to percentage changes in health expenditures, population, medical care prices, real disposable income, the age index, and third-party payments. *Epo*, *Epr*, *Ey*, *Ea*, and *Etp* refer to the elasticity of expenditures with respect to each of the variables and are assumed equal to 1 for all but *Etp*, the elasticity of which is estimated below. *X* refers to the residual factor that cannot be accounted for by the five variables. Presumably, it reflects biomedical research or technological change.

The actual data show the following results:

$$(1 + 31.50) = (1 + .75)(1 + 3.28)(1 + 1.21)(1 + .13)$$

$$(1 + 2.0(.54))(1 - .17).$$

We can also convert the total increase into percent per annum rise in expenditures accounted for by each of the variables:

$$1.078 = (1.012)(1.032)(1.018)(1.002)(1.016)(.996).$$

In applying the residual model it was necessary to quantify elasticities of health expenditures with respect to each of the five factors considered. We postulated that the elasticity with respect to the three factors of population, aging, and price was equal to 1, and focused on identifying the elasticity with respect to the remaining factors of income and third-party payments. With those we can now account for the increase in health expenditure by the residual model.

We postulate linear forms of relationship between the adjusted expenditure and the two variables of income and third-party payments. Income is the per capita real disposable income, whereas third-party payments constitute the proportion of total expenditures made by third parties. Table 12-2 summarizes the results of three possible runs.

An examination of these results shows that both estimated elasticities seem to revolve around unity. The estimated income elasticity tends to confirm results obtained from individual data. The third-party payments elasticity seems to be higher than that obtained

Age	1975 per capita expenditure	% 1930 population	% 1975 population
Under 19	$ 183.19	38.8	35.0
19-64	419.56	55.8	54.5
65+	1,217.84	5.4	10.5

$$\frac{(.350)(183.19) + (.545)(419.56) + (.105)(1217.84)}{(.388)(183.19) + (.558)(419.56) + (.054)(1217.84)} = 1.13$$

Table 12-1.   Factors Contributing to the Increase in Health Expenditures, Fiscal Years 1930-75[1]

Factors	Total percent change in each of the variables	Percent of total rise attributed to each factor
Total rise	+3,150	100.0
Population	+75	16.0
Price	+328	42.0
Income	+121	23.0
Aging	+13	3.0
Third-party payments	+200	21.0
Residual	−17	−5.0

[1] In computing these percentage increases, Social Security estimates for calendar year 1929 are used to represent fiscal year 1930. This use of the estimates is made possible because the basic data used in compiling the Social Security estimates for calendar year 1929 are from the Committee on Costs of Medical Care study that relates to a twelve-month period during 1928-31.

Sources: M.S. Mueller and R.M. Gibson: "National health expenditures, fiscal year 1975." *Soc. Sec. Bull.* 39:3-20, February 1976; and B. Cooper, N. Worthington, and M. McGee: "Compendium of national health expenditures." U.S. Government Printing Office, Washington, D.C., 1976.

in previous studies.[8, 9] We can use prior information, for example, assuming an income elasticity of 1, to eliminate the effect of real income on the dependent variable and then regress on third-party payments only.

This method calls for our prior knowledge (or assumption) of the elasticity of either income or third-party payments with respect to adjusted health expenditure. If we assume an income elasticity of 1, then the effect of income on expenditure can be subtracted from the dependent variable and a regression on third-party payments alone can be performed to elucidate the effect of these payments in terms of regression coefficient and elasticity. With such an assumption, the regression produces an elasticity for third-party payments (calculated at the mean) of 0.54. Because of the assumed elasticities applied in the analysis, we ran a series of regressions based on different assumptions about the elasticity of either income or third-party payments to indicate the sensitivity of the results. The resulting elasticities are:

Assumed income elasticity	Resulting third-party payments elasticity
.50	.99
.60	.90
.70	.80
.80	.71
.90	.62
1.00	.54
1.10	.45

Assumed third-party payments elasticity	Resulting income elasticity
.30	1.19
.40	1.10
.50	1.00
.60	.91
.70	.81
.80	.72
.90	.62
1.00	.54
1.10	.45

Source: Reference 5.

Despite the apparent sensitivity of the third-party payments elasticity to the assumed level of income elasticity, the estimate of the residual is relatively stable. This stability occurs because the sum of the two elasticities is confined to a range of 1.49 to 1.55; thus, the total change in health expenditures explained by these two factors remains relatively constant.

Table 12-3 shows the results of a comparison of our findings with those of Fuchs.[7] Fuchs found that the residual is positive for 1947 to 1967, suggesting that over these twenty years new technology and biomedical advances added to, rather than reduced, health expenditures. Our finding differs from that of Fuchs by showing a negative rather than a positive impact. But the time periods differ, and this may explain the difference in the two results. Our separate treatment of third-party payments may also make some difference. If we take account of the interaction of quantity demanded and price change, as proposed by Fuchs, our residual estimate would show a somewhat

Table 12-2. Regression Results Obtained by Use of Adjusted Health Expenditure Per Capita as the Dependent Variable (n=46)

Runs	Income	Third-party payments	R^2
Run 1:			
Coefficient	.1031	–	.953
Elasticity	1.37	–	
t	29.8		
Run 2:			
Coefficient	–	5.206	.942
Elasticity	–	1.34	
t	–	26.8	
Run 3:			
Coefficient	.0580	2.432	.976
Elasticity	.77	.63	
t	7.75	6.40	

t (5%, 30) = 1.70.

Table 12-3. Factors Contributing to Growth of Total Health Expenditures

Factors	1930-75 annual rate of change (percent)	Fuchs's study 1947-67 annual rate of change (percent)
Total health expenditures	7.7	8.0
Accounted for by:		
Growth of population	1.2	1.6
Aging of population	0.2	–
Rise in price	3.2	3.7
Growth of real income	1.8	2.3
Growth in third-party payments	1.6	–
Decline in quantity demanded due to relative price change	–	–0.2
Unexplained residual	–0.5	+0.6

Source: Reference 7.

smaller impact of biomedical research or technology on health expenditures, but the impact from 1930 to 1975 would still be negative.

The residual, as computed, is highly sensitive to basic data used to measure each of the components of the model. We applied alternative sources of data for income, for example, with a resulting change in the size of the residual. To use another illustration, we applied alternative weights of the distribution of population by age to compute the adjustment for aging. For the period 1930-75, however, alternative adjustments did not change the size of the residual.

Biomedical advances have not uniformly affected health expenditures for the different diseases. Table 12-4 shows the expenditures by disease category in 1930 and 1975 and the residual impact of biomedical research on the expenditures. The impact of biomedical research, as we have measured it, deals only with the changes that have occurred in total direct health expenditures for specific diseases. After adjusting the total changes in expenditures by population, prices, income, third-party payments, and age-distribution changes, we attributed the remainder of the increase (or decrease) to biomedical research. Expenditures on a disease or other illness class, however, are a function of both its prevalence and the costs of treatment. Therefore, changes in expenditures could result either from a research finding that led to a reduction in the number of cases of a disease or from an improvement in the treatment technique applied to the disease. In any case, the residual includes a number of factors additional to biomedical research.

For infective and parasitic diseases, biomedical research, as we have computed the residual, exerts a considerable negative impact on expenditures, at the rate of —4 percent per year, owing to the effect of primary prevention measures that greatly reduced the incidence of many communicable diseases, particularly tuberculosis. Biomedical research also appears to have had a negative effect on expenditures for diseases of the respiratory system, reflecting, in part, the decrease in the incidence and duration of influenza and the amount of care demanded. In addition, diseases of the digestive system and the oral cavity, salivary glands, and jaws, diseases of the skin, and diseases of pregnancy, childbirth, and the puerperium have experienced a decrease in expenditures that we attribute to the impact of biomedical research. This reduction partly reflects a substantial difference in the treatment provided to patients with these diseases. Expenditures on accidents and diseases of the nervous system have also been negatively affected by biomedical research, but the explanation for this phenomenon is not a clear-cut one. Part of the reduction may be due to the difficulty in achieving comparability between the 1975 and 1930 definitions of these diseases; we attempted it but were not fully successful in this study.

The expenditure categories that appear to have been positively affected by biomedical research include cancer, diseases of the circulatory system, cerebrovascular diseases, mental disorders, and endocrine and metabolic diseases. Circulatory diseases and stroke tend to be concentrated in the older age groups and, with the elimination of many of the childhood diseases, these diseases become increasingly important in terms of incidence and prevalence. Also, the improvements in technology that have yielded such innovations as hospital coronary care units equipped with sophisticated equipment to monitor patients' progress and the breakthroughs in surgical techniques that enable the prolongation of life have had an important effect on total costs. The same experience is occurring with the surgical techniques and treatments used for cancer patients and the improved ability to diagnose and treat diabetes and other endocrine and metabolic disorders. The increase in expenditures on mental disorders may not reflect an increase in institutionalization, but rather an increase in the number of specialists used in treating mental illness and elimination of many social barriers that previously prevented the recognition and acceptance of the mentally ill.

Table 12-4.   Health Expenditures by Disease Category and the Impact of the Residual

Disease category	1930 health expenditures (millions)	1975 health expenditures (millions)	1975/1930	Percent per annum increase due to the residual
Infective and parasitic diseases	$340	$2,027	5.96	-.04
Neoplasms	40	5,279	131.98	.03
Endocrine, nutritional, and metabolic diseases	55	3,337	60.67	.01
Diseases of the blood and blood-forming organs	15	667	45.07	.003
Mental disorders	180	9,411	52.28	.02
Diseases of the nervous system and sense organs (except eye diseases)	92	2,811	30.55	-.01
Eye diseases	156	4,648	29.79	.01
Diseases of the circulatory system (except cerebrovascular disease)	98	13,384	136.57	.03
Cerebrovascular disease	18	2,633	146.28	.03
Diseases of the respiratory system	583	7,571	12.99	-.02
Diseases of the digestive system (except dental)	217	6,787	31.28	-.004
Diseases of the oral cavity, salivary glands, and jaws	494	7,777	15.74	-.003
Diseases of the genitourinary system	138	5,575	40.40	.00
Complications of pregnancy, childbirth, and the puerperium	169	3,387	20.04	-.01
Diseases of the skin and subcutaneous tissue	77	2,120	27.53	-.01
Diseases of the musculoskeletal system and connective tissue	125	5,113	40.90	.00
Congenital anomalies	11	432	39.27	.00
Certain causes of perinatal morbidity and mortality	11	64	5.82	-.04
Symptoms and ill-defined conditions	45	3,180	70.67	.01
Accidents, poisonings, and violence	233	6,846	29.38	-.006
Other	35	6,316	180.46	.03

Sources: 1930 data: A. Berk and L.C. Paringer: "Costs of illness and disease, fiscal year 1930." Public Services Laboratory, Georgetown University, Washington, D.C., May 1977; 1975 data: L.C. Paringer and A. Berk: "Costs of illness and disease, fiscal year 1975." Public Services Laboratory, Georgetown University, Washington, D.C., January 1977.

With few exceptions, the impact of research on expenditures for various diseases is not unexpected, in view of the changes in medical practice and disease incidence between 1930 and 1975.

BIOMEDICAL RESEARCH AND HEALTH EXPENDITURES, 1900-30

The findings for the period 1930-75, especially in those disease categories where expenditures were lowered by biomedical research, suggest that a larger negative impact would be found for the period 1900-30. A larger share of the diseases in the population during the early 1900s were communicable and infectious. Death rates from these diseases were high. Infant deaths in particular were substantially higher in the 1900s than in the 1930s, and there was a far greater reduction in expenditures for perinatal morbidity and mortality from 1900 to 1930 as a consequence of new medical knowledge than the reduction *experienced* from 1930 to 1975.

However, the analysis of health expenditures over the period 1900-30 does not suggest that biomedical research affected the expenditure level significantly. When income was measured by disposable income, the computation produced a residual of +1 percent; when income was measured by GNP, the result showed a residual contribution of —3 percent. Table 12-5 lists the increase in each of the factors and the share of health expenditure rise accounted for by each factor for the total period and annually. Only a slight overall effect of medical advance on health expenditures can be noted.

What is the reason for this finding when savings in medical care expenditures were assumed to be a result of the drop in death rates and the drastic declines in major infectious and communicable diseases? The finding reflects that other characteristics of the use of medical services were countereffective during the thirty-year period. The impact of biomedical research on health expenditures is affected not only by the incidence of sickness and terminal illness, but also by (a) the relative use of health services in the two periods; (b) the relative family budgets for health services; (c) the types of health services used; and (d) the kinds of treatment prescribed.

We examined each of these factors for the years 1900 and 1930 and assessed how the changes that took place may have operated to affect the way in which improved medical knowledge could influence spending for health care.

Relative Use of Health Services
Despite the extent of sickness and the large size of families in 1900, about 1 in 10 families reported no expenditures for health

Table 12-5.   Factors Contributing to the Increases in Health Expenditures, 1900-30

Factors	Total percent rise	Percent of total rise attributable to each factor	Annual percent change
Total health expenditure	574	100	5.45
Population	61	25	1.37
Price	127	43	2.34
Income	51	5	1.17
Aging	10	22	0.27
Third-party payments	9	4	0.23
Residual	2	1	0.04

Source: Reference 5.

purposes in a major survey of New York City budgets conducted during the first decade of the 1900s for the Russell Sage Foundation.[10] By the years 1928-31, all but 3 percent of the families reported some expenditures for medical care; this percentage dropped to 2 percent in the largest cities.[11]

Early budget studies do not uniformly report a sizable share of families without expenditures for health care. In a Southern cotton mill community in which 21 families were surveyed, all families had received some medical care.[12] A survey of working class families in Fall River, Massachusetts, reported that one of the 14 families interviewed had had no medical care.[12] In Greenwich Village (New York City) from 1903 to 1905, 169, or 84.5 percent, of the 200 families surveyed reported expenditures on medical care; the remaining 15.5 percent had no expenditures.[13]

Relative Family Budgets
for Health Services

When incomes averaged about $700 to $800 or less annually, the margin for medical care was small. Choices among goods and services had to be made, and a number of families opted for spending on food, housing, and other purposes. For families who had no health expenditures, improvements in medical knowledge could effect no savings such as those postulated to result from biomedical advances. Instead, the amounts for care would more likely be applied to care for those who had not received care earlier.

Spending on sickness and death on the average in 1901, as reported in a Bureau of Labor Statistics survey of U.S. families, amounted to $20.54, or 2.7 percent of total family expenditures.[14] (Average family income that year was $827.19, and average family size was 5.31 persons.) Such an expenditure level in 1930 prices would be the equivalent of $46.68. In contrast, the Committee on Costs of Medical Care for 1930 (1928-31) reported family medical care spending as averaging $108.14, more than twice the real resource use of 1901.[11] Clearly, more family resources were going to health care by 1930 than at the turn of the century. The 1900 level, even on the average, was so low as to suggest that family members who were ill were "left to succumb to the attacks of disease without adequate medical aid."[10]

Types of Health Care

Savings in medical care costs as a consequence of biomedical research would result from reduction in certain illnesses if other health care needs did not replace those for which medical care was purchased earlier. However, medical care in 1900 was quite different from today's medical care. Sick persons in 1900 were most often cared for in the home and they turned to pharmacists for remedies. A midwife or practical nurse was used for attendance in childbirth. In 1900, women could "seldom be persuaded to go for a confinement" to a hospital.[13] Dentistry was rare for most families; indeed, only a small percent had expenditures for dental care. However, when there was need for dental care and dangers of infection were great, the costs were high.

Types of Treatment Prescribed

Even when professional help was sought in the early 1900s, the limited knowledge of specific therapies gave rise to treatments, by the more scientifically oriented of the physicians, that looked to improved diets, more exercise, and a better environment in the home and neighborhood. Physicians' training at that time emphasized their lack of capacity to treat and cure. Therefore, improvements in knowledge that gave rise to medical services where none were indicated before would tend to increase rather than reduce medical expenditures.

In 1900, the treatment for tuberculosis basically was good nutrition and fresh open air. Osler wrote: "The requirements of a suitable climate are a *pure atmosphere, an equable temperature* not subject to rapid variations and a maximum amount of sunshine."[15] Special sanitoria for the treatment of tuberculosis were then being organized, but most patients were cared for at home.

Perhaps tuberculosis care was especially associated with diet and environmental conditions. But a quick examination of the treatments outlined then show that such emphasis on approaches to treatment by diet, exercise, and environment was not limited to tuberculosis.

Of the treatment of typhoid fever, Osler wrote: "Careful nursing and a regulated diet are the essentials in the majority of the cases. . . ." For diarrhea of children, Osler indicated that hygenic management was of the first importance: "The effect of a change from the hot stifling atmosphere of a town to the mountains or the sea is often seen at once in a reduction in the number of stools and a rapid improvement in the physical condition."[1 5] Even in the case of myocardium disease, part of the treatment reported was diet and exercise, part was drugs in the form of digitalis, and part was the use of stimulants such as aromatic spirits of ammonia and sulphuric ether. "When the pulse is hard and firm," Osler wrote, "nitroglycerin may be cautiously administered." In the case of cancers—even though there is a clear statement of the incurable nature of the disease—the treatment, except for relief of pain by use of morphia, was given in terms of diet and the washing out of the stomach to combat vomiting.[1 5]

Given the facts about medical care of 1900, it is not unreasonable that some persons, even with serious illness, did not seek care, and those who did found the better physicians cautious of prescribing medications. Considerable changes by 1930 resulted in an increase in effectiveness of medical care and a higher demand for care, including care in hospitals.

A MARKET MODEL

Our second approach to the question of impact of biomedical research was to apply a model of the underlying demand and supply characteristics of the market and use this model to quantify the extent to which biomedical research explains the variation in health expenditures. The model is basically the same as that applied earlier in assessing the share of mortality and morbidity changes attributable to biomedical research (see Chapter 4).

In formulating the model, the earlier conceptual framework of Booms and Hu[1 6] was followed here, as in the case of mortality and morbidity. The endogenous variable health expenditures (Y) is estimated using the following equation:

$$Y = P \cdot Q = h \text{ (INC, SOC, ENV, FIN, PROV, TECH)}$$

where P = price, Q = quantity, and these in turn equal the function of economic (INC), societal (SOC), environmental (ENV), financial (FIN), and medical care characteristics (PROV and TECH). This equation was estimated in log form. Table 12-6 presents the regres-

Table 12-6. Empirical Results for Expenditure Regression, 1930-75 (Elasticity Estimates Adjusted for First-order Autocorrelation)

Dependent variable	INC	SOC	ENV	FIN	PROV	TECH	Constant	R^2	Unexplained percent share
Expenditures									
Elasticity coefficient	0.58	−0.06	−0.09	0.16	0.75	0.07	−1.59	.970	
(t-value)	(6.94)	(−3.10)	(−1.20)	(3.40)	(2.83)	(2.05)	(−2.80)		
Percent share	37	−1	2	20	26	13			3

sion results and each factor's relative contribution to changes in health expenditures. The results presented in the table have been adjusted for first-order autocorrelation, since the Durbin-Watson statistic indicated serious autocorrelation in ordinary least squares (OLS) estimates. This procedure, however, makes interpretation of the t values somewhat less precise than t values on coefficients estimated bv the OLS method.

As indicated in Chapters 4 and 8, to assess the relative contribution of each factor, an equation was employed, which divides the average annual increases of the dependent variable into portions attributable to each independent variable as follows:

$$100\% = \frac{e_1 \Delta INC}{\Delta Y_i} \cdot \frac{e_2 \Delta SOC}{\Delta Y_i} \cdot \frac{e_3 \Delta ENV}{\Delta Y_i} \cdot \frac{e_4 \Delta FIN}{\Delta Y_i} \cdot \frac{e_5 \Delta PROV}{\Delta Y_i} \cdot \frac{e_6 \Delta TECH}{\Delta Y_i} \cdot \frac{U}{\Delta Y_i}$$

where $i = 1,2$, the e's are the estimated elasticities, the Δ's signify average annual percent changes in the variables, and U is the unexplained difference.

Changes in real income, characteristics of providers, and third-party payments contributed 83 percent of the increases in real per capita health expenditures with a far smaller share, 13 percent, of the expenditure increases attributed to biomedical research effort.

Review of the model when applied to health expenditures suggested that an important factor affecting use of health services was omitted, namely, health status of the population. Presumably, the main users of medical care are the sick. Accordingly, a modification was made in the equation to include mortality rates as a health status measure and to exclude providers of care as a variable as a more indirect measure of factors affecting use of services.

The new regression results shown in Table 12-7 gave new emphasis to the lack of robustness in the regressions when the dependent variable is expenditures. Many of the factors determining changes over time are highly correlated. We expected a serious multicollinearity problem that would make precise estimation of the individual coefficients difficult. Our test run with a new equation incorporating mortality rates as a proxy for a health status variable mirrored history, but in terms of analysis of the question, it is troublesome. The regression results suggest that expenditures rise with improved health status, or, more specifically, lower death rates, over the period 1930-75, but the variable coefficients are insignificant for the years 1900-75.

The coefficient of the biomedical research variable is insignificant for all but one computation for the period 1900-75, and that for an

Table 12-7. Health Expenditures Regressions: Alternative Measures of Health Care Providers and Health Status (Elasticity Coefficients Adjusted for First-order Autocorrelation)

	1900-75 Dependent variables: per capita health expenditures					1930-75				
Independent variables:										
Income	.896 (9.50)	.931 (9.33)	.877 (9.31)	.856 (8.34)	.853 (8.15)	.582 (6.98)	.466 (6.42)	.420 (6.54)	.412 (6.85)	.529 (7.09)
Health insurance	.029 (.499)	.125 (2.53)	.022 (.418)	.178 (3.31)	.169 (3.07)	.163 (3.40)	.179 (6.00)	.111 (3.61)	.103 (3.71)	.120 (2.95)
Environmental factors	-.294 (3.84)	-.256 (3.00)	-.306 (3.77)	-.290 (2.31)	-.178 (2.06)	-.091 (1.20)	.176 (2.65)	.081 (1.18)	.099 (1.66)	-.056 (.94)
Societal factors	.016 (.92)	.026 (1.42)	.011 (.633)	.02 (1.15)	.025 (1.41)	-.055 (3.10)	-.030 (1.95)	-.040 (2.93)	-0.048 (3.66)	-.065 (4.14)
Providers										
Doctors and nurses Per capita	.845 (2.50)	.886 (2.80)				.75 (2.83)		.637 (3.30)		
Nurses per capita				.145 (2.24)	.132 (2.05)				.605 (4.25)	.83 (4.79)
Death rates	.004 (.026)		-.072 (.49)	.123 (.798)	—	-.956 (5.66)		-.964 (6.32)	-.807 (5.34)	
Biomedical research	.063 (1.61)	.116 (2.97)	.048 (1.11)	.081 (1.97)	.070 (1.74)	.072 (2.05)	.057 (2.04)	.016 (.585)	.003 (.121)	.034 (1.03)
n	76	76	76	76	76	46	46	46	46	46
Intercept	-3.32	-2.70	-2.94	13.26	-2.86	-1.58	2.076	1.94	.406	-4.08
R^2	.963	.956	.972	.959	.952	.980	.985	.991	.993	.980

Note: Coefficients with *t* ratios in parentheses.

equation in which the providers of care are excluded as a variable impacting on demand for care is excluded. Even for the period 1930-75, the coefficients for biomedical research are insignificant in three of the five equations.

Elasticity coefficients varied as well with different measures of biomedical research. When biomedical research in the model is measured as the weighted average of the stock of biomedical PhD's, drug patents, and medical instrument patents, the coefficient is negative; it is positive when measured by biomedical PhD's (lagged ten years), or drug patents (lagged seven years), or new medical journals by initial year of publication (lagged one year). The results of these regressions are shown in Table 12-8.

Because of the instability of findings and the relatively small magnitude of the elasticities, we have assumed, in later estimates, that health expenditures are neither increased nor decreased, on balance, by biomedical advances.

Table 12-8. Empirical Results Using Real Per Capita Personal Health Care Expenditures as the Dependent Variable, 1930-75 (Elasticity Coefficients Adjusted for First-order Autocorrelation)

Variable	Weighted average index	Ph.D.'s, lagged 10 years	Drug patents, lagged 7 years	Biomedical journals
		Optional measures of biomedical research		
Constant	−2.16	−1.59	−1.72	−2.04
(*t*)	(−2.57)	(−2.80)	(−2.96)	(−5.06)
INC	0.66	0.58	0.61	0.62
(*t*)	(8.07)	(6.94)	(7.23)	(10.21)
% share	41	37	39	39
SOC	−0.05	−0.06	−0.05	−0.06
(*t*)	(−2.82)	(−3.10)	(−2.87)	(−3.64)
% share	−1	−1	1	−1
ENV	−0.16	−0.09	−0.13	−0.13
(*t*)	(−2.06)	(−1.20)	(−1.66)	(−1.96)
% share	4	2	3	3
FIN	0.15	0.16	0.15	0.08
(*t*)	(3.04)	(3.40)	(2.98)	(2.36)
% share	19	20	19	10
PROV	1.13	0.75	0.86	1.00
(*t*)	(2.75)	(2.83)	(3.21)	(5.26)
% share	39	26	30	34
TECH1	−0.04			
(*t*)	(−0.31)			
% share	−4			
TECH2		0.07		
(*t*)		(2.05)		
% share		13		
TECH3			0.05	
(*t*)			(1.30)	
% share			9	
TECH4				0.12
(*t*)				(4.77)
% share				8
R^2	.972	.970	.969	.990

INC   = real per capita income (in 1967 prices) net of personal health expenditures
PROV = weighted average of the stock of doctors and nurses
FIN   = share of third-party payments in total medical care expenditures
TECH1 = weighted average of the stock of biomedical Ph.D.'s, drug patents, and medical instrument patents
TECH2 = biomedical Ph.D.'s lagged ten years
TECH3 = drug patents lagged seven years
TECH4 = new biomedical journals by initial year of publication lagged one year
SOC   = unemployment rate lagged two years
ENV   = work injury rate

REFERENCES

1. Lave, J., and Lave, L.: Hospital cost functions. Am Econ Rev 60: 379-395, June 1970.

2. Salkever, D.: A micro-economic study of hospital cost inflation. J Pol Econ 80: 1144-1166, November-December 1972.

3. Davis, K.: The role of technology demand, and labor markets in the determination of hospital costs. *In* The economics of health and medical care, edited by M. Perlman. John Wiley & Sons, New York, 1974, pp. 283-301.

4. Klarman, H., Rice, D., Cooper, B., and Statler, H.L.: Sources of increase in selected medical care expenditures, 1929-1969. American Public Health Association Journal 60, June 1970.

5. Mushkin, S.J., Paringer, L.C., and Chen, M.M.: Returns to biomedical research, 1900-1975: an initial assessment of impacts on health expenditures. *In* Technology and the quality of health care, edited by R.H. Egdahl and P.M. Gertman. Aspen System Corporation, Germantown, Md., 1978, pp. 105-120.

6. Feldstein, M.: The rising cost of hospital care. Information Resources Press, Washington, D.C., 1971.

7. Fuchs, V.R.: Essays in the economics of health and medical care. National Bureau of Economic Research, New York, 1972, p. 63.

8. Anderson, R., and Benham, L.: Factors affecting the relationship between family income and medical care consumption. *In* Empirical studies in health economics, edited by H.E. Klarman. Johns Hopkins University Press, Baltimore, Md., 1970.

9. Newhouse, J.: A model of physician pricing. Southern Econ J 37, October 1970.

10. Chapin, R.C.: The standard of living among workingmen's families in New York City. Charities Publication Committee, New York, 1909.

11. Falk, J., Rorem, R., and Ring, M.: The costs of medical care: a summary of investigations on the economic aspects of the prevention and care of illness. University of Chicago Press, Committee on the Costs of Medical Care Publication No. 27, January 1933.

12. U.S. Bureau of Labor: Women and child wage earners—family budgets. U.S. Government Printing Office, Washington, D.C., 1910-1913 (19 volumes).

13. More, L.B.: Wage earners' budgets: a study of standards and cost of living in New York City. Greenwich House Series of Social Studies, No. 1, Henry Holt and Company, New York, 1907.

14. U.S. Department of Labor: Cost of living, 18th annual report. U.S. Government Printing Office, Washington, D.C., 1903.

15. Osler, W.: The principles and practice of medicine. D. Appleton and Co., New York, 1901.

16. Booms, B.H., and Hu, T.: Towards a positive theory of state and local public expenditures: an empirical example. Public Finance 26: 419-436, 1971.

Chapter Thirteen

Summing Up the Burden of Illness

A summing up of the information on burden of illness suggests a look back over the decades at what biomedical science has achieved as well as a look ahead at future priorities in research. Single-year estimates of the burden of illness are now familiar. Indeed, for many years, estimates of illness burdens were prepared by the separate voluntary agencies and compiled periodically by the National Health Education Committee.[1] In this way, the public and the Congress had estimates on how much the major illnesses were costing and often, on how many persons were afflicted. Where the costs were high, additional research on medical expenditures would presumably help to lower the burden. At least, this was the basis for the lobbying of the disease-specific interest groups.

Costing of individual diseases has a long and impressive history. Economists, including some of the nation's most distinguished, such as Irving Fisher, made such estimates as early as the first decade of the twentieth century.[2] Actuarial valuations also came to be applied drawing on earlier conceptual work by Farr,[3] Petty,[4] and others. Dublin contributed to this work, first by preparing estimates of the cost of tuberculosis[5] and later, in 1930, by producing with Lotka estimates of capital values of males by age group in a volume that is now regarded as a classic.[6]

In 1966, Rice advanced the entire process by developing a technique for costing in which estimates were prepared for all diseases identified in the two-digit ICDA Code so that the total burden shown for each disease was constrained by the aggregate for all.[7] This approach marked an important step forward. Prior to the Rice study, the potential overlapping cost burdens and double counting problems were unclear.

However, that study and the subsequent study by Cooper and Rice for a later year[8] did not undertake to compare the burdens of illness over time. The estimates for the two years examined (1963 and 1972) were, in fact, not comparable on a number of scores: drug expenditures were counted in 1972 but not 1963; household value was estimated for housewives in 1972, but in 1963, women were assumed to earn the same amount as domestic servants; hospital costs by disease were assumed to be uniform in 1963 but were varied in 1972; and so forth. The National Institutes of Health sought consistent estimates of burden of illness over a span of years. Dr. Herbert B. Woolley of the National Institutes of Health thought that comparison of estimates across years might shed light on such questions as: Has the real burden of illness gone down? And for what diseases? Has the cost of premature death been reduced? Have disability losses due to absence from work been cut, and has availability for work opportunity been enhanced?

The present summing up of disease burdens from one period to another permits an examination of those questions. It also seeks to review burden estimates in terms of targets for research in the years ahead. The counts of burden of illness are examined as a basis for target setting bearing in mind the public's view of disease priorities that place cancer and blindness at the top of the list of dread diseases[9] despite the fact that these diseases do not rank first as causes of death.

We earlier indicated what I choose to call "Congress's rule," which matches funds to total deaths. If deaths are more numerous for one disease than another, the need is plain. It is the reduction in cost of those deaths that are more numerous by providing resources for research that can give some promise of reducing deaths. The exploration of the correlation between deaths and funding of research in Chapter 6 is for a recent year. But there is even clearer evidence of congressional and administration action on research in the changing pattern of disease and death over the years. Much research of the early years of the twentieth century was directed to problems of infective and parasitic diseases and childbirth (both maternal and infant deaths). As we have observed, national defense and economic objectives, as well as health concerns, guided research decisions. Yellow fever, hookworm, malaria, and tuberculosis claimed considerable research resources, both public and private.

Comparison of the illness burden in one period with the illness burden in another does not yield the easy accounting of medical advance that was intended. For example, the number of deaths in the population in 1930 fell below the number in 1900, but the population age distribution had changed. More, rather than fewer, deaths were among those of working age with the potential, compared to infant deaths, of sizable loss in earnings. Moreover, classification of deaths by disease changed from one ICDA code to another, reducing comparability of death data.

Sickness experience defied easy analysis. Data for the early years of the century were far from adequate. The earliest sickness surveys reflected differences in perception about illness, the lack of medical knowledge, and the important economic impact of the lack of insurance and sick leave benefits on sickness rates. Even a careful assessment of incidence of sickness in 1930 and in 1975 emphasized the reporting of fewer cases of disease in 1930 than 1975. Comparisons of health expenditures were complicated even more by demographic, social, and economic differences from one period to another as well as by changes in medical knowledge that made medical care more productive in 1975 than in 1930 and more productive in 1930 than in 1900. It is interesting to speculate what the demand for health care would be today if all financial conditions were as they are now, including widespread use of third-party payments, but the state of medical knowledge was that of 1900.

Despite all the complexity, the comparative estimates underscore that cost of death from infective and parasitic diseases declined between 1900 and 1975. Even health expenditures per capita on a constant price basis for these diseases and for perinatal diseases were lower in 1975 than 1930. Thus the comparative data on illness burdens do show that economic resources have been released from the production of health services for diagnosis and treatment of infectious and communicable diseases that biomedical research played a major role in preventing and curing. The comparisons also document the shifting patterns of major disease problems toward the degenerative diseases. And the comparative data by two-digit ICDA Code, when used in terms of relative rankings or percentage distributions rather than absolute cost burdens, provide considerable insight into the changing patterns of diseases and deaths over the past seventy-five years. These relative values are discussed in a subsequent section.

TRENDS IN BURDEN OF ILLNESS

What has happened over the past period to the burden of illness? If any phenomenon is characteristic of modern life, it is the almost endless rise in the cost of being sick. The increased cost of medical care makes the headlines almost daily. National expenditures for physician, dental, hospital, and related health services reached in excess of $160 billion in 1977, four times the 1965 level. According to the projections of the Public Services Laboratory for the year 2000, these expenditures will top $1 trillion by the year 2000 (in year 2000 dollars).[9]

The indirect cost of sickness, that is, the cost of premature death and the loss in product due to sickness in the population, has also risen, but the rise has been far less pronounced than that of outlays for direct health care. Figure 13-1 shows the current dollar costs of sickness for the years covered by the present study, adding together the direct cost for health care, the amounts that are paid to hospitals, physicians, dentists, and other providers of care, and the indirect cost of loss of product due to sickness and premature death.

A considerable share of the historic cost increases is attributable to inflation. In 1900, medical care expenditures in the dollars of that year totaled less than half a billion. In 1975 prices, that expenditure is over ten times as large or over $5 billion. Similarly, 1930 expenditures in the dollars of that year amounted to $3.6 billion; in 1975 prices, these expenditures were 4.5 times as much or $15.6 billion. In constant dollars, the year 2000 estimated direct health expenditures would be a little over $400 billion rather than the estimated $1-trillion outlay in year 2000 dollars.

As indicated earlier in this book, there are marked differences between the prices of 1900 and today. In 1900, hospital costs ranged generally from $2 to $3 a day. By 1930, the per diem cost as reported to the Committee on the Cost of Medical Care was $5. Today, costs of hospitals approach $200 a day.

We have adjusted the estimates of wage-loss due to both premature death and sickness by an index of average earnings, including self-employment earnings. The indirect cost estimates for the first period of the century are raised even more than direct health outlays by the price adjustment. Earnings rose in response not only to consumer prices but also to productivity improvement. For the period ahead, the year 2000 estimate of indirect costs assumes a productivity rise per annum of 2 percent, which is somewhat under the historic trend value (Figure 13-2).

What do these trends suggest? A quick synopsis indicates the following:

- In the thirty-year period 1900-30, direct costs multiplied 4.5 times; in the subsequent forty-five-year period, they rose almost eightfold.
- Real indirect costs rose far less rapidly than direct costs.

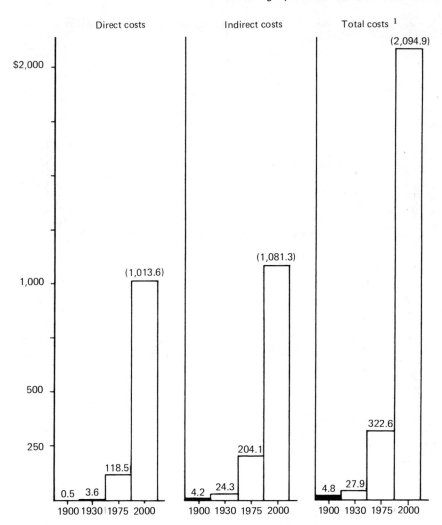

[1] Totals may not add due to rounding.

Source: Reference 9; and A. Berk and L.C. Paringer: "Costs of illness and disease, 1900." Public Services Laboratory, Georgetown University, Washington, D.C., August 1977, revised 1979.

Figure 13-1. Current Dollar Costs of Illness for Selected Years (in billions)

- The future prospect is for a further sizable rise in direct costs even on a constant price basis.
- Costs of premature death and sickness, all things considered, have demonstrated remarkable stability over the forty-five-year period 1930-75 and are projected to continue this pattern for

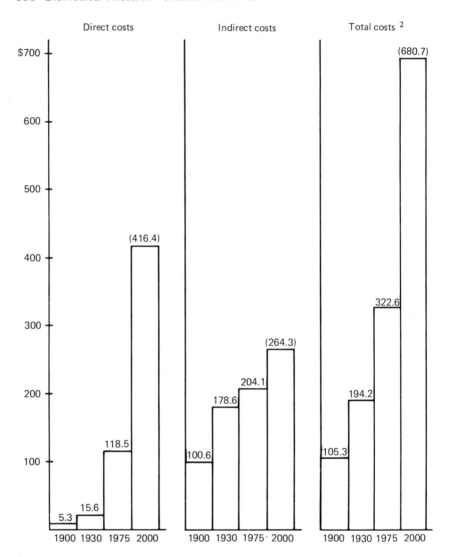

[1] Assuming constant labor force participation rates and including household values. Direct costs deflated by the medical care price index and indirect costs deflated by an index of average earnings. Productivity increase of 2 percent assumed. Alternative medical care price indexes yield year 2000 direct costs of $429.9 billion and $694.1 billion.
[2] Totals may not add due to rounding.
Sources: Reference 9; and A. Berk and L.C. Paringer: "Costs of illness and disease, 1900." Public Services Laboratory, Georgetown University, Washington, D.C., August 1977, revised 1979.

Figure 13-2. Constant 1975 Dollar Costs of Illness for Selected Years[1] (in billions)

the twenty-five years ahead, 1975-2000. As the population grows, this means lower and lower costs per capita.

INDEXES OF BURDEN OF ILLNESS

The estimates of disease and injury burdens provide information additional to mortality and morbidity data about the relative status of different diseases. (The relative values for the major diseases are summarized in Table 13-1.)

Some urge use of such burden estimates for priority setting in health research fund allocations. Certainly, the data in their detail (Tables 13-2, 13-3) shed light from a different perspective on the question of relative importance of certain disease problems. For example, the high cost of mental illness, particularly hospital costs, suggests consideration of the feasibility and productivity of added resources for mental health. Mortality data do not adequately define the importance of that disease. Dental diseases rank high in health expenditures and use of practitioner services; again, mortality data do not reflect this.

Table 13-1. **Percent Distribution of Economic Burden of Illness, by Disease, Selected Years 1900-75 (Earnings Loss Due to Deaths Valued at Discount Rate of 2.5 Percent)**

Diseases arrayed by size of total economic burden, 1975	1975	1930	1900
Diseases of the circulatory system	17.9	10.9	6.6
Accidents, poisonings, and violence	17.6	13.5	6.0
Neoplasms	8.7	3.9	1.0
Diseases of the digestive system	7.7	11.3	5.4
Diseases of the respiratory system	6.9	13.8	19.9
Mental disorders	6.3	2.8	2.3
Complications of pregnancy, childbirth, and puerperium and Certain causes of perinatal mortality	4.9	10.7	8.7
Infective and parasitic diseases[1]	1.8	16.0	32.3
All other	28.2	17.1	17.8

[1] Infective and parasitic diseases are shown in this array only for purposes of comparison with earlier years.

Sources: L.C. Paringer and A. Berk: "Costs of illness and disease, fiscal year 1975." Public Services Laboratory, Georgetown University, Washington, D.C., January 1977; A. Berk and L.C. Paringer: "Costs of illness and disease, fiscal year 1930." Public Services Laboratory, Georgetown University, Washington, D.C., May 1977; and A. Berk and L.C. Paringer: "Costs of illness and disease, 1900." Public Services Laboratory, Georgetown University, Washington, D.C., August 1977, revised 1979.

Table 13-1 shows the distribution of the cost burden of illness for the years 1900, 1930, and 1975 by major disease category. It focuses better than do absolute quantities on the relative changes that have occurred in concentration of costs among diseases. Infective and parasitic diseases claimed 16 percent of economic costs in 1930 and 32 percent in 1900. By 1975, infective and parasitic diseases accounted for less than 2 percent of total economic cost. Burdens of diseases of the respiratory system similarly have declined, but not as dramatically. In 1900, 20 percent of the total economic cost of illness was attributable to respiratory diseases; that percentage declined to under 14 percent by 1930 and to under 7 percent by 1975. Some increases above the 1975 figure are anticipated in the future, owing to the greater number of women today who are smokers.

Diseases of the circulatory system have increased in importance over the decades of the twentieth century as a contributor to the burden of illness. By 1975, the share of economic costs attributed to circulatory diseases rose to 18 percent as compared to 11 percent in 1930 and under 7 percent in 1900.

Costs of accidents are becoming relatively more important. In 1900, 6 percent of all economic costs of illness was attributable to accidents; by 1930, that percentage had more than doubled, with a further rise in the share of costs attributable to accidents in 1975, bringing that share close to 18 percent.

The economic burden of neoplasms and of mental illness has risen sharply over the decades. In 1900, 1 percent of the economic burden of illness was attributed to neoplasms and 2 percent to mental illness. By 1975, the percentages had risen to almost 9 and 6 percent, respectively.

Annual growth rates of these cost burdens perhaps serve best to underscore the difference among the diseases. The total economic burden of infective and parasitic diseases rose considerably slower than other disease categories in both the period 1900-30 and 1930-75. The economic burden of diseases of the circulatory system, accidents, poisonings, and violence, neoplasms, and mental disorders rose faster than average. The direct costs for circulatory diseases, however, rose far more than average in the forty-five-year period 1930-75, followed closely in growth rate by neoplasms. The growth rate for both diseases in the earlier period was below average. The growth rate of direct health expenditures clearly exceeds that of indirect costs, but the rate of increase varies markedly among the diseases, as shown in Table 13-4.

Mortality costs continue to be high. Accidents, poisonings, and

Table 13-2. Percent Distribution of the Cost Burden of Death and Sickness, by Disease, Selected Years, 1900-75 (Earnings Loss Due to Deaths at Discount Rate of 2.5 Percent)

Diseases arrayed by size of total economic burden, 1975	Cost of premature deaths			Cost of sickness		
	1975	*1930*	*1900*	*1975*	*1930*	*1900*
Diseases of the circulatory system	22.4	12.9	6.6	15.1	8.3	3.8
Accidents, poisonings, and violence	30.2	14.6	6.2	9.8	14.2	4.5
Neoplasms	14.8	4.9	0.9	1.9	1.2	0.4
Diseases of the digestive system	4.7	10.2	3.8	5.9	9.3	5.4
Diseases of the respiratory system	4.3	13.1	19.1	14.8	14.9	27.1
Mental disorders	1.5	.6	.3	15.1	11.7	11.8
Complications of pregnancy, childbirth, and puerperium and Certain causes of perinatal mortality	8.3	11.1	3.2	.3	2.5	2.4
Infective and parasitic diseases	1.5	17.1	36.6	2.7	17.0	22.3
All other	12.3	15.5	23.3	34.4	20.9	22.3

Diseases of the genitourinary system and diseases of the musculoskeletal system and connective tissue omitted from Table 13-2 rank third and fourth in sickness costs in 1900.
Sources: See Table 13-1.

violence outrank other costs of deaths, accounting for a cost of $44 billion, or almost one-third the total cost of death in 1975. Diseases of the circulatory system rank second in total cost of death, amounting to $32 billion (when a discount rate of 2.5 percent is used). These deaths tend to be deaths of men at the peak of their earning power and thus are costly. Together the cost of accidental deaths and of deaths attributable to circulatory diseases account for more than half of the total. The third disease in order of cost of death is neoplasms. Without an allowance for pain, disfigurement, or other social costs, neoplasms account for almost $22 billion of mortality costs in 1975, or almost 15 percent of the total. In contrast, in 1900, neoplasms accounted for less than 1 percent of cost of death.

Cost of sickness is distributed among diseases in a way that departs from the distribution of cost of death. Mental illness claims 15 percent of cost of sickness followed by diseases of the circulatory system and diseases of the respiratory system.

The large share of costs of death and of illness attributable to environmental or social causes, such as the costs of accidents and mental illness, cannot but raise questions about the relation of cost burdens to medical care policies and scientific research. In contrast, a large share of research funds has gone for cancer research, which accounts for a small part of current health outlays (less than 5

Table 13-3. Percent Distribution of Cost of Direct Use of Health Resources

Diseases arrayed in order of size of total economic burden, 1975[1]	Total health expenditures			Hospital expenditures			Physician expenditures[1]		
	1975	1930	1900	1975	1930	1900	1975	1930	1900
Diseases of the circulatory system	13.5	3.4	9.7	16.7	2.3	4.4	12.0	5.1	10.9
Accidents, poisonings, and violence	5.8	7.5	6.6	9.1	7.1	9.5	6.6	11.0	5.8
Neoplasms	4.5	1.3	2.2	8.9	1.9	4.8	3.0	2.0	2.1
Diseases of the digestive system	12.3	22.7	16.4	11.0	11.0	6.4	4.9	8.1	6.7
Diseases of the respiratory system	6.4	18.6	17.3	7.0	8.5	3.5	11.5	26.9	37.9
Mental disorders	7.9	5.8	4.4	15.4	25.4	21.1	4.4	0.7	1.1
Complications of pregnancy, childbirth, and puerperium and Certain causes of perinatal mortality	2.9	5.8	7.2	6.8	11.2	10.0	0.9	6.2	10.1
Infective and parasitic diseases[1]	1.7	10.8	15.1	2.0	15.1	24.6	2.0	11.6	15.1
All other	45.0	24.1	21.0	23.1	17.5	15.7	54.7	36.6	10.3

[1] Dental care in 1975 accounts for over half the share attributed to diseases of the digestive system; in 1930, to three-fourths the total. Infective and parasitic diseases are shown in the array only for purposes of comparison with earlier years.

Sources: See Table 13-1.

Table 13-4.   Average Annual Growth Rate in Burden of Illness, 1900-75

Diseases ranked in order of importance in 1975	*1900-30*	*1930-75*
	Total economic burden	
All diseases	5.9	5.4
Diseases of the circulatory system	7.6	6.5
Accidents, poisonings, and violence	8.6	6.0
Diseases of the digestive system	8.3	4.6
Neoplasms	10.4	7.2
Mental disorders	6.6	7.2
Infective and parasitic diseases	3.6	.5
All other	5.5	5.4
	Growth in direct health expenditures	
All diseases	6.3	7.7
Diseases of the circulatory system	2.5	11.1
Accidents, poisonings, and violence	6.3	7.5
Diseases of the digestive system	7.0	6.7
Neoplasms	4.0	10.9
Mental disorders	6.9	8.8
Infective and parasitic diseases	4.8	4.0
All other	6.9	7.7
	Growth in indirect health expenditures	
All diseases	5.8	4.7
Diseases of the circulatory system	8.0	5.9
Accidents, poisonings, and violence	8.8	5.9
Diseases of the digestive system	8.8	3.2
Neoplasms	11.3	6.9
Mental disorders	6.5	6.4
Infective and parasitic diseases	3.5	−.3
All other	5.3	4.2

percent) and even a smaller share (2 percent) of the economic cost of sickness.

Although outlays for health care have gone up markedly during the twentieth century, advances in knowledge about public health, sanitation, and the life sciences have certainly had an impact on health expenditures. As indicated earlier, certain diseases have been prevented, and as a consequence, outlays for these diseases became unnecessary. But as the capacity of medicine has increased, so too has the demand for health care, and this effect has been amplified by the development and growth of third-party payments and higher living standards.

Priorities in terms of distribution of health expenditures have changed greatly. This change suggests the progress that the research community has made historically in conquering costly disease. In 1900, the four most costly diseases in order of relative health expenditures were diseases of the respiratory system; diseases of the digestive system; infective and parasitic diseases; and diseases of the musculoskeletal system and connective tissue (not shown in Table 13-3). Together these four diseases accounted for approximately 59 percent of total 1900 health expenditures. By 1930, little progress had been made in reducing costs; the four diseases accounted for 56 percent of the total, but by 1975, the proportion of costs for the four had dropped by more than half or to 29 percent of the total.

If the question is reversed and the costly diseases of 1975 are compared with the experience of earlier years, we find that diseases of the circulatory system and digestive system far outrank other diseases in direct cost (Table 13-3). Together with mental diseases and respiratory diseases, the four diseases account for 40 percent of the total in 1975. Neoplasms that rank so high in cost of death rank fairly low in health expenditures of 1975 among the seventeen disease classifications of the International Disease Code, accounting for less than 5 percent of health expenditures in that year. In 1900 and 1930, neoplasms were responsible for even a smaller share of the health costs (1 to 2 percent). Circulatory diseases and mental disorders together represented only 14 percent of total health expenditures in 1900 and even a smaller share of expenditures in 1930.

The contrasts from period to period in hospital expenditures are even sharper. Hospital expenditures today account for upward of 40 percent of total outlays, and the annual growth rate has exceeded that of other components of health care. It is largely to control hospital use and hospital pricing that constraints are now proposed. The cost of hospital care today approaches a $200 per diem room rate, and the total bill even for a two- or three-day hospital stay often exceeds $1,000. Circulatory diseases and mental disorders followed by diseases of the digestive system, accidents, poisonings, and violence, and neoplasms account for over one-half of the total hospital expense in recent years. The earlier years were very different. Infective and parasitic diseases, mental disorders, diseases of the digestive system, and complications of pregnancy accounted for the major share of hospital outlays. Indeed, 46 percent of hospital costs in 1900 fell into two disease categories: infective and parasitic diseases and mental disorders. By 1930, the concentration of hospital costs for these two diseases had somewhat decreased.

Physician services in 1975 predominate in the circulatory diseases,

diseases of the respiratory system, and accidents. A far larger share of physician services originated in 1930 for respiratory diseases, with infective and parasitic diseases ranking second, followed by accidents.

The shifts in disease patterns and relative importance of these diseases as cost burdens have been influenced by the advances in the life sciences and new methods of prevention, treatment, and diagnosis. The doubters of the effect of biomedical research should ask themselves the following question: What is the reason for the relative downward movement in economic burden where there have been marked successes in biomedical sciences and for the upward trends where there have not been successes? Another effect of biomedical research is that preventive and therapeutic measures have altered medical practices. For example, one change has been the growth of the medical center with its complex array of staff and equipment. Another change is the reduced need for home visits as the infectious diseases have been brought under control.

BIOMEDICAL ADVANCES AND IMPACT ON BURDEN

We have attempted a first cut at a classification system of burden-reducing and burden-increasing impacts of research:

A. *Burden-reducing Impacts*
- Reduction in sickness rates (e.g., preventive immunizations)
- Decreases in period of sickness (e.g., improved therapies such as antibiotics, development of immunizations for viral and other infectious diseases)
- Reduction in time required for treatment (e.g., technology of treatment of dental cavities)
- Reduction of errors in diagnosis (e.g., improved laboratory testing)
- Improved access to treatment (e.g., improved screening techniques)
- Improved surgery and anesthesiology (e.g., heart disease, congenital anomalies)
- Improved treatment of hypertension, Parkinson's disease, and mental disorders
- Reduction of errors in treatment (e.g., Rh factor, early ambulation after childbirth and surgery, advances in drug testing and testing of rehabilitation devices and techniques)

Better marketing of care, organization of productive care, and greater economy in the use of expensive equipment and facilities also are products of research.

B. *Burden-increasing Impacts*

- Better understanding of some diseases (e.g., earlier diagnosis and identification of disease conditions resulting in care where none was provided earlier)
- Prolongation of impaired lives (e.g., kidney dialysis, use of pacemakers)
- Improved, yet more complex, testing equipment (e.g., scanners, ultrasound imaging)
- Development of additional tests of disease for purposes of (a) establishing diagnosis, and (b) testing efficacy and progress of treatment (e.g., blood tests for potassium)
- More complex therapies (e.g., chemotherapy in cancer cases)
- More development and application of prosthetics (e.g., improved artificial limbs)
- Extension of periods of high-cost treatment (e.g., cardiac intensive care units)
- Additional margins for error in treatment due to the complexity of treatment

REAL GAINS FROM RISING OUTLAYS

The shift that has taken place from indirect to direct costs has received far less attention than the ever mounting size of the nation's health bill. Even as medical care costs have risen in recent years, the death rate for the U.S. population has slowly declined. So has time loss from work due to illness or injury. The tangible benefits that have begun to appear thus have to be balanced against the direct health outlays.

In 1900, almost 90 percent of the total burden of illness represented the loss in earnings and product due to sickness and premature death. The relatively small share remaining was accounted for by payments to physicians, pharmacists, and other providers. By 1930, direct outlays amounted to 13 percent of the total, and again, the major share of the estimated burden of illness was represented by the loss of product due to sickness and premature death.

The year 1975 shows the marked change in the distribution of the burden of illness. Product loss due to sickness and premature death dropped to under two-thirds of the total and direct health outlays rose to well over one-third. We project the distribution of sickness burdens to be about evenly distributed by the year 2000 between cost of premature death and disease and direct outlays for health care. It is estimated that the two types of cost will reach $1 trillion each, for a total $2-trillion burden of illness in the year 2000 at year 2000 dollar values (Figure 13-1).

Conversion of the burden estimates for each of the periods to 1975 dollars does not reverse the earlier finding (Figure 13-2). On the contrary, at constant 1975 prices, indirect costs, if anything, are a smaller rather than a larger share of the aggregate. The year 2000 projections in 1975 dollars suggest that direct cost will account not for half, but for over 60 percent of the total burden of illness.

It is real changes in mortality and morbidity that give rise to optimism about the future. The age-adjusted death rate, which corrects for the changing age composition of the population, fell to 6.4 deaths per 1,000 in 1975 and even lower in 1976. Especially noteworthy is the change in the death rates for males fifty-five to sixty-four years of age. Between 1969 and 1975, male death rates in this age group decreased by 12 percent, for an average of 2 percent per year. This decline stands in sharp contrast to the ten-year period beginning in the mid-1950s that actually witnessed a rise in the death rate for this age group.

Death rates among those of the prime working ages are down even more sharply. Rates of death from both heart disease and cancer have recently declined for those in the twenty-five to forty-five age group, and a further decline is expected. (The cancer death rate for this age group is now above the heart disease rate.) Accident death rates are also down. Only the suicide rate has moved up steadily. Work-loss days and days lost from work by those not able to participate in the work force due to illness and injury also are declining.

INDIRECT COST TRENDS AND THE CHALLENGE TO MEDICINE

Stability in death rates for over a decade (1955-65) was grist for the mill to those who would challenge the efficacy of medicine and the gains from medical science. The argument was repeatedly advanced that medical care had reached some limit in its capacity to prolong life and enhance the quality of life.[10] This argument was central to Fuchs's moderate thesis on assessment of choices in health care, given the failure of medicine for the period beginning in 1955 to make additional headway toward prolongation of life. The argument was critical to the extreme skepticism of Illich about the potential gain from additional resources allocated for health.[11]

Death rates have now turned down, suggesting that the economic cost of death is declining. While the causes for the decline are unclear, the challenge to medical science, assuming fact catches up with rhetoric, must necessarily be attenuated. Some attribute the decline in death rate, especially for circulatory diseases, to the newer efforts at holistic medicine, to more exercise, reduced smoking, and better nutrition. Others credit the control of hypertension, open heart surgery, emergency paramedical care, and cardiac intensive care units. For other diseases with lower death rates, there is the same division of credit. Certainly, the reduction in the speed limit to fifty-five miles per hour had some influence on death rates from auto accidents for the years 1975-76. Medicare and Medicaid may also have made a contribution to reduction in death rates and disability by easing access to care for aged persons and the poor.[12] (The cancer case stands out by way of contrast to circulatory diseases as a major cause of death with increasing, rather than decreasing, cost of death, despite the size of the biomedical research and health care budget devoted to the disease.)

It would be a gross exaggeration to claim a *large* reduction in economic cost of death. Changes in death rates among those in the productive years of life are not likely to be large. The expert testimony to further improvements in mortality for the younger ages (see Chapter 3) is certainly indicative of new gains and lowered cost, but the percentages tend to be small. As we indicated earlier, past historic progress in reduction of deaths, which has concentrated deaths in the upper age groups, sets a real limit on future gains.

While the challenge to medicine is premature, this does not mean that the current emphasis on the importance of life styles to health should be questioned. Preventive health care by improved diet, exercise, and reduced smoking and use of alcohol means improved health. Research has at least partially established that such preventive care means longer life and less sickness.[13, 14] Far more research, however, is needed in this area.

Cost of sickness is also estimated to be off from the levels these costs would reach without the projected improvement in work loss and withdrawals from the work force due to sickness. Research has yielded a new attitude toward long-term institutional care that has released individuals into the community and the work force instead of prescribing extended hospital stays. Better personal adjustments with high cure rates are associated with community rather than institutional care. Mental hospital patient censuses are down in consequence, as are other long-term hospital populations. Work-loss days are on the decline, though far from a steep decline.

The trend for most indicators of morbidity, however, moves in the opposite direction—up—adding fuel to the challenge of medicine. Restricted-activity days, bed days of care, and percent of individuals with limitations of activity are all up over the years for which National Center for Health Statistics data are available (see Chapter 7).

If death rates are down, sickness in the population may be expected to increase. The consequential phenomena of the impaired life and of chronic illness, point in that direction. Years ago, the impaired life consequences of declining death rates were refuted by the better health of those who were spared from disease, for example, the child who did not fight a bad case of diphtheria. Today, the impaired life consequences are of a different order. To the extent that the postponement of death is in the older ages, more impairment may be expected.[15] We do not know the relative distributional impact between improved health status and more impairment as a consequence of modern medicine. Far more information is needed. The rhetoric continues, however, claiming that at present, newer therapies mean short-term life extensions, with low quality of life, and at very high costs. Little is known about the overall balance.

BURDEN OF ILLNESS ON THE ECONOMY

We have estimated the burden of illness thus far in terms of (a) direct health expenditures; (b) cost of work-time loss due to absence and inability to work; and (c) cost of premature death. Direct expenditures are a part of the gross national product (GNP) or of the aggregate flow of goods and services. But the work-time loss and loss of productivity due to absence, inability to work, or premature death are not part of the valuation of GNP. On the contrary, it is because of the work-time loss and loss in production that the GNP is lower than it otherwise would be. To relate the work and productivity loss to GNP, it is necessary, first, to adjust the GNP figure by the amount of the loss.

Health expenditures were earlier shown as a percentage of GNP. In 1900, health expenditures amounted to 3 percent of GNP; this percentage grew to almost 4 percent in 1930, to 5.8 percent in 1963, and to 8.6 percent by 1977. A further rise of health expenditures to almost 12 percent of GNP is expected by year 2000 (Figure 13-3). However, to add together the several types of economic burden and relate the total to GNP, GNP has to be adjusted as indicated above.

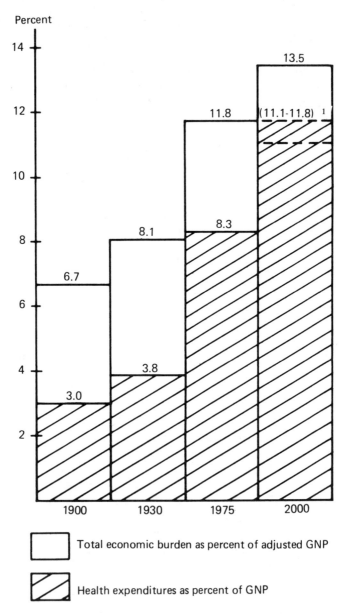

Percent

Total economic burden as percent of adjusted GNP

Health expenditures as percent of GNP

[1] Reflects projections using the aggregate and disaggregated approaches.

Sources: Reference 9; and A. Berk and L.C. Paringer: "Costs of illness and disease, 1900." Public Services Laboratory, Georgetown University, Washington, D.C., August 1977, revised 1979.

Figure 13-3. Economic Burden of Illness as a Percent of GNP for Selected Years

The burden of disease and injury for 1900 may be estimated as the sum of health expenditures, cost of work loss due to absence from work and inability to work and the single-year cost of premature death. These costs added together and computed as a percent of an adjusted GNP figure for year 1900 (with GNP increased to show the addition if there were no loss in work time or product due to sickness and premature death) are shown in Table 13-5, together with similar estimates for 1930, 1975, and 2000. Tables 13A-1, 13A-2, and 13A-3 in the appendix to this chapter show the data in greater detail for disease.

In 1900, the economic burden of illness and injury measured for comparison with GNP aggregated to $1.3 billion. That total reached $180.6 billion by 1975 and is projected at $1,401 billion by year 2000.

The cost of death used throughout this book is a different type of estimate than that required here. The concept used throughout is that the cost of deaths in a year represents not only earnings loss that year due to premature death but also loss of earnings in the years remaining of a normal life expectancy and work expectancy given the age and sex of the persons who die prematurely. The estimate thus is not confined to a single-year loss in work time and earnings. Here, however, to relate the cost of death to the annual flow of goods and services produced in the economy, it was necessary to confine the cost of death to the amount of work time and product loss in a single year. The estimates presented in Tables 13-5 and 13-6 are computed in this way.

The total economic burden of illness in 1975 is estimated to claim almost 12 percent of the adjusted GNP or of the national flow of goods and services. For the year 2000, a further growth in the share of adjusted GNP is projected; the economic burden of illness is estimated to reach 13.5 percent. In contrast, for the beginning of the century, the total economic burden is estimated at 6.7 percent or below one-half the relative burden, year 2000.

Are these shares too large a drain on GNP? There is no ready answer. The burden of illness, when assessed in terms of the nation's flow of goods and services, shows the considerable burden of illness and premature death. The share of costs attributable to the cost of wage loss and loss in production is declining (Figure 13-3).

The magnitude shown, however, is so large as to raise questions about controlling the growth. By the year 2000, unless far greater gains are made in controlling direct costs and in preventing unnecessary sickness and premature deaths, the share of GNP claimed by the

Table 13-5.   Economic Burden of Illness, in Billions, Selected Years, 1900-2000

Disease category by fiscal year 1975 ranking	2000	1975	1930	1900
Total[1]	$1,401.2	$180.6	$8.2	$1.3
Diseases of the circulatory system	193.5	26.6	.6	.1
Mental disorders	133.5	18.2	.7	.1
Diseases of the digestive system	149.3	18.2	1.1	.1
Diseases of the respiratory system	125.9	16.3	1.2	.3
Diseases of the nervous system	94.7	13.2	.5	.1
Accidents, poisonings, and violence	105.6	13.1	.9	.1
Diseases of the musculoskeletal system	94.7	12.5	.4	.1
Neoplasms	61.8	7.4	.1	[2]
Diseases of the genitourinary system	66.5	7.4	.3	.1
Infective and parasitic diseases[3]	29.6	3.6	1.1	.2

[1] Includes unallocated totals.

[2] Less than $50 million.

[3] Infective and parasitic diseases added even though they rank lower than other categories of disease to permit comparison with 1900 data.

Sources: Reference 9; see Table 13-1.

burden of illness will have more than doubled. The twentieth century will thus witness extraordinary change in the shares of the nation's output claimed by sickness and death. It is possible, however, to reinterpret the figures not as a drain but as a potential increment in goods and services—additions that might be achieved by prevention of disease and injury within one or another disease category. The potential gains may be assessed disease category by disease category. If steps could be taken to prevent circulatory diseases, mental disorders, and diseases of the digestive system, the three most costly diseases, the share of adjusted GNP claimed by the economic burden of sickness and premature death would be reduced from 11.8 percent of GNP to 7.7 percent, a decrease which would amount in 1975 GNP values to $62.8 billion and in the values of 1977, to far larger sums. A 50-percent reduction in the economic burden of these three major diseases would add $31.4 billion to the value of goods and services available for other purposes.

Important steps to check the incidence of sickness in the work force by new prevention measures and to postpone death to an advanced age would go a long way toward cutting those costs. Some gains have recently been made but the rate of advances will have to be greatly accelerated. But some scientists believe that the rate of

Table 13-6. Economic Burden of Illness as a Percent of Adjusted Gross National Product[1]

Disease category by fiscal year 1975 ranking	*2000*	*1975*	*1930*	*1900*
All diseases	13.5	11.8	8.1	6.7
Diseases of the circulatory system	1.9	1.7	0.5	0.5
Mental disorders	1.3	1.2	0.7	0.5
Diseases of the digestive system	1.4	1.2	1.1	0.7
Diseases of the respiratory system	1.2	1.1	1.2	1.5
Diseases of the nervous system	0.9	0.9	0.5	0.3
Accidents, poisonings, and violence	1.0	0.9	0.9	0.4
Diseases of the musculoskeletal system	0.9	0.8	0.4	0.5
Neoplasms	0.6	0.5	0.1	0.1
Diseases of the genitourinary system	0.6	0.5	0.3	0.4
Infective and parasitic diseases	0.3	0.2	1.1	1.3
Adjusted GNP, in billions[1]	10,406	1,533	101	19

[1] Gross national product for the fiscal years to which has been added the cost of morbidity and premature mortality during the single year.

Sources: Reference 9; see Table 13-1.

introduction of new toxic substances in the industrial environment is far outstripping the capacity of the medical profession to develop preventives.

COST ESTIMATES EXPANDED

We have presented the estimates of the burdens of illness over the decades from 1900 to year 2000, applying a traditional accounting of those burdens. Certain characteristics of the estimates of the cost of premature deaths probably warrant some further elaboration. Cost of premature death for each of the designated years generally is estimated assuming that the value of future earnings is appropriately discounted at 2.5 percent per year. In the preceding section, cost of premature death is estimated for a single year only, the year of death, and no account is taken of subsequent earnings loss so that earnings are not discounted. Future work-force participation earnings for 1900 and 1930 are not tied to the actual future experience. Rather, the estimates are prepared in a manner consistent with that of the year 1975, namely, the figures are estimated as if the future beyond 1900 and 1930 were not known any more than the future for years of the 1980s and beyond are known. Labor force participation rates and earnings thus are those of the year of the estimate.

Productivity over the years ahead, however, is assumed to rise 2 percent per annum as an adjustment for real earnings' trends.

Essentially, two types of questions are at issue about that traditional accounting. The first is the range of cost originating in disease and injury that is not included as part of the traditional accounts. The second is directed to the essential meaning of "burden of illness."

A word is in order about this second issue, which is discussed at greater length in Chapter 15. The traditional measure of burden of illness depends on vital statistics that have come to be familiar over the years. Deaths, death rates (infant mortality, maternal deaths per 1,000 births), life expectancy at different ages, survival rates by age, and so forth are all part of the customary vital statistics package. As we have indicated, sickness surveys were made as early as the 1910s and sickness data were collected in the 1890 census. It was clear that death rates alone did not define health status of the population; information was needed on sickness. Several measures of sickness came to be applied. Vital statistics were extended to include such measures as prevalence rates of illness, days of illness—disabling and nondisabling in the population—days confined to bed, and work-loss days. These existing data were not designed to measure the impact of medical care or biomedical research and they serve the purpose poorly. Much new work is going forward to substitute measurement of functional states and quality of life for earlier indexes or to supplement those conventional measurements.[16] The burden of illness importantly depends, for those with a chronic disease, on the capacity to function on a daily basis in "normal" economic and social life. The challenge to biomedical research lies primarily in achieving such functionality and to biostatisticians in measuring this functionality.

We attempt, as well, to quantify the cost of illness that falls outside the health sector of the economy. At best, the costs quantified are only a segment of the added resources due to illness or injury. For consumers, for example, both the quality of consumption and quality of being are altered by illness. Two families with the same income and access to goods experience very different degrees of enjoyment if the members of one family are ill and the members of the other are well. Quality of life is impaired for those who are sick and their families. A true count of burden of illness should assess changes in consumer expenditure patterns as a result of illness and put a shadow price on the altered quality of living. However, to do so requires detailed analysis outside the scope of the present study. We did estimate the cost of transportation for the 1,675 million trips to health care facilities in 1975. We also included the costs to consumers of property damage due to mental illnesses, in particular, alcohol and other drug abuse (Table 13-7).

Government outlays originating in illness and injury also were priced. The types of expenditures made are many, ranging from extra school costs to added costs of waste disposal processes to antitrust and insurance commission enforcement.

As part of this study we have estimated a number of cost items that are excluded from the traditional accounts. What we have accounted for, however, falls short of what needs to be done to round out the accounting. More specifically, we have estimated (*a*) the cost of debility or loss of product or higher cost of product due to the sick worker at work; (*b*) the value of time spent in receiving care or assisting patients; (*c*) governmental and industrial outlays made on account of the disabled or sick that are not included

Table 13-7. An Expanded Estimate of the Burden of Illness, 1975

	Burden of illness (in billions)
Total	$419.6-640.3
Traditional count of burden of illness	322.6
Direct health expenditures	118.5
Cost of premature death (at 2.5-percent discount)	146.2
Loss in work time and product due to sickness	57.8
Cost of debility	42.0-51.3
Acute temporary conditions	34.5-41.5
Impairments following major illness	0.7-2.8
Static impairments	5.5
Other losses in industrial accidents	1.3-1.5
Nonhealth sector cost of illness	29.2-37.8
Consumer outlays (e.g., transportation, property losses)	3.9-4.3
Government expenditures (e.g., extra education costs, counseling, aid to handicapped, costs of antisocial behavior)	8.0-14.5
Time costs of health care	4.5-6.2
Industry	12.8
Costs of pain	25.8-228.6

Sources: See Chapter 10; L.C. Paringer and A. Berk: "Costs of illness and disease, fiscal year 1975." Public Services Laboratory, Georgetown University, Washington, D.C., January 1977; S.J. Mushkin and J.S. Landefeld: "Non-health sector costs of illness." Public Services Laboratory, Georgetown University, Washington, D.C., January 1978; and S.J. Mushkin, C. Resnick, and J.S. Landefeld: "The cost of pain." Public Services Laboratory, Georgetown University, Washington, D.C., June 1978.

in the current definition of health expenditures; and (*d*) the cost of pain. For most, if not all, of the items for which we have prepared supplementary estimates, a dollar price is given based on actual costs incurred, or market prices. For debility, time loss and earnings losses are used, paralleling the count for disability as indicated in Chapter 10.

Pain is valued using optional shadow prices. Estimates are based on the use of medical care that originates in a pain symptom, on the amount spent by consumers on painkillers, and on the price of pain clinics. We also priced pain in terms of the value given to pain and suffering in court awards.

Cost burdens excluded from the traditional counts are many and varied. Some of these costs are economic and are wholly compatible with the concept of human capital on which the traditional measurements rest. Others are psychological and social costs that some would assess in terms of some aggregate measure of willingness to pay to reduce a statistical probability of being confronted with a disease problem either as a patient, or as a family member, or as part of a community. Others attempt the estimation using some shadow prices for each of identified cost items as they impact on individual, family, or community.

Burden of illness data as an indicator of relative need for remedial action, whether through biomedical research or some other health program, can be misleading if important burdens are omitted.

We have included in this exercise items of mental health costs and of drug addiction and alcoholism that are not part of the usual accounts. Cost of disfigurement is not valued nor is stress. Much sickness is thought to originate in stress, but sickness also causes stress of a variety of kinds, for example, stress in the person afflicted with disease and stress in family and friends. Other cost burdens may be those of family conflict, divorce, alienation, and suicide, all of which have been associated with disease problems.

Intergenerational impacts of disease conditions are of great importance. We have counted the cost of school absences due to sickness as part of the added governmental outlays; we have not estimated the price to children of disturbed household arrangements when serious illness strikes.

We earlier referred to the work of Abt who perhaps more than others has quantified certain social and psychological costs.[17] In his article on the cost of cancer, he identifies, as we indicated earlier, groups who incur social or psychological costs as a consequence of association with terminal cancer. For the cost items identified he developed market or shadow prices. Only those psychological and social costs quantified as $1 million or more and separately identified are shown here.

Psychological and social costs	Patient	Family	Friends and co-workers	Providers of care	Total
			(In millions)		
Mental	$35	$ 55	$30		$120
Sexual loss	75	75			150
Antisocial behavior		210			210
Suicidal behavior (guilt, anxiety, etc.)	35	65			100

The emphasis of the Abt estimates is on the dying cancer patient and the cost of dying, including the cost to the patient of isolation. Indeed, almost half the psychological or social costs fall into this category. We have not included these costs. In some measure, they are already in the economic estimates of the cost of premature death and morbidity. The cost items identified above, however, total $580 million.

Out of those $580 million, $210 million, in turn, represent two types of antisocial behavior. The first is the loss of school progress, which, in turn, is measured by the loss in lifetime earnings of the children of cancer patients. The second and far smaller share (5 percent of the total) is attributed to the delinquency and crime of children whose lives are disrupted by the death of a parent.

The estimates of social and psychological cost have been presented to underscore that the state of research on burden of illness is not favorable to early application of burden estimates in determining research priorities. The economic costs of cancer estimated in this report at $19 to $28 billion are compatible with earlier economic cost estimates but they are widely at variance with the psychological-social cost accounting.

Relevant to an understanding of the allocation of research funds and measurement of outcomes, it is important that research proceed on the two issues identified earlier: functional status measurement and better accounting of costs of disease. Policy officials can be aided in their quest for accountability only if information from such research becomes available.

Table 13A-1. Total Economic Burden of Illness, in Millions, Fiscal Year 1975

Disease category	Total	Direct cost	Indirect cost		
			Total	Morbidity	Mortality (single year only)
All diseases[1]	$180,574	$118,500	$62,074	$57,846	$4,228
Infective and parasitic diseases	3,622	2,027	1,595	1,559	36
Neoplasms	7,403	5,279	2,124	1,105	1,019
Endocrine, nutritional, and metabolic diseases	5,134	3,337	1,797	1,695	102
Diseases of the blood and blood-forming organs	978	676	302	281	21
Mental disorders	18,201	9,411	8,790	8,751	39
Diseases of the nervous system and sense organs	13,210	7,459	5,751	5,706	45
Eye diseases[2]	(5,022)	(4,648)	(374)	(374)	2
Diseases of the circulatory system	26,616	16.017	10,599	8,744	1,855
Cerebrovascular diseases[2]	(3,262)	(2,633)	(629)	(353)	(276)
Diseases of the respiratory system	16,314	7.571	8,743	8,542	201
Diseases of the digestive system	18,159	14.564	3,595	3,438	157
Diseases of the oral cavity salivary glands, and jaws[2]	(8,123)	(7,777)	(346)	(346)	2
Diseases of the genitourinary system	7,395	5.575	1,820	1,770	50
Complications of pregnancy, childbirth and puerperium	3,582	3 387	195	193	2
Diseases of the skin and subcutaneous tissue	2,523	2,120	403	399	4
Diseases of the musculoskeletal system and connective tissue	12,477	5.113	7,364	7,351	13
Congenital anomalies	879	432	447	437	10
Certain causes of perinatal morbidity and mortality	65	64	1	—	1

Symptoms and ill-defined conditions	4,519	3,180	1,339	1,260	79
Accidents, poisonings, and violence	13,109	6,846	6,263	5,669	594
Other	7,262	6,316	946	946	—
Unallocated	19,126	19,126	—	—	—

[1] Totals may not add due to rounding.

[2] Included in previous total.

Source: L.C. Paringer and A. Berk: "Costs of illness and disease, fiscal year 1975." Public Services Laboratory, Georgetown University, Washington, D.C., January 1977.

Table 13A-2.   Total Economic Burden of Illness, in Millions, Fiscal Year 1930

| | | | | Indirect cost | |
Disease category	Total	Direct cost	Total	Morbidity	Mortality (single year only)
All diseases[1]	$8,188.6	$3,644.0	$4,544.6	$4,181.2	$363.4
Infective and parasitic diseases	1,092.4	339.7	752.7	708.8	43.9
Neoplasms	127.9	40.0	87.9	48.2	39.7
Endocrine, nutritional, and metabolic diseases	122.4	54.6	67.8	57.0	10.8
Diseases of the blood and blood-forming organs	72.6	14.8	57.8	54.9	2.9
Mental disorders	672.9	180.4	492.5	489.1	3.4
Diseases of the nervous system and sense organs	518.9	257.2	261.7	252.8	8.9
Eye diseases[2]	166.7	155.8	10.9	10.9	[2]
Diseases of the circulatory system	556.4	106.8	449.6	347.7	101.9
Cerebrovascular diseases[2]	99.5	9.2	90.3	64.4	25.9[2]
Diseases of the respiratory system	1,238.4	583.4	655.0	621.5	33.5
Diseases of the digestive system	1,125.1	710.7	414.4	390.1	24.3
Diseases of the oral cavity, salivary glands, and jaws[2]	496.7	493.8	2.9	2.9	[2]
Diseases of the genitourinary system	333.8	138.2	195.6	159.7	35.9
Complications of pregnancy, childbirth, and puerperium	278.9	169.3	109.6	104.3	5.3
Diseases of the skin and subcutaneous tissue	132.8	76.9	55.9	55.3	.6
Diseases of the musculoskeletal system and connective tissue	391.0	124.8	266.2	265.5	.7
Congenital anomalies	11.5	11.4	.1	—	.1
Certain causes of perinatal morbidity and mortality	11.3	11.3	.0	—	.0

Summing Up the Burden of Illness 391

Symptoms and ill-defined conditions	82.7	44.9	37.8	32.6	5.2
Accidents, poisonings, and violence	873.9	233.5	640.4	593.7	46.7
Other	546.1	546.1	—	—	—

[1] Totals may not add due to rounding.
[2] Included in previous total.

Source: A. Berk and L.C. Paringer: "Costs of illness and disease, fiscal year 1930." Public Services Laboratory, Georgetown University, Washington, D.C., May 1977.

Table 13A-3.   Total Economic Burden of Illness, in Millions, 1900

Disease category	Total	Direct cost	Indirect cost		
			Total	Mortality (single year only)	Morbidity
All diseases[1]	$1,251	$544	$707	$76	$631
Infective and parasitic diseases	243	80	163	22	141
Neoplasms	17	12	5	3	2
Endocrine, nutritional, and metabolic diseases	5	1	4	1	3
Diseases of the blood and blood-forming organs	4	1	3	[3]	3
Mental disorders	98	23	75	1	74
Diseases of the nervous system and sense organs	58	22	36	2	34
Diseases of the circulatory system	88	51	37	13[2]	24
Diseases of the respiratory system	274	91	183	12	171
Diseases of the digestive system	123	86	37	3	34
Diseases of the genitourinary system	82	23	59	10	49
Complications of pregnancy, childbirth, and the puerperium	53	37	16	1	15
Diseases of the skin and subcutaneous tissue	8	4	4	[3]	4
Diseases of the musculoskeletal system and connective tissue	102	55	47	[3]	47
Congenital anomalies and Certain causes of perinatal morbidity and mortality	1	1	—	0	—

Symptoms and ill-defined conditions	8	4	4	1	3
Accidents, poisonings, and violence	68	35	33	5	28
Unallocated	18	18	—	—	—

[1] Totals may not add due to rounding.

[2] Diseases of the circulatory system includes cerebrovascular diseases.

[3] Amounts are less than $.5 million.

Source: A. Berk and L.C. Paringer: "Costs of illness and disease, 1900." Public Services Laboratory, Georgetown University, Washington, D.C., August 1977, revised 1979.

REFERENCES

1. National Health Education Committee: Facts on the major killing and crippling diseases in the United States today. National Health Education Committee, New York, 1959.

2. Report of the National Conservation Commission, Vol. 3, U.S. Senate Document No. 676, 60th Congress, 2d sess., Washington, D.C., February 1909.

3. Farr, W.: Journal of the Statistical Society, 1853.

4. Quoted in Dublin, L.I., and Lotka, A.J.: The money value of a man. Ronald Press, New York, 1946.

5. Dublin, L.I., and Whitney, J.: On the cost of tuberculosis. Journal of the American Statistical Association 42, December 1920.

6. Dublin, L.I., and Lotka, A.J.: The money value of a man. Ronald Press, New York, 1946.

7. Rice, D.P.: Estimating the cost of illness. Department of Health, Education, and Welfare, U.S. Government Printing Office, Washington, D.C., 1966.

8. Cooper, B., and Rice, D.: The economic cost of illness revisited. Soc Sec Bull 21, February 1976.

9. Mushkin, S.J., et al.: Cost of disease and illness in the United States in the year 2000. Public Health Rep 93: 497-588, September-October 1978.

10. Fuchs, V.R.: Who shall live? health, economics, and social choice. Basic Books, New York, 1974.

11. Illich, I.: Medical nemesis. Pantheon, New York, 1976.

12. Friedman, B.: Mortality, disability, and normative economics of medicare. *In* The role of health insurance in the health services sector, edited by Richard N. Rosett. National Bureau of Economic Research, New York, 1976.

13. Belloc, N.B.: Relationship to health practices and mortality. Preventive Medicine 2: 67-81, 1973.

14. Belloc, N.B., and Breslow, L.: Relationship of physical health status and health practices. Preventive Medicine 1: 409-421, 1972.

15. Gruenberg, E.M.: The failure of success. Milbank Memorial Fund Quarterly 55: 3-24, winter 1977.

16. Mushkin, S.J., and Dunlop, D., editors: Health: what is it worth? Pergamon Press, Elmsford, N.Y., 1979.

17. Abt, C.: The social costs of cancer. Social Indicators Research 2: 175-190, 1975.

Chapter Fourteen

Objectives and an Accounting

Demands for accountability for expenditure of public funds have contributed to a search for methods to determine the profitability of biomedical research. The quest for accountability has encouraged evaluation of biomedical research expenditure despite the general skepticism about analyses of research programs. Even Niskanen, once the OMB top official on analysis and evauation, wrote: "Most 'systems analyses' of research programs I believe have been, and will be, rather sterile."[1]

BIOMEDICAL RESEARCH OBJECTIVES

One explanation for the difficulty in assessment of biomedical research is the multiplicity of objectives that characterize such research. Objectives run from the advance of science as an intellectual pursuit to the highly practical purpose of reducing time spent in a surgical or medical procedure. Even a partial listing of objectives would include the following:

- Advancement of scientific knowledge
- Reduction in mortality and morbidity
- Improvement in functional states or in quality of patient life
- A healthier and more vigorous population
- Correction of historic health inequities
- Reduction in environmental health hazards
- Greater productivity of medical procedures and processes, and of health personnel

- Improved international relations
- Support of national defense
- Greater productivity of work force and economic growth

In the orthodoxy of evaluation processes for each of these objectives, a number of criteria are required that capture the content as completely as possible. (Criteria for criteria of assessment are outlined in the following chapter.)

As a trial and a partial undertaking, outlined here are some criteria for assessing each of the illustrative objectives:

Objectives	*Criteria*
Advancement of scientific knowledge	Number of Nobel or other scientific awards received Number of articles published in scientific journals Number of scientific articles cited by others
Reduction in mortality and morbidity	Reduced death rates Increased life expectancy Reduced disability days Reduced restricted-activity days
Improvement in functional states or in quality of patient life	Number and percent of those with disease fully functioning (see Chapter 15) Quality-adjusted years of life
A healthier population	In the absence of positive criteria for assessing health, certain process variables might be used, such as: Proportion of population participating in exercise programs Proportion of population participating in nutrition improvement programs Proportion of population who are no longer smoking
Correction of historic health inequities	Again process variables may be used that would give approximations of the amount and

	portion of research devoted to special health problems of minority groups, e.g., blacks, Indians
Reduction in environmental health hazards	Number of toxic substances identified Reduction in number and percent of deaths from environmental hazards (air, foods, occupational diseases)
Greater productivity of procedures and personnel	Changes in time spent carrying out medical, surgical, and dental procedures Number of patients per practitioner
Improved international relations	The criteria might run from reduced death, disability, or debility rates to improved foreign press comments on the United States
Support of national defense	Percent of wounded who recover Deaths averted Disabilities averted
Greater productivity of work force and economic growth	More years of work Higher marginal product of added workers Less loss of output of those at work Increased national product

This list of criteria for assessing how much progress is made toward the several identified objectives of biomedical research conveys the range of measurement problems in achieving accountability.

Estimates have not been made of biomedical research by objectives. This is partly so because a formulation of research objectives is still in the developmental phase. The tentative listing outlined here may have little to do with any statement of objectives that is subsequently formulated by the National Institutes of Health or by the general research community in response to the Secretary of DHEW's request for long-range plans for medical research.

THE INVESTMENT IN
BIOMEDICAL RESEARCH

What has been the investment in biomedical research? As we have indicated earlier (Chapter 2), about $45.1 billion was spent cumulatively for health research by industry, government, private voluntary agencies, and foundations and academic institutions from 1900 to 1975. An additional $10.5 billion was spent during the period 1976-77, raising the total to $55.6 billion in current dollars through fiscal year 1977.

A lag exists between resource inputs into biomedical research represented by expenditures and intermediate products in the form of publications or patents received, and presumably, there is still a longer lag between an expenditure for research and an effect on health status of the population. No one expects immediate returns, but the question remains: How long is the lag between research and development expenditures and product? We assume here a ten-year lag between expenditures and outputs, which is the lag we applied earlier in this volume for assessing mortality and morbidity gains from biomedical research.

Several qualifications about the lag period require emphasis. The actual lag between conception of an idea, to invention, to trials, to widespread application may be expected to have varied historically. If the historic sickness data tell us anything, they point to a long lag at the turn of the century between new knowledge and application. Smallpox cases appeared in the early 1900s and for years afterward despite the availability of the vaccine by the mid-1800s. Similarly, diphtheria anti-toxin was developed in 1890 but immunization on a significant scale did not begin until 1920. Perhaps the poverty of many in the population, lack of access to medical care, and lack of information about what medical care might do are among the factors contributing to lags, particularly those of varying duration over time. Yet the information about lags in health care technology or productivity is most deficient. The studies that give us data are few.[2] They deal with special cases and there are wide differences in experience with these cases. The ten-year lag is clearly an assumption made for working purposes. It may be somewhat short, or long, and it undoubtedly varied as an average over the years of the twentieth century.

The cumulative period of research outlays that interest us in terms of assessing the investment made in research and development, given a ten-year lag, is that between 1890 and 1965. Expenditures in the early years were low and we have not bothered to estimate them for the period of 1890 to the early 1900s, except by assuming 1900 outlays for each of the years of the decade earlier; change in the level of expenditures for those early years would make little difference in the final results.

The cumulative investment in biomedical research does not give us a full accounting of what the cost of research was in opportunities forgone. We account for those opportunity costs by asking: What would be the value of the investment in research and development if we added interest to reflect what would have been earned as a yield had the sums not been spent for research and instead had been invested in other enterprises or activities?

We estimate the opportunity costs of the research and development funds at $96 billion for the years through 1977, at almost $30 billion through 1965, with interest only added for the period 1965-75 (Table 14-1), and at $73 billion for the period 1900-75. The interest cost forgone entering into the opportunity cost computation is calculated here year by year at the long-term federal rate.

As an alternative computation, we have also estimated the present value of research and development at 1975 price levels using the biomedical research price index computed by Westat, supplemented by a regression of the GNP deflator and the Westat research and development price index for the earlier years. The 1975 price calculations were made to develop a cumulative research and development outlay that is compatible with the benefit amount. In

Table 14-1. **Biomedical Research Expenditures, Total in Current Dollars and Opportunity Cost, Selected Periods, in Billions**

Period	Biomedical research, cumulative total		Opportunity cost of biomedical research expenditures, including interest[1]	
	Current dollars	Constant dollars	Current dollars	Constant dollars
1900-77	$56	$78	$96	$102
1900-75	45	68	73	88
1900-65	13	26	30[2]	42[3]
1930-65	13	26	29[2]	41[3]

[1] Interest cost computed based on long-term bond rate 1918-77; for years for which such data are not available, the municipal bond rate was used. (This selection may understate somewhat the real interest cost for the period in which the tax-exempt status of municipal securities was significant—1913-18.)

[2] Compound value of investments in biomedical research from 1900 and also 1930 to 1965 plus interest foregone 1965-75. The opportunity cost of interest is calculated by compounding interest annually at the average annual rate on long-term government bonds.

[3] Interest foregone is estimated at 2.5 percent in view of the price adjustment.

determining the interest charges to add to biomedical research at constant 1975 prices, we have used 2.5 percent, or the social preference rate.

In the absence of detailed data, estimates have been prepared that do not precisely reflect the expenditures made. While there is reason to believe that the overall magnitude is reasonable, the division of the total by the period leaves much to be desired. As one possible adjustment, given private foundation support of research in the period before 1930, the opportunity cost of that earlier period may be $100 million or so too low.

Products of research applied in the United States but developed in other countries are not included in the dollar counts; nor are benefits received in other countries from research in the United States added to the benefit valuations. There is no reason to assume that these balance out. We know that much medical knowledge was borrowed from Germany, England, and other countries especially in the years prior to World War II and prior to the building of a sizable scientific community in the United States.

MULTIPLE OBJECTIVES AND INVESTMENT IN THE HEALTH CONDITIONS

The opportunity costs incurred for biomedical research encompass all research objectives. Accordingly in concept, at least, a share of costs should be assigned to each of those objectives.

A major objective for which an adjustment might be made is basic research. Basic research is concerned with scientific advance and the intellectual challenge of such advance rather than a direct health mission such as reduction in mortality or morbidity.

The share of health research that goes toward basic research is far from negligible. The president's 1980 budget analysis places the obligations for basic research of the National Institutes of Health for 1978 at $1.2 billion of a total research obligation, or 46 percent of the $2.6 billion proposed for the National Institutes of Health.[3] While the National Institutes of Health do much of the basic research on life sciences through the intermural and extramural programs, other groups, such as industry and voluntary agencies, conduct some basic research. Truth, knowledge for its own sake, is the goal. For the scientists engaged in the nation's biomedical research effort, the primary rewards given by the professional and institutional organizations are for contributions to basic science. The National Institutes of Health's outstanding record for Nobel prize winners underscores this reward system.

We shall assume for purposes of illustration that about one-quarter of the total annual health research outlay or about $1.4 billion in 1977 went for such basic research. This is, on average, far below the share estimated in the 1980 budget for the National Institutes of Health, reflecting the larger overall concentration on applied problems. The standard for a payoff on basic research dollars is the excellence of the research as evidenced by scientific recognition, and scientific publications. Outstanding contributions might be made in the area of genetics or molecular structures without any link between research expenditures and health status of the population. Basic research is not mission-bound in ways that would augment other national purposes, such as public health goals, economic goals, or even national defense goals.

If, over the twentieth century, about one-quarter of health research funds went for basic research, then about one-quarter of the estimated opportunity costs of research ($18 billion through 1975, $24 billion through 1977, and about $7.5 billion through 1965) can be assigned to intellectual scientific pursuits and their outcomes. From one point of view, the sum for basic research should be deducted in arriving at the payoff related to health missions. From another, no deduction should be made in anticipation of results from the unharnessed basic research, as suggested by Brooks.[4] In a recent article, he made the point this way: "The frequently demonstrated usefulness of 'useless' research is sometimes used as an argument against any kind of social guidance of research. Like the 'invisible hand' of the classical free market, it is argued that the autonomous working of the intellectual free market of ideas will produce socially optimal results at the least cost." But this concept, Brooks goes on to say, "scarcely seems viable in a polity in which a large fraction of the resources invested in the enterprise of science comes from the public, and in which the total investment is as large as it is in the modern industrial states."

Additionally, both international collaboration and defense objectives call for investment in biomedical research that is not appropriately or completely measured by reductions in mortality and morbidity in the United States. In particular, the Foundation for International Technological Cooperation has recently been established to strengthen the scientific and technical problem-solving capacities of developing countries and to focus increased attention of U.S. scientific resources on problems of concern to the developing countries. But international health concerns are not new to the biomedical research community. Some share of the investment in biomedical research has gone for international collaborative purposes, beginning with the conquest of yellow fever and the construction of the Panama Canal. Certain areas of research and development are specially identified as targets for the period ahead, including the development of new vaccines for tropical diseases, such as malaria, study to determine cause of failure of vaccines and chemotherapy in tropical countries, and an attack on diarrheal diseases that continue to be major causes of infant mortality and morbidity in developing countries. Safe, acceptable, effective, and cheap contraceptives are also identified for research priority with emphasis on the appropriateness of the contraceptive to multiple cultures and conditions.[5]

The relation of health research to military medicine has even a longer history. The Hygiene Laboratory and the Public Health Service were generally charged in World War I with major health responsibilities, including supervision of vaccines, manufacture of vaccines, development of substances for treatment of venereal diseases, and the like. The Public Health Service was given responsibility to provide hospital facilities for the care and treatment of discharged sick and disabled military personnel.

World War II witnessed the creation, as a parallel to the National Defense Research Committee, of the Committee on Medical Research representing the Army, Navy, and Public Health Service, with public representatives as well. Among its other tasks, the Committee on Medical Research had responsibility for recommending the need for and the character of contracts for research with universities, hospitals, and other agencies, and for making recommendations on the needs and results of research on medical problems related to national defense. The committee's successes can be identified by its achievements, including the development and widespread use of penicillin, sulfonamides, gamma globulin, adrenal steroids, and cortisone.

The share of biomedical research devoted to military medicine has varied noticeably over the years as had the amount spent for international cooperation. While the total investment in biomedical research could be adjusted with detailed study to relate expenditures to objectives of these programs, the alternative of making no adjustment seems preferable for the present purposes, given the complexity of the factual analysis.

ACCOUNTING FOR INDUSTRY'S BIOMEDICAL R&D

A very different problem arises conceptually in analyzing industry's share of biomedical research. Determination of how much to spend for industrial research is guided by market tests of profitability. Given the bottom profit line, there is no reason to construct somewhat artificial cost-benefit analyses that really are intended to be second-best administrative substitutes for market decisions. The fact that industry invests in biomedical research is evidence of the gains that are received or expected from the outlays made.

The National Institutes of Health annually publishes information about the amount of funds spent by source and by performer for health research and development. For 1977, industry is estimated to have provided $1.6 billion for health research and development.[6] The share of the total provided by industry has remained fairly constant in the last several years, varying from 26 percent of the total research and development bill to 29 percent. During these same years, the share of research funds of the National Institutes of Health has grown from 34 percent to 41 percent.

The 29 percent of total funds provided by industry for health research and development requires, from one perspective, no further justification for accountability. These funds have passed the market test of profitability that produced the decision to spend for research and development. While industry's share has varied over the years, exceeding historically the current 29 percent for some periods and possibly falling behind in others, it would not be unreasonable to assume that between 25 and 30 percent of the cumulative outlays for biomedical research, or $7 to $9 billion up to 1965 and $24 to $29 billion of the cumulative opportunity cost through 1977, has passed the profitability test of the market. Industry's share thus can be analyzed separately from other components of research and development.

The continuing investment by industry in biomedical research and development suggests that research investments are profitable.

The private returns on research and development investment by industry are an incomplete count of the gains. Social returns also accrue. The additive social returns attributable to private investment may even exceed the private returns. There are two ways of assessing these social returns. A private firm by its research and development tends to reduce the cost of a product (or improve the quality for a given cost). The price reduction represents a gain to consumers as part of the social return on new inventions that does not show up directly in the private rate of return of the firm that has achieved lower cost. Still a different way of viewing social returns centers on the characteristics of the cost of invention and the inventive process. Firms cannot always recoup, as their own profit returns, the saving that takes place in a second- or third-generation inventive effort.

Competitive firms may build on the certain knowledge, produced by the initial research and development, that the problem could be solved successfully. Nor can the firm with the initial invention achieve the lower cost that is characteristic of subsequent developmental efforts. The level of research and development of one firm thus benefits other firms in the industry.

If we consider only the immediate private return on R&D investment, social gains will be neglected. While we have found no study directly related to the comparisons of private and social rates of return in industries undertaking biomedical research, we have the evidence from other industrial research and development studies that total social returns are two to two-and-a-half times as great as private returns.

The coefficients for change in industrial output related to change in expenditures for research and development in industry are not unlike the coefficients derived in this study for biomedical research's impact on mortality and morbidity. Minasian's estimate (corrected by Mansfield for an omission) was a 0.08-percent change in output with a 1-percent change in research expenditures; Mansfield in a 1965 study derived a somewhat higher elasticity figure, 1.2.[7] The elasticity coefficients we have computed for change in mortality with changes in biomedical research range from —.10 to —0.5 percent; that is, with a 1-percent increase in research and development activity, there tends to be a 0.5-percent to .10-percent decrease in mortality. The signs of the coefficient differ for the two areas because the output in industrial cases is positive, while in the case of health we are forced to use, in the absence of positive health measures, a negative accounting for gains, such as reduced death rates. The coefficient for biomedical research in the health case measures research activity; in the industrial analysis, dollars for research are used. In each of the instances, no spillover effects are counted in the elasticity coefficients.

Nordhaus, in a conceptual study of the inventive process, estimates the social rate of return at about 2.5 times the private one for industrial research, suggesting the need for governmental or other intervention to assure a proper allocation of resources.[8] Mansfield, in a more recent study, compiled data analyzing the private and social rate of return from investments in seventeen innovations.[9] The findings are shown in Table 14-2.

The findings generally suggest high returns on investment in these seventeen innovations. The median estimated social rate of return is about 56 percent. The private rates of return (before taxes) average about half this rate, or 25 percent. But, as the figures indicate, there

Table 14-2. Social and Private Rates of Return from Investment in Seventeen Innovations

Innovation	Rate of return (percent)	
	Social	Private
Primary metals innovation	17	18
Machine tool innovation	83	35
Component for control system	29	7
Construction material	96	9
Drilling material	54	16
Drafting innovation	92	47
Paper innovation	82	42
Thread innovation	307	27
Door control innovation	27	37
New electronic device	Negative	Negative
Chemical product innovation	71	9
Chemical process innovation	32	25
Chemical process innovation	13	4
Major chemical process innovation	56[1]	31
Household cleaning device	209	214
Stain remover	116	4
Dishwashing liquid	45	46
Median	*56*	*25*

[1] Based on investment of entire industry.

Source: Reference 9.

is large variation. In the case of six innovations, the private rate of return was less than 10 percent, while for five innovations, it was more than 40 percent. In about 30 percent of the cases, the private rate of return was so low as to suggest that, given full knowledge of payoff ahead of time, the firms would not have invested. The social rate of return in these cases was quite high, however, indicating that the innovations were worthwhile. The median social rate of return is 2.2 times the private return in the Mansfield study.

If social returns on industrial biomedical research are 2.2 times or more private returns, expenditures for biomedical research of at least 2.2 times the level now made by industry would be justified. This is especially so given the high rates of return found by Mansfield. Assuming industry's biomedical research expenditures have averaged 25 to 30 percent of the total health research costs over the years (plus accumulated interest forgone), industry invested $7 to $9 billion through 1965 and $24 to $29 billion through 1977. These sums presumably passed the market test of profitability. And if social returns on private research and development are 2.2 times as great as private returns, $15 to $20 billion through 1965 and $53 to $64 billion through 1977 are justified as worthwhile in terms of payoff.

THE PARTIAL ACCOUNTING

Those who challenge the worthwhileness of investment in biomedical research have many arguments to counter in addition to the public's obvious enthusiasm for such research. We have not attempted to consider those arguments at length here. Rather, we have tried to lend some direction to the question of biomedical research investment by identifying several objectives of such research and following through to the implications about profitability given these objectives.

The ground we have covered may be summarized by a brief tabular presentation. It shows how, given that basic health research is a contribution to knowledge rather than a means toward a health-related mission, and given the social returns on industry's health research, the accumulated investment in health research and development that remains to be defended as profitable is not large (Table 14-3). Only $8 to $19 billion of the cumulative total $96 billion opportunity cost of research from 1900 to 1977 is not accounted for, and the same applies for only $2 to $7 billion of the almost $30 billion opportunity cost for research and development through 1965. But there are important objectives that lead to governmental support of health research and development, including military purposes and international relations, which perhaps could account for all the remaining dollars invested.

Table 14-3. Opportunity Cost of Biomedical Research and Some Benefit Offsets

	Opportunity cost,[1] in billions, of health research and development		
	1900-77	*With no lag*[2]	*With 10-year lag*[3]
Total	$96	$73	$30
Basic research (25 percent of total)	24	18	8
Industrial research			
Private returns only (25 to 30 percent of total)	24-29	18-22	7-9
Total social returns (2.2 times private returns)	53-64	40-48	15-20
International military and other objectives		Not available	
Residual to account for profitability	8-19	7-15	2-7

[1] With interest on investment computed at long-term Treasury interest rates.
[2] Opportunity cost, 1900-75.
[3] Opportunity cost, 1900-65.

However, in a sense, this method of dealing with the profitability of health research and development sidesteps the central question. The test of worthwhileness of industrial research based on market decisions fails to probe the real usefulness of the development of new drugs or prosthetic appliances. The underlying purpose of these inventions is to reduce sickness and postpone death. Similarly, the accounting for basic health research as an intellectual exercise without ties to a health mission of one kind or another gives at best only a partial view of the question of research and development support and priorities in such support. Of real importance is the essential impact of research and development on the health status of the population and the quality of patient life.

BENEFITS AND COST OF R&D

In several earlier chapters, we have quantified the value of the reduction in premature death and in work-time loss due to sickness and analyzed the shares of those values attributable to biomedical research, recognizing that many factors have influenced the improvement in mortality and work loss, and that at best, mortality improvement and reduction in work loss are only partial measures of the benefits of research and development. The major estimates of benefits derived in the earlier chapters are summarized here (Table 14-4).

The figures are intended to quantify what biomedical research has achieved by way of reduction in deaths and prevention of sickness. The quantification is made at a time when some investigators have computed the contribution of biomedical research and challenge a favorable finding. Reductions in deaths, for example, are historically a consequence of better nutrition, according to McKeown; new medical treatments and research findings have had little to do with those health gains.[10]

Not only is the contribution of biomedical research to improved health challenged, but there are some who argue that new treatments resulting from biomedical research in fact impair health, increase deaths, and, at best, extend life for a very brief period at great expense. Costs of care are raised by the new technology flowing from biomedical research, the argument goes, without real health gains.

There is, some believe, a new unease about science and research, an unease that has opened up the issue of controls. Perhaps a new stage has been reached, in which an increasing segment of the public is growing concerned about science and technology. Scientists themselves are beginning to accept some approaches to accountability. The concept of limits to scientific inquiry is addressed by the

Table 14-4. Summary of the Value of Reduction in Illness and Premature Death Attributable to Biomedical Research, 1900-75 and 1930-75

	Total value of reduction in sickness or postponement of premature death	Value attributable to biomedical research
	In billions	
Total	$481	$145-167
Saving achieved in 1975 deaths compared to 1930	221	44-66
Saving achieved in 1975 objective sickness rates compared to 1930	260	101
Total	936-1,211	300-480
Saving achieved in 1975 deaths compared to 1900	725	218-290
Saving achieved in 1975 objective sickness rates compared to 1900	211-486	82-190
	In trillions	
Assets in human capital created:		
Total, 1930-75	2.9-3.2	0.8-1.1
Labor force addition in 1975 by reduction in deaths since 1930	2.0-2.3	0.4-0.7
Reduction in long-term disability since 1930	0.9	0.4
Total, 1900-75	6.8-8.3	2.1-3.3
Labor force addition in 1975 by reduction in deaths since 1900	5.7-7.2	1.7-2.9
Reduction in long-term disability since 1900	1.1	0.4

scientific community not in an atmosphere of criticism, but one of acceptance.

There is good reason to believe that new medical knowledge and new therapies have contributed to reduction in deaths and sickness. The methodology that produced the findings of little gain due to research is grossly deficient. It fails to consider the many changes in diagnosis and therapy that have taken place over the years.

A number of diseases that were very prevalent in the early 1900s have largely been conquered by a combination of factors, to be sure, but new knowledge and therapies are important among them. Syphilis that claimed 2 million persons' capacity to function around the first decade of this century, has largely been brought under some measure of control. Malaria in the United States has largely been wiped out.

The analyses carried out here establish the share of reduced deaths and reductions in work-time losses attributable to biomedical research. These analyses, carried out over a substantial time period, have been subjected to professional peer review. A number of versions have been tested, and in the analysis of biomedical research as a factor in reduced mortality, at least, have been found to have robust results.

The analyses carried out addressed principally the shares of reduction in deaths and sickness attributable to biomedical research. In the course of these analyses, other factors were studied, such as the effect of income levels, social stress, environmental hazards, and provision of care.

The findings are summarized briefly here.

A. Impact of biomedical research on the reduction in premature deaths
Period 1930-75

Period 1900-75

B. Impact of biomedical research on the reduction in the objective sickness rates
Period 1900-75 and 1930-75

Shares attributable are estimated at 20 to 40 percent
20 to 30 percent of the mortality reduction
30 to 40 percent of the mortality reduction

Share attributable is 39 percent

39 percent

The estimates indicate several characteristics of biomedical research and health status.

The longer the time period, the larger the share of gains attributable to biomedical research. Only a single figure is shown for sickness. This is so, not because the principle is likely to be different, but because of data problems that prevent a division of the period into two blocks a year.

- The share of reduced mortality attributable to biomedical research over the forty-five-year period is 20 to 30 percent of the total.

- The share of changes in sickness attributable to biomedical research is larger than that for deaths provided the data are corrected to exclude changes in economic capacity to be sick and changes in perception and understanding of illness.

Having estimated the shares of reduced death rates and sickness attributable to biomedical research, the process was set in motion to adjust the value of reduced mortality and morbidity so as to arrive at the benefits from research.

The several estimates derived of the value of reduction in illness and premature death for the periods 1900-75 and 1930-75 are summarized in Table 14-4. The estimates of benefits are essentially of two types: The first set of estimates are comparisons of single-year gains in reduced death rates and sickness between two points in time (shown in billions). The second set are comparisons for multiple years; they measure changes attributable to the sum of the years between two points in time (shown in trillions). The first set presents the value of economic benefits as a consequence of the reduction in death rates since 1930 (or 1900). The question for which a value figure was derived is: What is the difference in value (cost) of premature death between the actual experience in 1975 and a hypothetical experience for 1975, calculated as the 1930 death rates applied by age and sex to the 1975 population and labor market circumstances and then valued at the present (1975) value of future earnings given the age and sex of the working population? The figure shown answers this question. There are also added estimates of the value of the reduction in sickness. The reduction in value of sickness represents a summation of the cost of temporary absences from work and of long-term sickness, including withdrawal from the work force and institutional care due to sickness. Actual reported numbers of work-loss days (temporary and long run) are adjusted to show the difference in work-loss cost between the actual 1975 year and a hypothetical 1975 year in which 1930 (1900) sickness rates are assumed. Reported 1900 and 1930 work-loss data are adjusted for the objective sickness rates that remove the bias in sickness statistics attributable to changes in perception of illness, economic capacity to be sick, and knowledge about health care. The adjusted numbers are computed to take account of the number of employed persons in 1975 and the value of earnings per sick day in 1975.

The second column of figures shown in Table 14-4 is derived from the first. For deaths, the figures for 1930-75 are shown in a range that assumes that 20 to 30 percent of the reduced value is attributable to biomedical research. The figures for 1900-75 assume, as the corresponding numbers, 30 to 40 percent. Saving in sickness costs attributable to biomedical research (1930-75) is computed at 39 percent of the total. The range for 1900-75 is due to adjustment of the sickness rates for 1900 to take account of (a) what appears to be underreporting of the institutional population in 1900, and (b) persons or population not in the numbers showing the work-force reduction due to sickness.

The estimates shown in trillions essentially are asset numbers that are based on a calculation of change in the labor force size between what it was and what it would have been in 1975 if death rates of earlier decades had been obtained. For the hypothetical labor force changes, the present value of future earnings are used to measure value differences (by age and sex). Estimated nonlabor costs are added to maintain capital-labor ratios. Savings in long-term disability costs also are estimated for the institutional population and the population withdrawn from the labor force due to illness. The present value of future earnings is computed for the estimated years of disability of these groups. Having derived benefits in reduced deaths and lower work-time losses, the next step is to estimate the shares attributable to biomedical research.

While the shares of mortality and sickness improvement attributable to biomedical research are not large, the net benefits of biomedical research turn out to be surprisingly high. This is so because the value of each death averted we estimate at $76,000 and the value of a work year of sickness averted, at $12,250. The high economic value of a life saved (even when limited to valuation for those in the work force) and of a working year of life raises benefits well above the cost of research.

In line with our earlier estimates, we assume a ten-year lag between biomedical research expenditures and benefits in reduced deaths or sickness. The cumulative cost of research (including interest, 1900 through 1975) would be $30 billion. This $30-billion estimate is the equivalent of 400,000 lives saved, or 2.4 million sickness years averted. In other words, if it can be shown that 400,000 lives have been saved over the period 1900-75 as a consequence of research, the gains would equal the full cost with an assumed lag of ten years. There is no single right way of measuring the net gains; no simple rule of comparison exists.

Benefits from biomedical research are four to six times the cost of the research for the period 1930-75 (Table 14-5).

The research and development investment figures are adjusted to include interest forgone as a consequence of the use of the resources for such research. No further correction is made for length of

Table 14-5. Benefits from Biomedical Research and Research Costs

Measure of benefits	*Benefits less R&D costs, in billions*	*Benefits: ratio to R&D costs*
Value of reduced death and sickness (see Table 14-4)		
1930-75 $145-$167	$115-$137	4-6 times
1900-75 300-480	227-407	10-16 times
		Internal rate of return
Value of year-by-year direct changes in death and sickness		
1930-75		46%
1900-75		54
Year-by-year changes in GNP attributable to reduced deaths and sickness		
1930-75		48
1900-75		62

investment because the cumulative total changed very little in the early years of the century. Research and development outlays were comparatively small prior to 1930. Early-year costs are not high but benefits are, yielding a ratio of benefits to costs of ten to sixteen times for the period 1900-75.

The benefit amounts less costs are sufficiently high as to suggest profitable investment. After the costs of research and development are met, benefits reach $115 to $137 billion given the simulations of 1930 and 1975. For the longer time period, the net benefits reach $407 billion.

Still a different way of showing the relationship of benefits to costs is to compute an internal rate of return. For the years 1930-75, the internal rate of return is calculated at 46 to 48 percent, with the small difference reflecting a different method of calculation. For the period 1900-75, the internal rate of return is estimated at 54 to 64 percent. These rates of return are defined as rates of discount that will set the present value of net benefits or of benefits minus cost equal to zero,[a] or, in other words, the rate at which benefits and costs are made equal.

[a]The formula for computation is usually expressed as

$$\sum_{t=1}^{n} \frac{B_t - C_t}{(1+r)^n} = 0.$$

To calculate the internal rate of return, year-by-year estimates had to be generated requiring new sets of simulations additional to those shown in Table 14-4. In one computation of an internal rate of return, the yearly change in death and sickness rates is computed to measure benefits. In computing the value of these benefits, changes in age-adjusted death rates are applied to the total population per annum multiplied by the 1975 value per death (with the 1975 value lost per death calculated at a 2.5-percent discount rate). This figure is then reduced to reflect only the share of reduction in deaths attributable to biomedical research. In determining the cost of sickness to add to the cost of death, the change in the sickness rate per employed person from year to year is multiplied by the size of the employed population and by the value of product lost per sick day at 1975 levels. The cost of sickness is further adjusted to reflect only that share of reduced sickness attributable to biomedical research.

Still another simulation is run in which the internal rates of return are computed based on the effect of changes in deaths and sickness rates on the growth rate of GNP. The starting point for these computations is the change in the 1975 work force due to reduction in death rates alternatively from 1900 to 1930 and changes in long-term disability measured by days of institutional care and of withdrawals from the work force. The estimates show a 10 percent higher work force in 1975 than there would have been if death rates of 1930 had prevailed throughout the period 1930-75; they show a 29 percent higher work force in 1975 than the work force that would have prevailed at 1900 death rate levels. These changes in work force are converted to changes in GNP product based on earning rates. Similarly, changes in disability days are priced at 1975 levels.

The internal rate of return is above 45 percent assuming a biomedical research benefit valuation starting with 1930 and approximately a 25 percent higher return if the valuation starts with 1900. The internal rate of return thus is of a magnitude about that of the average social rate of return for industry's investments in research and development (see Table 14-2). This appears to be so despite the high level of basic, nonmission-oriented, life science research.

QUALIFICATIONS

The relating of benefits to cost in the health area is fraught with problems, as we have repeatedly indicated throughout this volume. The carrying out of the political arithmetic should not in any way detract from the conceptual and theoretical difficulties that have been enumerated. The largest issue is the valuation of human life and the differentials that exist in present methods of counting that attribute lower values to women and blacks and understate the value of children. The cost of death and cost of a year of work-time loss due to sickness are derived from such valuation. Human values cannot simply be shadow-priced and added up for gains and losses as one does costs on a water project, an energy plant, or a program of environmental safeguards. With due recognition of the range of benefit and cost assumptions that influence the findings, we round out computations on cost of illness by making the comparisons. These are subject to limitations of concept and measurement.

We have not considered the full range of research and development impacts on health status. Many aspects of health status in addition to premature death and loss of work time of those in the working ages are of concern. Certainly, research findings that would aid in diagnosis, treatment, and cure of disease of children are important outcomes of research, yet in the economic cost we have calculated this type of research output is omitted. Research that would reduce the suffering from diseases of the elderly also have human meaning of benefit value that should be reflected in the amount of benefits. We have not done so. Nor have we estimated the changes that have occurred in debility of the population and, accordingly, in the economic value of those changes. Clearly, some changes have lowered cost, such as the reduction in malaria, tuberculosis, pellagra, and the eradication of smallpox. In other instances, stress may be increasing the hazard of debility. And those who have had a partial "cure," for example, from heart disease, may also be contributing to more rather than less debility in the population. We have not added to economic cost burdens the psychological or social costs of disease.

Other qualifications warrant some emphasis. We have set aside as neutral in its impact the effect of biomedical research on health expenditures. Our study findings suggest that there are conditions in which biomedical sciences augment medical costs but there are also circumstances in which new knowledge reduces costs. On balance, our estimates suggest that over the forty-five-year period 1930-75, biomedical research has had little net impact on medical costs.

In the counts of improvements in death rates, we have not taken into consideration what the rates would have been in the absence of improved medical knowledge. The benefits thus tend to be understated. Environmental factors are assumed to increase exposure to toxic substances and to increase death rates; however, the higher death rates in some instances are masked by higher cure rates. Changes in environmental conditions over the past seventy-five years are difficult to document in many cases. Certainly, in some respects, there have been gains. In other instances, however, health status has become worse.

We have set aside adverse effects and costs associated with prolongation of life, such as the higher retirement costs and the use of nursing homes. And we have not paid attention to the net impact of changes in cause of death that may substitute more painful and prolonged illness for sudden deaths.

The qualifications are listed to suggest that the economic costs of premature death and of loss of work time are, at best, limited objectives of biomedical research, and that the quantifications based on these limited objectives give us only a partial answer about the contribution of biomedical research.

The omissions are typically of the kind that tend to reduce the size of the benefits from biomedical research. This is not universally so but it seems to be the case for many of the items. If, on balance, benefits neglected would increase the value of biomedical advances despite the size of the benefit-cost ratios, the findings would be even more favorable.

AN ACCOUNTING BY DISEASE

The estimates of gains from biomedical research have been aggregate figures for deaths and sickness from all causes. What can be said of gains by disease category? Essentially, the method of analysis that yields the estimates on the share of reduced sickness and of premature mortality attributable to biomedical research is not disease specific. On the contrary, the analysis deals with the total of all diseases.

Unless biomedical research activities can be associated with particular outcomes by broad disease category, it will not be feasible to answer questions about returns on biomedical investments by ICDA (two-digit code) disease categories.

We estimated earlier the savings attributable to biomedical research based on a simulation of 1930-75 death and sickness rates. A comparable set of estimates was prepared for the period 1900-75. The basic estimates of cost of death, saving in those costs, and the estimates of cost of sickness and saving in sickness costs were carried out by disease category. The figures, as presented in Table 14-6, give the estimates derived, except the share of savings attributed to biomedical research is kept uniform for each disease category despite the likelihood that in reality the shares attributable to biomedical research are very uneven by diseases; more progress has been made in preventing and curing some diseases than others. However, at this

Table 14-6. Total Savings Attributable to Biomedical Research, in Billions

Disease category	1900-75 simulation		1930-75 simulation[2]	
Total[1]	$299.37 to $479.83		$145.64 to $167.76	
Infective and parasitic diseases	118.35 to	174.16	63.15 to	69.23
Neoplasms	−2.66 to	−3.17	−1.17 to	−1.40
Endocrine, nutritional, and metabolic diseases	0.28 to	0.95	−1.57 to	−0.99
Diseases of the blood and blood-forming organs	0.76 to	1.27	5.22 to	5.45
Mental disorders	9.20 to	21.88	3.73 to	3.72
Diseases of the nervous system and sense organs	14.76 to	24.31	−3.32 to	−2.70
Diseases of the circulatory system	10.68 to	18.11	−6.42 to	−4.91
Diseases of the respiratory system	71.75 to	116.38	23.44 to	27.56
Diseases of the digestive system, oral cavity, salivary glands, and jaws	12.96 to	21.62	23.53 to	26.53
Diseases of the genitourinary system	23.58 to	37.28	9.27 to	10.96
Complications of pregnancy, childbirth, and puerperium	4.59 to	7.88	10.92 to	11.62
Diseases of the skin and subcutaneous tissue	0.93 to	1.76	2.98 to	3.04
Diseases of the musculoskeletal system and connective tissue	6.19 to	14.59	−11.04 to	−10.98
Congenital anomalies	7.56 to	10.08	−1.41 to	−1.11
Certain causes of perinatal morbidity and mortality	2.80 to	3.73	4.38 to	6.58
Symptoms and ill-defined conditions	14.46 to	19.80	−2.10 to	−1.67
Accidents, poisonings, and violence	4.08 to	9.39	26.05 to	26.86

[1] Totals may not add due to rounding.

[2] Derived from A. Berk and L.C. Paringer: "Economic costs of illness, 1930-1975." Public Services Laboratory, Georgetown University, Washington, D.C., May 1977.

point in the research on biomedical returns, we do not have data that differentiate returns by broad disease code.

Interestingly, despite the approximation that comes from use of a single estimate of shares of saving by disease attributable to biomedical research, the total estimates of saving vary markedly. In some instances, these figures are negative, suggesting an increase in cost rather than a saving; in others, a net saving is indicated.

Returns by disease category are approached here indirectly and most approximately by applying the estimates derived for all diseases combined to each of the individual two-digit codes of ICDA.

R&D by Disease

To begin with, research and development expenditures by disease code are estimated. We have already indicated the difficulty of converting the research and development investments by disease. A major effort by a consultant firm to achieve such parceling out has reportedly yielded little. Perhaps the closest approximation to disease-category-by-disease-category outlays for research and development is to use death data, supplemented to take account of the typical reversal of cancer and heart disease positions on number of deaths and research and development support. Table 14-7 allocates the research and development dollars in each of the selected years by number of deaths, except the relative positions of heart diseases and neoplasms are reversed. Limitations of the estimates are suggested by the relatively small sums shown for mental illness, a result of the arbitrary allocation by number of deaths.

R&D and Economic Cost Burdens

In terms of benefits from research and development expenditures, a quick comparison that helps to identify some of the problems in

Table 14-7. Estimated Biomedical Research Outlays, Selected Years, 1900-75

	1900	1930	1963	1975
Disease category	*(in thousands)*		*(in millions)*	
Total[1]	$157.0	$10,018.0	$1,561.0	$4,640.0
Infective and parasitic diseases	47.6	1,032.9	17.2	37.6
Neoplasms	19.5	2,829.1	847.6	2,464.8
Endocrine, nutritional, and metabolic diseases	0.6	277.5	33.2	109.0
Diseases of the blood and blood-forming organs	0.3	70.1	4.5	12.5
Mental disorders	0.5	46.1	4.1	22.7
Diseases of the nervous system and sense organs	7.2	216.4	14.2	41.3
Diseases of the circulatory system	3.9	913.6	252.4	876.0
Diseases of the respiratory system	30.5	1,060.9	96.5	261.7
Diseases of the digestive system, oral cavity, salivary glands, and jaws	6.0	727.3	62.3	175.4
Diseases of the genitourinary system	12.9	933.8	25.8	66.8
Complications of pregnancy, childbirth, and puerperium	0.9	114.2	1.2	0.9
Diseases of the skin and subcutaneous tissue	0.2	16.0	1.9	4.6
Diseases of the musculoskeletal system and connective tissue	0.6	24.0	3.3	12.1
Congenital anomalies	–	109.2	18.4	32.0
Certain causes of perinatal morbidity and mortality	8.5	444.8	50.0	68.7
Symptoms and ill-defined conditions	9.6	272.5	19.4	74.2
Accidents, poisonings, and violence	6.8	937.7	109.0	379.6

[1] Totals may not add due to rounding.

allocation is that between biomedical research expenditures and the economic burden of illness. Table 14-8 shows the percent of the economic cost of a disease represented by estimated biomedical research expenditures. With the exception of neoplasms, the largest percentage in 1975 was under 2. In some instances, the smallness of the percentage may be due to the error in allocation of research and development monies. We have already identified the special problem with the allocation to mental disorders. Similar difficulty may arise in connection with pregnancies.

By 1975, research and development expenditures reached an average of 1.4 percent of the total economic burden of illness. In earlier years, research and development averaged less than one-tenth of 1 percent. By disease class, as indicated earlier, few of the disease categories approach the average. In 1975, neoplasms, circulatory, and

Table 14-8. Estimated Biomedical Research Outlays as a Percent of Total Economic Cost Burden by Disease, 1930, 1963, and 1975

Disease category	1930	1963	1975
Total	0.04	1.14[1]	1.4[1]
Infective and parasitic diseases	0.02	0.55	0.66
Neoplasms	0.26	5.70	8.78
Endocrine, nutritional, and metabolic diseases	0.05	1.24	1.44
Diseases of the blood and blood-forming organs	0.03	0.75	0.83
Mental disorders	0.01	0.05	0.11
Diseases of the nervous system and sense organs	0.02	0.24	0.25
Diseases of the circulatory system	0.03	0.78	1.52
Diseases of the respiratory system	0.03	0.81	1.17
Diseases of the digestive system, oral cavity, salivary glands, and jaws	0.02	0.64	0.71
Diseases of the genitourinary system	0.07	0.81	0.77
Complications of pregnancy, childbirth, and puerperium	0.02	0.07	0.02
Diseases of the skin and subcutaneous tissue	0.01	0.23	0.17
Diseases of the musculoskeletal system and connective tissue	0.01	0.10	0.09
Congenital anomalies	0.02	0.48	0.54
Certain causes of perinatal morbidity and mortality	0.02	0.46	0.57
Symptoms and ill-defined conditions	0.05	0.78	0.79
Accidents, poisonings, and violence	0.02	0.58	0.67

[1] Total economic costs include unallocated costs. Excluding unallocated costs increases percentage in 1963 to 1.16 percent and in 1975 to 1.53 percent.

endocrine are the three disease categories for which estimated research and development is equal to or in excess of the average for all diseases. For all other disease categories, the percentage spent for research and development appears to have been less than 1.4 percent of the total economic burden. When the data are compared for selected years, we find that there is not a uniform increase in the percentages of total economic cost devoted to research and development. On the contrary, for some disease categories, there has been a fall-off of the percentage albeit rather small. The research and development outlays being used for these comparisons include all health research funds, public and private.

CURRENT YEAR RETURNS ON R&D

The wide range in benefit values should not distract from the finding that biomedical research investment has been profitable, and has yielded returns large by any investment standard.

But, it is objected, the gains estimated happened long ago and what we really are concerned with are the present returns from research and development expenditures made now. Historically, the gains were larger than they are now. Does this mean that the analyses of values attributable to biomedical research in years past are not useful as a guide for the future? The returns are not unfavorable, as some persons assume. The opportunity cost of research and development outlays that may have had an impact on mortality and work loss in 1975, when adjusted to take account of the yield at the actual rate on long-term government bonds, amounted to $3.4 billion. The returns on these investments in reduced deaths attributable to biomedical research during 1975, assuming a ten-year lag between investment and product, total $302.6 million; the returns in reduced sickness are $267.8 million, making a total benefit return of $570.4 million. This return is on an investment of $3.4 billion. Along with the $3.4 billion for research and development, mortality declined and work-loss days declined by an amount estimated to save $570.4 million. The savings accrue each year from 1975, making an annual return of 16.7 percent as the percent return on investment; it is not an internal rate of return that would tend to equalize the $3.4 billion with $3.4 billion benefits. Indeed, the rate is considerably below the internal rates of return reported earlier. It is not an inconsequential return, however, nor one unfavorable by other investment standards.

There is little reason to question the growing difficulty of acquisition of biomedical knowledge. The very gains already made have had this effect. However, it is most difficult to predict or value the output of biomedical research ahead of time. And the economic and social environment in which a new biomedical research finding is introduced is so much more complex than earlier that the gains, while incremental, could be sizable. Perhaps a major challenge that lies ahead is to develop criteria for more adequate assessment of biomedical knowledge and to collect all the information required for such an assessment. This will result in a balanced and rounded picture of the extent to which biomedical research has achieved what it set out to do.

REFERENCES

1. Niskanen, W.A.: Comments on the evaluation of Federal research and development programs. Paper given to the Executive Institute Series at the Civil Service Commission Seminar, Arlington, Va., March 1968.

2. Battelle Columbus Laboratories: Final report on analysis of selected biomedical research programs to President's biomedical research panel. Battelle Columbus Laboratories, Columbus, Ohio, January 1976.

3. Special Analyses. 1980 Budget Document. U.S. Bureau of the Budget. U.S. Government Printing Office, Washington, D.C., January 1979.

4. Brooks, H.: The problem of research priorities. Daedalus, spring 1978, p. 177.

5. Foundation for International Technological Cooperation: Status report. Planning Office, January 17, 1979.

6. U.S. Department of Health, Education, and Welfare: Basic data relating to the National Institutes of Health. National Institutes of Health, Washington, D.C., 1978.

7. Mansfield, E.: Industrial research and technological innovation. Norton, New York, 1968.

8. Nordhaus, W.D.: Invention, growth, and welfare; a theoretical treatment of technological change. MIT press, Cambridge, Mass., 1969.

9. Mansfield, E., et al.: Social and private rates of return from industrial innovations. Q J Econ 91:221-239, 1977.

10. McKeown, T., Record, R.G., and Turner, R.D.: An interpretation of the decline of mortality in England and Wales during the twentieth century. Population Studies 29, November 1975, pp. 391-422.

✳ *Chapter Fifteen*

New Directions

The summary of calculations of the burdens of illness over the century 1900-2000, coupled with the preliminary findings on priorities and the reduction of those burdens that are attributable to biomedical research, serve to underscore three questions:

- What are the most important and relevant gradations in levels of health and well-being that represent outcomes or benefits of health programs?
- What is the value of desirable outcomes? What would the public be willing to pay for improved chances of being at a higher functional level when afflicted with a chronic disease? How can this willingness be measured practically?
- Given public preferences, how should health funds, including biomedical research funds, be distributed among disease problems?

The tools for assessment presented in earlier chapters clarify the need for further exploration. New directions are required to achieve a clarification of the gradations in levels of health achieved by biomedical advances and medical care in which such advances are embodied. The more traditional measurement of reductions in deaths or days lost from work due to disability are not adequate for the task without supplementation.

The desirability of shifting the basis of measurement from traditional human capital terms to measures of consumer preference for biomedical research has repeatedly surfaced in previous discussions, which emphasized the failings of the human capital counts and, in particular, the underevaluation of women, minorities, and children, the uncertainty attributable to the discount rate selection, and the omission of certain costs such as pain.

Of special concern is the way in which measurements can be applied to determine relative priorities among biomedical research problems or disease categories. Implicit in the analyses described in earlier chapters is that relative burden, or relative cost, of diseases is an important criterion for determining priorities. However, we have shown that the Congress tends, with some exceptions, to be guided in its appropriations decisions by the relative number of deaths from each disease. We have also shown how the priorities would change with optional methods of assessing the extent of the disease problem.

New directions can be taken on priorities that recognize the importance of reflecting gradations in levels of health or quality of well-being and that build into the process a surer reflection of the preferences of consumers for different health research emphases.

GRADATIONS OF LEVELS OF HEALTH

The record of past progress in medicine is familiar. Death rates have declined and illness from infective and parasitic diseases has been markedly reduced.[1] A number of the early major killers and cripplers in the United States—including smallpox, typhoid, diphtheria, malaria, hookworm, and pellagra—have been largely wiped out. Particularly impressive in the record of progress is the dramatic reduction in infant and early childhood deaths and in maternity deaths. An epoch of miracle medicine was ushered in with antibiotics that helped to reduce the duration of sickness and mortality further, including the death rates of the adult population.

However, most health policies and research activities now are designed to alleviate a disease condition or to provide "half-way technologies"[2] that allow a person with a disease to function, but they do not cure the disease. The major research Institutes of the National Institutes of Health deal mainly with chronic diseases, such as heart disease, cancer, and chronic obstructive lung diseases. Their mission is basic research and development of new therapies to treat and control chronic conditions.

Early statistics on mortality and morbidity that have come to be used as outcome measures were developed mainly as general indicators of the health of the nation or community. However, they do not capture the essential impacts of biomedical research or provide

operational need-assessment or evaluation criteria for health programs. Alternative measures of health status are needed.

The need for new criteria and measurements for health policies in
place of mortality and traditional morbidity data has stimulated
much research on health status. Studies of new measures of health
status and functionality are being carried out in increasing numbers.
These studies importantly include the work of Fanshel and Bush,
who formulated measures of functional years (well years) or value-
adjusted life expectancy.[3] The measure is derived by weighting
functional level expectancies to yield a scalar value. Zeckhauser and
Shepard have adopted a quality-adjusted life year as an evaluative
criterion.[4] Wylie and White earlier developed the Maryland Disability
Index for measuring the effectiveness of rehabilitation services.[5]
Densen and associates applied to nursing home care[6] the "Index of
Activities of Daily Living" developed by Katz[7] for measuring the
functional status of the elderly and chronically ill. The National
Cancer Institute has applied a "Sickness Impact Profile" (SIP) to
clinical trials, as a component in a quality of life assessment.[8]

Measurements run the gamut from a few selected indexes of the
capacity of individuals to function to complex sociomedical and
health indicators to quality of life.[9] The simple measures rely on a
few measures of functionality that are easy to collect and interpret.
The more complex measurements seek to incorporate gradations of
physical, psychological, and social dysfunction. In addition, they
often include time-specific states of function that yield transition
probabilities based on time spent in a defined condition and
subsequent prognosis. The number of components of these complex
indexes vary, and as that number increases the indexes become more
technical and complicated.

CRITERIA USED TO JUDGE
MEASUREMENTS OF HEALTH STATUS

Choosing among the many measurements of health status that have
or might become available, by use of a variety of techniques and
application of a variety of concepts, can be a monumental task. The
choice will be guided by the desired use of the measure. A health
status index is needed that can measure which treatments are most
effective. It should serve as a guide in health policy choices. Among
other things, an effective measure is one that is easy to comprehend
and to explain to others and unlikely to be misunderstood or
misinterpreted. In addition, an effective measure is one for which

data can be collected without inordinate expense. The following are desirable attributes of an index of health and function:

Simplicity: The measure should be easy to understand and to present to policymakers.

Comprehensiveness: The measure must assess as fully as possible the degree to which intended public purposes are being met by resource allocations or program decisions.

Ability to isolate impacts: The measurement index should change only if a change in health or functional states occurs due to intervention. In addition, it should record adverse as well as positive impacts.

Ability to identify target groups: Measurements need to facilitate the identification of impact on special target groups, for example, changes in functional capacity of children.

Reproducibility: Information should be collected in a sufficiently simple manner to facilitate repeated samples. Each time the procedure is reproduced it should gather the same type of information so that it can be compared to other groups of individuals or to the same individuals in different time periods.

Low cost: Collection of information needs to be kept at a cost commensurate with the usefulness of the data.

Reasonability: Measures need to be equally acceptable to all the diverse groups whose interests are involved in the health policy, for example, consumers, policy officials, health providers, and research scientists.

In addition to these criteria, there is the issue of commonality among diseases. Each disease has special characteristics that lead practitioners and research scientists to measurements of progress toward prevention or control in terms of those special attributes. In the case of lung diseases, this may mean measurements related specifically to lung function; in the case of heart diseases, results of EKGs may be important.

To use measures for choice about health policy, the functional status indexes must be comparable across diseases and usable from one health problem to another. Only by such a single set of measurements can options be compared. Thus, the commonality of measures of outcome in terms of functional states must be stressed. Precision in measuring outcomes with regard to each disease clearly will be lost; however, the sacrifice allows applicability of the index to a wide range of purposes and with lower initial cost.

EXAMPLE OF A DESIRABLE
FUNCTIONAL INDICATOR

An example of a functional measure that meets many of the criteria follows. Developed initially for use in an evaluation scheme for lung diseases, the functional states identified appear to meet the need for a set of indicators about health that reflect the real outcomes of current health programs and are useful for policy analysis and evaluation.[10]

1. *Cured or in Remission*
   This category includes persons considered to be cured of diseases subsequent to a recommended intervention. They can perform all major activities that are normal for their age and sex, and have no remaining detectable signs of the disease.
2. *Fully Functioning Despite Disease or Impairment*
   This category includes persons with disease or impairment who engage in such activities as keeping house, working, shopping, attending school, church, or clubs, and engaging in sports or other recreational activities.

   To be considered fully functioning despite disease or impairment, the person must be free of pain most of the time and must not be affected in ways that are an embarrassment to the patient or a cause for rejection by friends, acquaintances, or employers. Persons may be included in this category even if they have some minor limitations in mobility or are on medication that requires a limited number of hours a week away from work or school.
3. *Functioning with Some Limitations*
   This category, as defined by the National Center for Health Statistics, includes persons who are:
   a. unable to carry on major activities in which persons of their age and sex normally engage
   b. limited in the amount or kind of major activity performed
   c. not limited in major activity but otherwise limited in athletics, extracurricular activities, church, hobbies, shopping, civic projects, or other usual activities
4. *Capable of Self-Care but Major and Other Activities Severely Limited*
   This category includes persons with disease or impairment who are capable of self-care (eating, dressing, bathing, etc.), but who are unable most of the time to leave their home and are unable to work (including keeping house), shop, go to schools, church or

clubs, or engage in sports and other recreational activities. Persons included in this category can care for themselves, but their mobility is limited to the point that they need help in leaving their homes.

5. *Not Capable of Self-Care*

This category includes persons in institutions and requiring care by others because their physical or mental capacity is so impaired that they are unable to perform all or most self-care activities (eating, bathing, dressing, going to the toilet, etc.).

Persons are included in this category if they are in institutions for long-term care (nursing homes) or are in extended-care facilities, even if they might otherwise be able to care for themselves. Persons are also included in this category if they require assistance from professional nurses or paid homemakers for an extended period, or if such assistance is provided by family members or friends who devote substantial time to such care.

Data on the functional states of a population would permit comparisons between the results of current practices without a new intervention and the changes in status attributable to interventions. To illustrate the uses of quantification of functional states, Table 15-1 represents the assumed distribution of the functional states of the population with a disease before a new program intervention or new therapy and after two optional procedures. The costs of each alternative, as well as the prevalence of functional states, is presented. (It is assumed that there is no difference in death rates among the options.)

The illustration underscores some problems of choice. The differences in cost are large in relation to the differences in impact. A first $100 million of added cost yields a 10 percentage point gain in numbers cured and a 20 percentage point gain in those fully functioning, and it moves all persons with the disease to *at least* a self-care position. The program or policy official choosing whether to intervene by the first method with an expenditure of $100 million can judge the importance of the change. The second intervention also costs $100 million. It changes those with the disease 10 percentage points from limited to fully functioning compared to intervention 1, but at the cost of more persons requiring care by others. The decision on which intervention is better depends on the relative valuation placed on changes in functional states. What value should be placed on moving from limited functioning to fully functioning? What value should be placed on moving from requiring care to self-care? The officials responsible for fund allocation must decide which intervention is better, and they must be accountable to the public for their decisions.

Table 15-1. Proportion of the Population with a Disease of Six Months' Duration, by Functional Status Before and After Intervention

Intervention	Cost of intervention (in millions)	Percent cured	Percent fully functioning despite disease[1]	Percent with limited functioning[2]	Percent confined but capable of self-care	Percent confined and requiring care by others
Before intervention	—	10	10	50	20	10
After intervention:						
Intervention 1	$100M	20	30	40	10	—
Intervention 2	$100M	20	40	30	5	5

[1] Bothered little or not at all.

[2] Activity limitation.

This example can be expanded in many ways to incorporate more information. The time under consideration can be varied. Outcomes for a designated patient group may be assessed over intervals of specified months, or there may be follow ups through longitudinal studies over a long term. Cross-sectional outcome and analysis may be sought in which the intent is to assess the likely change in the functional status of a population group—those healthy and those with disease—given diverse programs and different commitments of health resources. The existence of severe pain, or disfigurement due to the available therapies, can be added to the functional state measurements. Functionality might be shown separately by age of individual, with special reference to children. While each characteristic provides more information, it also adds complexity, making it more difficult to display and evaluate. Therefore, the use of additional information must be balanced against additional complexity.

In contrast to indexes of quality of life or of functional years, such as those mentioned earlier, [3, 4] quantification of functional states permits public officials to identify the types of changes occurring in function through the interventions. The changes are not "buried" by incorporation into an overall index.

The concept of functional states, while requiring new data collection, relies to a maximum extent on pre-existing data from the National Center for Health Statistics and restricts the additional data collection required to an essential minimum. This is an extremely desirable attribute because it is more efficient; it reduces the costs and takes advantage of past research and data collection. Another advantage is that, in concept, functional state measurement has various evaluation applications that range from clinical testing of therapies to analysis of optional congressional policies on health benefits under a health insurance program. Commonality of measurement would permit the compilation of data, for example, on the change in distribution of the patient population among functional states due to a chemotherapy agent for cancer, or greater success in curtailing smoking behavior, or greater compliance with physician-prescribed regimens in hypertension, or health services quality controls under various monitoring plans.

If a single, composite index is considered more useful than the separate criteria, the indexes of Bush and Zeckhauser or others becomes most appropriate. Alternatively, efforts can be made to translate days at each level of functioning into a single index by asking groups of individuals, for example, how many days of dependent bed care they would accept in order to achieve a higher level of functioning. The number of days of dependent bed care in essence becomes the common unit of measurement. (In a trial, with a limited number of respondents from the health professions, most indicated a willingness when ill to accept ten days of dependent care to gain one fully functioning day and five days of confinement to bed while capable of self-care for one day of full functionality. To one respondent, "each day has an equal value.")

Measured changes in the distribution of cases among functional states facilitate answers to such questions as: What difference does one therapy as contrasted with another make in functioning? For how long is there a difference? What, for example, is the probability of success as measured by a shift from bed care to fully functioning? Is psychological or emotional support in serious illness more (or less) important that physical medicine in terms of functional levels? What kind of medical care can make a difference in functional status? Does a particular eligibility test or method of payment for care encourage (or discourage) self-care and use of those health services that might make a difference in functional status?

Effectiveness criteria on functional states can supply adequate data to inform policy officials sufficiently for many purposes. Indeed, the quantities on specific measures of functional states often serve policy purposes better than any composite summary figure. For other purposes, however, composite estimates of health gains that can be compared with costs and that can provide the comparability of monetary measures from one program to another are highly useful.

CONSUMER PREFERENCES

In the past, "pricing" of health benefits has relied on measurement of human capital gained through reductions in disability or death; for example, see Weisbrod;[11] Mushkin;[12] Klarman;[13] and Rice and Cooper.[14] By analogy to physical capital, human capital has been measured in terms of gains in the length of time at work and the productivity while at work. The human capital approach is now being challenged both conceptually and practically. The facts about health intervention in recent years, when based only on death rates and disability indexes, do not give rise to much optimism about the benefits of further research and medical treatment. This does not mean that benefits will not be achieved; the measurements are simply not sensitive enough to the current and future changes.

It is also charged that the conceptual notion of human capital does not fit the basic economic idea of consumer satisfaction as a guiding mechanism in the economy; nor does it reflect the desire of individuals to improve their chances of survival (Schelling;[15] Mishan[16]) or of functioning fully when disease strikes. Indeed, the concept has been challenged as being appropriate only to a "slave state."

A method that fits the conceptual framework of economic efficiency analysis and consumer preferences better than human capital is the measurement of benefits as the sum of individuals' willingness to pay when well to reduce risks of sickness. What, for example, is the price individuals would pay to improve the ratio of quality-adjusted life years to total life years or longevity? Or, to draw an illustration from the more specific evaluation criteria discussed earlier, what would individuals pay to reduce the probability of spending years in bed, dependent upon others for care when illness strikes, in favor of greater self-care and self-dependency?

Willingness to pay, as a conceptual method of putting dollar values on benefits or program outcomes that can then permit benefit and cost comparisons, has gained in acceptance for application to health program analysis. However, operational application continues to pose real difficulties. A primary question is: What analytical approaches should be followed to give reality to the theoretical concepts, recognizing that many of these approaches remain controversial?

Different methods of determining willingness to pay have been presented by Clarke,[17] Lipscomb,[18] and Schulze and associates.[19] The various optional measures include direct response from consumers through surveys, imputations of value from market behavior, and the application of demand-revealing processes.

In all cases, the benefits that are being priced by determinations of willingness to pay are benefits to all persons in the population, specified in terms of a reduction in the risk, for example, of being confined to bed when chronic illness strikes. If the chance that 1 per 1,000 persons will be confined to bed with a chronic ailment next year could be reduced to 0.3 per 1,000 as a consequence of new biomedical research, what would each person and, in sum, all persons together be willing to pay to reduce the probability of bed confinement? The price that individuals would pay for a change in the probability of being in a less desirable state, or of being in that state for a longer time, is likely to vary according to age, income, and risk aversion.

SURVEYS OF PREFERENCES

In the literature on willingness to pay, three kinds of benefits flowing from health interventions have been distinguished, each of which requires pricing. These benefits are those to the individual, to the family, and to society.

Seemingly, the most direct method of determining individuals' preferences is to ask them by surveys. The question to be posed concerns the dollar value that the individual consumer would give up of other consumption for some defined reduction in the probability of impairment or illness in a defined period. Acton has pioneered in work on surveys along these lines, particularly in a study of the risk of heart attacks.[20]

A number of difficult issues are encountered in the survey method of deriving preferences. We cannot reasonably assume that the responses are accurate, or even that the hypothetical question is really understood. When eliciting willingness-to-pay responses for actual implementation of policy, there is no way to monitor the truthfulness of response or to penalize strategic behavior that involves representation of preferences. The validity of the survey instrument, stability of response, and replicability of result are of technical concern. Response behavior in surveys of willingness to pay is not well researched as yet. To date, the survey technique has not yielded a practical measurement tool that is acceptable for guiding policy officials in making decisions for the public.

Optional methods are available, however, to assess willingness to pay and consumer preferences about resource allocations in health programs. One such method is suggested by the work of Bailey.[21]

PRESENT MARKET VALUES AS MINIMUM WILLINGNESS TO PAY

Bailey obtains a lower bound for the "value of life" by measuring the discounted present value of the stream of lifetime earnings. The lower bound for the value of life, or an individual's willingness to pay for maintaining earnings for his or her family in the event of death, according to Bailey, is the discounted present value of the expected stream of lifetime earnings. The argument is advanced that if an individual were assured that on his or her death the family would continue to receive income equivalent to his or her earnings, this person would not purchase life insurance. Life insurance purchases, accordingly, are a market indication of the preference of the individual for protection for the family. They represent a lower bound and an underestimate when consideration is given to both the value of life above and beyond that of mere consumption and the amounts paid for life insurance as a premium for risk aversion.

Individuals manifest their aversion to risk by their behavior in a number of ways, including the purchase of insurance with a loading factor that calls for premiums in excess of claims paid.

Bailey measures the willingness to pay for risk avoidance by using estimates of wage differentials or premiums paid for increased risk based on the Thaler-Rosen study.[2 2] In attempting to separate the premiums for risk of death from premiums for risk of injury, he essentially asks: How much compensation is required to induce a worker to accept a .001 per year risk of permanent disability as compared to the .001 percent risk of death? In making this comparison, it is assumed, based on data from the Social Security Administration, that accidental death at work causes a loss of twenty-four years of work and earnings, and accidents resulting in permanent disability lead to an average of five years inability to work plus partial disability for the rest of the life. The amount of extra compensation for the risk of disability is considered by Bailey somewhat arbitrarily (based on the ratio of five years of disability to twenty-four years of work lost due to death) to be one-fifth or 0.2 of the compensation for the risk of death. Thus, a .001 per year extra risk of work disablement would require one-fifth the compensation for the same probability of death.

In contrast to Bailey's examples of accidental death and disability due to work injuries, general health and biomedical research policies are concerned with chronic illnesses in which years of illness may precede death, resulting in a larger number of impaired lives in the population. Instead of deaths among young persons, there is an increase in illness. Relatively young persons may live on with a chronic problem. For instance, instead of five years loss due to disability, consider a risk of 1 per 1,000 of living thirty or forty more years with an illness such as diabetes. This option may be considered less desirable than the option of five years of loss followed by a slightly impaired life. Thus, instead of a market value of .2 for the extra compensation due to premature death, the value could be perhaps .5 to .9 that of death. In the Bailey example, updated to 1978, the premium or wage differential for the risk of accidental death would be $180 per year at a probability level of 1 per 1,000 workers.

For any individual and as a group average, there are "function level expectancies," to use Chen, Bush, and Patrick's terminology,[2 3] or the distribution of remaining years of life among functional levels indicative of the transition experience, given existing medical knowledge and practices for defined disease conditions. Diabetes and cancer of the skin, with existing therapies (and assuming adherence to those therapies) at different ages, move along defined transition courses of functional states within somewhat defined time frames. The probabilities of the average length of each transition need to be quantified for known alternative therapies.

The concept of willingness related to market valuation of risk as measured by wage differences can be applied to the previous example of an analytical approach to quantification by functional states and, accordingly, to quantification of benefits from expenditures on improvement of knowledge about disease and therapies.

As shown in Table 15-2, suppose that $180 is the added compensation for a 1 per 1,000 probability of death. The corresponding average annual premium per accidental injury at the probability level of 1 per 1,000 would be $36, or one-fifth of $180. Some fraction or ratio of the $180 compensation for a 1 per 1,000 risk would represent the premium for the additional risk to individuals of functional states short of ultimate death. For example, the functional state "in bed, dependent upon others" may require a premium equal to nine-tenths of $180 at the probability level of 1 per 1,000; that is, the added compensation required for the risk of dependency in bed would be $162, compared to the 1 per 1,000 risk of death at $180 per year. The risk of having the disease, yet being able to function fully, might require a premium equal to two-tenths of $180 or require additional compensation equal to $36. The cost of the risk of a functional state would in each case be the added compensation required for the risk and the willingness to pay to avoid that added risk.

With information on the average probability of contracting a chronic disease that will affect functioning for a period, it is possible to quantify the benefits in terms of willingness to pay each year for improvement in functional state. It is also practical to quantify the present value of annual amounts that would continue for a substantial length of time by discounting those annual payments over the length of time the improved functional state is expected to last.

Table 15-2. Illustrative Premiums by Functional State at a 1 per 1,000 Risk Level

Functional state	Annual percentage of added death compensation	Premium for 1 per 1,000 probability
Death	100	$180
Confined to dependent bed care	90	162
Confined but caring for self	80	144
Partially functioning	50	90
Fully functioning	20	36

If, following Bailey, we accept the notion that an individual's willingness to pay to reduce the risk of loss in functionality is measured in relation to the earnings difference attributable to risk, there remains the problem of assessing willingness to pay for the other two classes of benefits identified by Dorfman: reduction in risk for family members and neighbors and net financial gain to society.[24] It may be argued that the willingness to pay for family members is linked to the consumption value of earnings. As indicated earlier, in the case of life insurance, the protection is for the surviving beneficiary. Except for survivors, there would be no need for life insurance and no risk of loss of consumption by survivors. The willingness to buy such protection depends on and may be measured by the present value of future earnings. Similarly, when the potential beneficiary is the family of a disabled wage earner rather than a survivor, willingness to pay for a reduction in the chances of the impairments may be considered as some share of the chief wage earner's income. Members of families certainly are willing to pay to improve chances of greater functionality of those they love. If we think of the family as a unit with a combined income, the wage adjustments made by the market for greater risk of illness or accident can be considered to measure benefit of improved functioning not only to self, but also to family.

The third class of benefits is the gain to society if the costs of chronic illnesses that confine patients to bed can be avoided and the lost resources that they represent, diverted to other more productive or desirable uses. Several measures of the price that persons would willingly pay for such net gains to society are feasible. One such measure is the net premium paid (premiums in excess of claims) for disability protection. These net premiums represent the "savings" individuals are willing to make available to others for the protection they receive for those premiums. Still another measure would be the cost of bed care averted that otherwise would have to be financed out of the common insurance pool, less health insurance premiums paid by the individual.

The use of market wage differences as the key to imputing values has weaknesses, as well as strengths. One weakness is that it depends upon markets that operate on an unfettered and competitive basis to establish wage differentials that reflect differences in risk. It presumes relatively informed wage earners. It does not take account of the likelihood that workers who take risky jobs are less averse to risks than others. Willingness, as measured, reflects existing earnings differentials between races and men and women. It has the tremendous advantage, however, of using pre-existing measures and complete abstracts from actual strategic behavior by individuals. Measurement of benefits of health programs in terms of earnings is familiar. Indeed, the computation of present value of future earnings of individuals is now routine in assessing health outcomes. But Bailey gives these measurements a different justification. The indicators are the same; the theoretical constructs, very different. Bailey applies earnings differentials as an indicator of willingness to pay. With risk compensation estimates, it is possible to quantify each functional state's value in relation to a defined rate of risk.

In summary, the valuation of changes in functional states would require a quantity estimate for (a) benefits to self of changes in those functional states; (b) benefits to family and friends, assumed to be measured by the same quantities as included in (a); and (c) benefits to society, measured either by net premiums for insurance in excess of benefits or by net remaining cost of hospital and other institutional care less premiums and charges paid by the individual (excluding employer and governmental payments).

Rough approximations, as indicated earlier, can be made. What is required is knowledge about changes in probabilities of a population's being in the different states with various forms of intervention. If quantification by disease is sought, difference among diseases in impact on functional states must be known.

DEMAND-REVEALING PROCESSES OF WILLINGNESS TO PAY

The conceptual framework formulated by Clarke overcomes the theoretical dilemmas that have long thwarted pricing a public good such as biomedical research. Two penalties are exacted for misrepresenting the true preferences: (a) the individual (or group) must pay an amount equal to the value forgone by others when his or her vote changes the outcome that otherwise would have been chosen, and (b) a lost benefit occurs if a solution other than the individual's preferred choice is decided upon. The conceptual framework is more complicated than may be implied here.

If individuals were asked to contribute to biomedical research at a price in terms of their preferences, we would have a record of those preferences and the risks relative to functional states that individuals are willing to pay to avoid by cures and treatments. However, we do not have that information. For one thing, the results of biomedical research are uncertain. The kinds of resources required to achieve prevention, cures, or disease control by functional state also are not known. To guide resource allocation by disease or Institutes requires more knowledge about how to produce changes, for example, in the probability of bed dependency or limited functionality. The option exists, however, within the bounds of existing knowledge, to substitute experts for the consumer in expressing preferences about functional states for resource allocation decisions.

Essentially, choices are sought—choices that reflect the relative scaling or priorities among classes of goods and services of which governmental support for biomedical research is only one part, and not a very large one. Asking consumers to record their willingness to pay for support of alternative packages of biomedical research presents many methodological problems, as indicated earlier. Instead, we might look to those groups who represent the public on biomedical research issues (namely, the various health agencies, such as the American Cancer Society, the American Diabetes Association, the American Heart Association, and the Epilepsy Foundation) to be representative of, and record the preferences of, those who contribute resources to them. The voluntary agencies have some expertise in the disease problems that are of concern to them and can call upon research scientists for further assistance. Like consumers, moreover, the voluntary agencies have budget limitations, so the choice of priorities will be subjected to the real-life situation of budget constraints. Public interest groups now use their dollars to influence appropriation priorities. We propose a more explicit participation plus penalties for misrepresentation.

Although knowledge about the technological production function of medical research is most inadequate, it should be understood best by agencies concerned about resources for research and the experts to whom they have easy access. These agencies have an understanding of the most likely research projects that would be undertaken by various scientists at different levels of funding. Thus, the voluntary agencies could be polled individually for their subjective opinions on the likely effect that different quantities of research effort would have on functional levels.

The questionnaire for such a survey would have to be developed, but the kind of information to be gathered may be illustrated by the following question: If the indicated amount of research money is allocated to research on the disease of special concern to your agency, what is your best estimate of the percentage of patients in the functional states described below?

In millions

Functional state	$0	$100	$200	$300	$400	$500
A. Cured	A_0[1]	A_1	A_2	A_3	A_4	A_5
B. Fully functioning	B_0	B_1	B_2	B_3	B_4	B_5
C. Limited function	C_0	C_1	C_2	C_3	C_4	C_5
D. Self-care	D_0	D_1	D_2	D_3	D_4	D_5
E. Not capable of self-care	E_0	E_1	E_2	E_3	E_4	E_5

[1] Represents percentage of patients in functional state A after spending $0 million.

The changes in percentages of patients in each functional state with changes in research expenditures would be combined in this process for all disease categories by weighting each column of entries for a research sum by the prevalence of the disease in the population. For example, if, with a $100-million research outlay for a disease such as chronic obstructive lung disease, 20 percent of the patients are estimated to be in a limited functional state at a cross-section of time and 40 percent to be capable of self-care, these percentages would be combined with reports from those concerned about cancer research, research in spinal cord injuries, and so forth, in accord with the relative prevalence of each disease. The result would be a composite distribution of the benefits in changes in functional state as a consequence of changes in the total budgeted funds for research based on the judgments of the voluntary agencies and their experts. These judgmental estimates would have to be scaled to the likely appropriations for biomedical research and a new estimate prepared of the expected changes in functional level. This process would be carried out by disease and for all diseases combined. The estimates of changes in the distribution of patients among functional states could be for some specified future time (for example, a five year period) or for a number of specified future dates.

To achieve reporting that is reasonably realistic, voluntary agencies could be "penalized" for gross inaccuracies in the percentage distribution of patients among functional states at different research budget levels, after a specified period. They could be required, as a condition for participation in the resource allocation process, to pledge, say, $1 of their budgeted funds for each $10 of research fund allocation that is diverted to research on the disease of special concern to them as a consequence of gross inaccuracy in the estimate of functional state distributions of patients.

The process for resource allocation is based on the general assumption that the returns to biomedical reasearch expenditure are decreasing returns. Additional outlays above some level are not expected to yield equal additional returns. At any time, projects most likely to pay off in terms of benefits will be undertaken first; those with somewhat lower probability of success will be assigned a lower claim on resources.

The expected payoff of enlarging funds for research on any disease would be measured by the change in the distribution of patients among functional states with changes in aggregate funding levels. For example, the change in expected payoff with research expenditures raised for a specific disease from $200 million to $300 million would be estimated as the difference in percentage distribution of patients by functional level. In the preceding illustration, the difference in each functional group would be as follows:

Functional Group	Hypothetical (percent)
A_3-A_2	10
B_3-B_2	20
C_3-C_2	− 5
D_3-D_2	−10
E_3-E_2	−15

Without a change in incidence of the disease, the number of new cases would not be altered by the various research funding levels. The improvement, if achieved, would show up in the gains in level of functionality.

AN EXPERIMENTAL RESOURCE ALLOCATION GUIDE

A somewhat different approach might be tested experimentally. This approach calls for application of a version of the recent theoretical work on demand-revealing processes.

We assume for purposes of this experiment that the forty or so voluntary health agencies are asked to record their preferences for the allocation of an incremental increase of funds among the Institutes of the National Institutes of Health. We assume the incremental amount to be $200 million, equivalent to something below 10 percent of biomedical research funds.[2 5] We assume further that the $200 million is the equivalent of about 50 cents for each $1 of funds available to the approximate forty voluntary agencies, in the aggregate.[2 6]

Each voluntary agency would be asked to record its preferences for the allocation of the $200 million among Institutes, subject to constraints. Two possible constraints might be:

1. Not more than 50 percent of all voting power can be allocated to one Institute.
2. The maximum voting power of a voluntary agency is the lesser of the following: (*a*) the volunteer agency's annual budget, or (*b*) the total amount that is being voted on for distribution.

Alternatively, the 50 percent constraint in item 1 might be removed and other rules set. Within these rules, choices would be made that would give the voluntary health agencies a more direct role in the allocation of research funds and that would, in concept at least, move the allocations closer to the efficiency of response to consumer choice.

In a trial by the staff of the Public Services Laboratory using hypothetical budget constraints, the $200 million add-on was allocated to Institutes. The votes were in accord, in concept at least, with an assumed voting pattern of specified voluntary agencies. The trial suggested that the distribution of total funds changes only fractionally, and the rank ordering, very little under the voting system. Although the trial was not representative of a real life vote, it clarified certain characteristics of the voting system. Each voluntary agency, reflecting its self-interest, tends to vote the maximum amount permitted by the rules to the Institute with which it is most closely associated. If the constraint were set below 100 percent, each health agency would tend to follow this vote strategically with a vote of funds to those other Institutes that in its view contribute most to its own mission.

An optional approach that comes closer, perhaps, to the demand-revealing process was suggested by some work done by Clarke. This approach permits the voluntary agencies to define alternative functional states and to accompany these definitions with "offers" of willingness to pay.[27] Decision might rest with the Office of Management and Budget, the president, and the Congress. But voluntary agencies as public interest groups would participate by explicitly indicating their financial contribution, and their readiness to accept a penalty if the "promises" of changes in functionality expected as a consequence of more research funds do not materialize.

Ways in which this method of setting priorities might work are illustrated. Initially, the Office of Management and Budget, after discussions with DHEW (NIH), would set forth an allocation of the research budget as it presently does. However, a voluntary agency, for example the March of Dimes, might intervene by indicating that a slight reallocation of funds would considerably improve the chances of fighting birth defects and that the agency would pay, for example, $100,000 for the change as well as subject itself to a penalty if the outcome in improved functionality, by reduction in numbers of birth defects, is not achieved. No other voluntary agency opposes the slight reallocation that the March of Dimes advances. If the proposed reallocation is adopted—and there is no opposition to its adoption— the penalty that otherwise might be assessed is removed.

If, in place of a slight change and no opposition (illustrated in example 1 in Table 15-3), there is a good deal of conflict among several voluntary agencies over priorities as formulated by the appropriation proposed, the situation is then very different. Each of three voluntary agencies indicates its willingness to pay to alter the proposed budget priorities decision. Agency A, for example, indicates that it is willing to pay half a million for option A, agency B indicates its willingness to pay $2 million for option A, or more funds for metabolic disease research and $1 million for option B, which calls for a large allocation of funds for multiple sclerosis research. Voluntary agency C indicates that it is willing to pay $4 million for larger allocations for MS but nothing for option A. Example 2 in Table 15-3 illustrates what the vote process might be when there are diverse views among voluntary agencies. In summary, a vote of $5 million is cast for more funds for MS research. A penalty is to be imposed if indeed the modification of a change in priorities is accepted as a result of the demand revealed.

Again, appropriations of $4 million are proposed by the Office of

Table 15-3. Voluntary Agencies' Explicit Participation in Priority Setting

	Example 1 *No conflict about priorities*			*Example 2* *Conflict about priorities*		
					Options (in millions)	
					A	*B*
Group	*Allocation proposed*	*Option (in millions)*	*Group*	*Allocation proposed (in millions)*	*More funds for metabolic diseases*	*More funds for MS*
March of Dimes	0	$.1	A	$2	$0.5	0
All others	0	0	B	0	2	$1
Total	0	.1	C	2	0	4
			Total	$4	$2.5	$5

Management and Budget; voluntary agency A would alter this proposal by adding $0.5 million for research on metabolic diseases. Voluntary agency B would add $3 million ($2 million for metabolic diseases and $1 million for MS research), and voluntary agency C would add $4 million for MS research. Agency C changes the vote by its expression of willingness to pay $4 million. In accord with the Clarke penalty, agency C would indeed be called upon to pay the difference between the amount other groups are willing to allocate for research on metabolic diseases, their appraised benefit of an added $2.5 million from research on metabolic diseases, and the indicated benefit expected by others from research on MS or $1 million. The penalty for the vote change thus would be the difference between $2.5 million and $1 million or $1.5 million.

The entire area of measuring functional states and quantifying preferences and demand for biomedical research is of extreme importance. It is worth grappling with concepts other than the traditional human capital approach to broaden the information that is made available to policy offices. The growing importance of special interest groups and the expanding role of these groups in the area of citizen participation also pose major problems. Greater effort is required not only to learn how to give these groups a piece of the action, but also to make them responsible for their advocacy.

REFERENCES

1. Public Health Service: Vital statistics of the United States, Vol. 2, sec. 5, Life tables. U.S. Government Printing Office, Washington, D.C., 1975.

2. Thomas, L.: The lives of a cell. Bantam Books, Inc., New York, 1975, p. 37.

3. Fanshel, S., and Bush, J.W.: A health status index and its application to health-services outcomes. Operations Res 18:1021-1066, November-December 1970.

4. Zeckhauser, R., and Shepard, D.: Where now for saving lives? Law Contemp Prob 405:5-45, autumn 1976.

5. Wylie, C.M., and White, B.K.: A measure of disability. Arch Environ Health 8:834-839, June 1964.

6. Jones, E.W., McNitt, B.J., and Densen, P.M.: An approach to the assessment of long-term care. *In* Health: what is it worth?, edited by S.J. Mushkin and D.W. Dunlop. Pergamon Press, Elmsford, N.Y., 1979, pp. 43-57.

7. Katz, S., et al.: Studies of illness in the aged. The index of ADL: a standardized measure of biological and psychosocial function. JAMA 185:914-919, November 1963.

8. Gilson, B.S., et al.: The sickness impact profile: development of and outcome measure of health care. Am J Public Health 65:1304-1310, December 1975.

9. Chen, M.M., and Bush, J.S.: Health status measures, policy, and biomedical research. *In* Health: what is it worth? edited by S.J. Mushkin and D.W. Dunlop, Pergamon Press, Elmsford, N.Y., 1979, pp. 15-41.

10. Mushkin, S.J.: Criteria for program evaluation. *In* Respiratory diseases: task force report on prevention, control, education. DHEW Publication No. (NIH) 77-1248, Washington, D.C., March 1977.

11. Weisbrod, B.A.: The economics of public health. University of Pennsylvania Press, Philadelphia, 1961.

12. Mushkin, S.J.: Health as an investment. J Polit Econ 70:129-157, October 1962.

13. Klarman, H.E.: Syphilis control programs in measuring benefits of public investments. *In* Measuring benefits of government expenditures, edited by R. Dorfman. Brookings Institution, Washington, D.C., 1965, pp. 367-414.

14. Cooper, B.S., and Rice, D.P.: The economic value of human life. Am J Public Health 57:1954-1966, November 1967.

15. Schelling, T.C.: The life you save may be your own. *In* Problems in public expenditure analysis, edited by S.B. Chase. Brookings Institution, Washington, D.C., 1968, pp. 127-162.

16. Mishan, E.J.: Evaluation of life and limb: a theoretical approach. J Polit Econ 19:687-705, July-August 1971.

17. Clarke, E.H.: Demand revelation and public goods. Woodrow Wilson Center, Smithsonian Institution, Washington, D.C., 1977; Social valuation of life- and health-saving activities by the demand-revealing process. *In* Health: what is it worth?, edited by S.J. Mushkin and D.W. Dunlop, Pergamon Press, Elmsford, N.Y., 1979, pp. 69-90.

18. Lipscomb, J.: The willingness-to-pay criterion and public program evaluation in health. *In* Health: what is it worth?, edited by S.J. Mushkin and D.W. Dunlop. Pergamon Press, Elmsford, N.Y., 1979, pp. 91-139.

19. Schulze, W., Ben-David, S., Crocker, T.D., and Kneese, A.: Economics and epidemiology: application to cancer. *In* Health: what is it worth?, edited by S.J. Mushkin and D.W. Dunlop. Pergamon Press, Elmsford, N.Y., 1979.

20. Acton, J.P.: Evaluating public programs to save lives: the case of heart attacks, R-950-RC; Measuring the social impact of heart and circulatory disease programs: preliminary framework and estimates, R-1697-NHLI. Rand Corporation, Santa Monica, Calif., 1975.

21. Bailey, M.: Safety decisions and insurance. Am Econ Rev 68:295-298, 1978; Earnings, life valuation, and insurance. Measuring the benefits of life-saving. University of Maryland, College Park, discussion papers, 1977-78.

22. Thaler, R., and Rosen, S.: Estimating the value of a life: evidence from the labor market. *In* Household production and consumption, edited by N.E. Terleckji, Columbia University Press, New York, 1976.

23. Chen, M.M., Bush, J.W., and Patrick, D.L.: Social indicators for health planning and policy analysis. Policy Sciences 6:71-89, March 1975.

24. Dorfman, N.: The social value of saving a life. *In* Health: what is it worth?, edited by S.J. Mushkin and D.W. Dunlop, Pergamon Press, Elmsford, N.Y., 1979, pp. 61-68.

25. Public Health Service: Basic data relating to the National Institutes of Health. U.S. Department of Health, Education, and Welfare, Washington, D.C., March 1978.

26. Based on estimates of voluntary agencies provided by the National Institutes of Health.

27. Based on comments on an earlier version of this chapter by E.H. Clarke of the Woodrow Wilson International Scholars Center.

Index

Abraham, C., 159
Abt, C., 268, 386
Accidents, 86, 169, 173, 214-15, 351
   and burden of illness, 370-71,
      374-75
   and cost of debility, 297, 309-12
   and cost of sickness, 280-81,
      286-87, 311
Acton, J., 269
Acute diseases, 201, 209, 212,
    295-302, 309
Adelman, I., 124
Administrative decisions, 15, 30, 43
Age, 21-23, 26-27, 162-69, 171, 174,
    178-79, 319. *See also* Life ex-
    pectancy
   by cause of death, 99-100, 169
   and cost of sickness, 275-78, 285
   and debility, temporary, 302-304
   and disability, 258, 262, 303
   in expenditure model, 345-47, 350
   maturation, and improved health,
    215, 218
   mortality rates, 80-87, 91, 94-100,
    103-110, 169, 177-78
   sickness rates and, 209, 212-13,
    232-33
Air pollution. *See* Environment
Albritten, R.B., 24
Allocation of resources, 15-18, 29-30,
    159, 174, 191, 193, 195-204, 404

guide to, 438-41
American Cancer Society, 436
American College of Surgeons, 3, 118,
    121-22
American Diabetes Society, 436
American Heart Association, 436
American Medical Association, 126
American Surgical Association, 3, 121
Andersen, R., 323, 331
Antibiotics, 119, 126-27, 148-49, 287,
    326
Assessment, 29, 396-97, 421, 423-25.
    See also Criteria; Indexes
   and costs/benefits of research,
    407-15
   by disease category, 415-19
   for industry's biomedical R&D,
    402-405
   and objectives of biomedical re-
    search, 395-97, 406-407, 419-21
Attitudes, 212-13, 222-23, 231-32,
    247-48. *See also* Perception of
    sickness
Auster, R., 4, 80, 124, 144-45
Axnick, N.W., 24

Bailey, M., 431-32, 434-35
Basic research, 46-47, 192-93,
    400-402, 406, 422
Baumel, W.J., 161
Bed days of illness, 221, 232-33, 258

Benham, L., 323
Biomedical advances
  and burden of illness, 375-76
  in expenditure model, 345-46,
    356-60
  and health expenditures, 346-53,
    353-56, 373
  effect on mortality/morbidity, 3-5,
    407-409
  in mortality rates model, 128,
    130-44, 146-49
  as objective, 395-96, 400-402
Biomedical Research Panel, 35, 48,
  330
Blood disease, 287, 338
Boston Edison, and sickness data, 210,
  223-24, 242-43
Brenner, H.M., 124, 146
Brooks, H., 63, 401
Burchenal, J.H., 29, 206
Burden of illness, 197, 268, 363-69,
  422
  and biomedical research, 35, 363,
    371, 375-76
  costs of, 383-87
  economic costs of, 369-75, 383-87,
    414, 417-19
  and economy, 379-83, 414
  and funds for research, 192, 195-96
  indexes of, 369-75
Burgess, P.L., 262
Bush, J.W., 24, 29, 206, 423, 428, 432

Cancer
  and burden of illness, 192, 371-73
  as cause of death, 99-101, 169,
    178-79
  and cost of death, 171-73, 178-80
  costs of, 171, 180, 268-69, 288-89
  and health expenditures, 329, 351
  mortality rates and, 90-94, 99-101,
    103-108, 178-80
  and NIH, 422
  research expenditures and, 192,
    417
  and research missions, 193-95
Carnegie Institution of Washington, 47
Carter, T.L., 15
CCMC study. *See* Committee on the
  Costs of Medical Care
Census, and sickness data, 99, 209-12,
  232-33

Chang, C., 259
Chapin, R.C., 321
Chen, M.M., 24, 432
Chronic diseases
  in biomedical research, 117, 201,
    244, 246, 315, 421-22, 432
  and health expenditures, 325-26,
    329
  mortality rates and, 90-94
  in sickness data, 209, 212
  as type of debility, 305-308
  and willingness to pay, 431-35
Circulatory disease
  and burden of illness, 370-71, 378,
    382, 418
  and cost of sickness, 281, 286-88,
    382
  health expenditures for, 325, 329,
    337-41, 351, 374-75
  research expenditures for, 200-201,
    418
Clarke, E.H., 430, 435, 439
Cochrane, D., 136, 249
Colds, 218-19, 295, 297-302, 313
Collins, S.D., 223
Committee on the Costs of Medical
  Care (CCMC)(1930), 111,
  209-210, 212, 215, 297-98,
  320-21, 324, 328, 333, 355, 366
Commonwealth Fund, 56
Communicable diseases, 47, 215-18,
  239-40, 351, 353
Congress, 363-64, 422, 439
Conley, R.W., 26, 308
Consumers, 50-51, 403, 421-22,
  429-31, 436. *See also* Burden of
  illness; Willingness to pay
Conwell, M., 308
Cooper, B.S., 18, 364, 429
Cost-benefit analysis, 13-15, 17-20,
  21-28
  definition of, 17-19
  new criteria for, 28-30, 396-97,
    423-25
Cost containment, 50, 53-54, 315-16
Cost-effectiveness analysis, 19-20, 24,
  28-30
Cost
  of accidents, 169-73, 370-71. *See
    also* Cost of premature death
  of cancer, 171, 180, 268-69,
    288-89

of death, 23, 171-73, 178-80, 200,
    365, 370-71, 381, 413-15. *See
    also* Economic cost of death
of debility, 28, 293-95, 301-302,
    304, 308-13, 385-86
of disease, 10, 15, 21-23, 53, 173,
    326-29, 383-87, 422
of health care, 11, 48-50, 284-85,
    315-18, 323-33, 345
of hospitals, 324, 331-34, 366, 374
of living, 323-24
of mental health, 385-86
of pain, 28, 386, 422
of physicians, 324
of premature death, 23, 174, 272,
    313, 366-67, 381, 383, 410
of production, 308-311, 312
Cost of sickness, 15, 18, 22-23,
    267-69, 376-79
    effect of antibiotics on, 326
    biomedical research and, 35-36, 53,
        253, 282-85, 363-66, 371, 378,
        384, 413-15
    and cost of debility, 293, 301, 311
    by disease, 171, 180, 279-81,
        285-90, 374-75, 415
    increase in, 276-78, 288-90
    and work-loss days, 269-72, 275
Cost per death, by disease, 199-204
Costs
    and biomedical research, 199-204,
        284-85, 315-16
    and burden of illness, 366, 376-79,
        382-87
    capital, 330-33
    definition of, 18, 267
    direct, 2-3, 15, 18, 22-23, 376-77
    and functional states concept,
        426-29
    indirect, 2-3, 15, 18, 22-23, 376-79
    mortality rates and, 11
    nonpayroll, 331-32
    opportunity, 9, 18, 27, 399-401,
        406-407, 419
    psychological, 113, 267-68, 386-87,
        414
    social, 14-15, 26, 28, 267-68,
        386-87, 414
Council on Wage and Price Stability,
    331
Cretin, S., 25
Criteria, for assessment, 29, 396-97,

423-25
Crosby standard, 112-13

Davis, J.M., 262
Davis, K., 331, 345
Death, causes of, 47, 85-94, 96-101.
    See also Diseases
    and economic cost of death,
        169-73, 178-80
    funds for research and, 191-92,
        214-15, 337-41, 351-53
    future causes of, 103-110
    preventable causes of, 110-13
Death rate. *See* Mortality rate
Death-Registration Area (DRA),
    97-100
Death-Registration States (DRS),
    97-100
Debility
    cost of, 28, 293-95, 301-302, 304,
        308-13, 385-86
    and funds for research, 196
    reduction, and biomedical research,
        60, 64
    types of, 295, 295-302, 302-304,
        305-308
Densen, P.M., 423
Dental disease, 195, 334-35, 369
DHEW (Department of Health,
    Education, and Welfare), 15, 38,
    40, 51, 397, 439
Diabetes, 103, 109, 432
Digestive diseases, 103, 109-110,
    298-99, 337-41, 351, 374-75,
    382
Direct costs, 2-3, 15, 18, 22-23,
    376-77
Disability, 23, 48, 50, 215, 221-22,
    241, 243, 258-63, 307-308. *See
    also* Debility; Sickness rate
Discount rate, 18, 22, 25, 161-65,
    177-78, 383, 422
Diseases, 206-208, 214-16, 239,
    286-88, 424, 426-28
    acute, 201, 209, 212, 244
        295-302, 309
    and biomedical research, 21-25,
        239, 243-44, 315, 326, 337-41,
        350-53, 408-409, 415-19,
        422-23
    and burden of illness, 363-65,
        369-75, 382, 418-19

Diseases, cont.
  chronic, 90-94, 117, 201, 209, 246,
    305-308, 325-29, 421-22,
    431-35
  and cost of death, 169-76, 178-80,
    415
  and cost of sickness, 171, 180,
    279-81, 285-90, 374-75, 415
  data on, 208-13
  effect on economic productivity,
    301, 308
  funds for research and, 16-17,
    47-48, 191-93, 195-97, 197-204,
    421, 436-38
  and health expenditures, 325-26,
    326-29, 337-41, 350-53
  and health status, 215-21
  in methodology for mortality rates,
    97-101
  and mortality rates, 85-94,
    103-110, 118-24, 148-49, 178,
    216, 353, 364-65
  mortality trends and, 85-94
  preventable, 111-12, 125, 148,
    243-44
  and research missions, 193-95
  willingness to pay and, 243-44
Dorfman, N., 434
Drug patents, 5, 62-71, 360
Drugs, 62-64, 70-71, 119, 126-27,
    132-37, 142-43, 148-49, 335-36
Dubos, R., 80
Duke Endowment, 56
Dunlop, D.W., 50, 262

Earnings, 160-69, 171, 178-80,
    276-78, 294, 306, 331-32, 366
Eckstein, O., 161
Econometric models
  of health expenditures, 345-46,
    356-60
  of mortality rates, 5-6, 118,
    127-37, 137-47, 240-42
  of objective sickness rates, 7,
    248-49
  of sickness rates, 240-42
  of work loss, 253-57
Economic cost
  of burden of illness, 369-75, 414,
    417-19
  of death, 159, 167-80, 378-79
  of disease, 2-3, 5-6, 21-25, 171,

    418-19. *See also* Direct costs;
    Indirect costs
  of premature death, 159
Economic cost of sickness, 14, 15-18,
    201, 267-69, 293
  in cost-benefit studies, 21-25
  definition, 267
  and disability measures, 205
  by disease, 279-81, 285-90, 369-75
  estimates of, 269-81
  factors influencing increase, 276-78
  and research expenditures, 43
Economic factors, 128-31, 137-39,
    221, 224, 228-33, 240, 254-57,
    356
Economic growth, 1, 180-84, 396-97.
    See also GNP
Economic productivity, 227-28,
    396-97
  effect of burden of illness on,
    376-77, 379
  and cost of debility, 293-95,
    301-302, 306-308, 312-13
  and cost of sickness, 267, 273, 275
Economy, 379-83, 414, 429-30
Education, 223, 232-42, 246, 256-57,
    259
Effectiveness criteria, 19-20, 24,
    28-30, 50-53, 429
Environmental factors, 36, 80, 107,
    117, 371, 383
  in econometric models, 128-31,
    137-39, 145-46, 240, 248, 356
  and health expenditures, 318-19,
    324-25
  and mortality rates, 80, 117,
    414-15
Environmental Protection Agency
    (EPA), 160
Epilepsy Foundation, 436
Expenditures
  drug, 335-36
  health, 45-47, 54-60, 80, 267,
    316-25, 345-56, 373-75, 379-81
  R&D, 37-43, 197-204, 398-400,
    402, 405, 414-20

Falk, I.S., 334
Fanshel, S., 423
Farr, W., 363
Federal government, roll of, 37-38,
    44-47, 55-58

Fein, R., 21, 162, 315
Feinstein, A.R., 52
Feldstein, M., 161, 331, 346
Finland, 118
Fisher, I., 88, 110, 209, 278-79, 363
Foundation for International Tech-
    nological Cooperation, 401
Freidin, R., 24
Friedman, B., 221-22, 259-62
Frost, W.H., 298, 300
Fuchs, V.R., 4-5, 124, 144-45, 300,
    316, 331, 346, 350, 377
Functional states, 1, 11, 206, 395-96,
    421, 423, 425-29, 433-38, 441
Functional years, 206, 423, 428
Funds for research, 13-18, 36-37, 42,
    44-47, 56-58, 191-92. *See also*
    Federal government; Research
    expenditures
  and burden of illness, 369, 371
  by disease category, 191-93,
    197-204, 416-17, 421-22
  guide to, 438-41
  and industry, 402-405
  and institutes, 436-38
  and mortality, 42, 47-48, 191-93,
    195-97, 200-201
  and NIH, 403

Galton, F., 130
Gifford, R.H., 52
Gilman, H., 162
GNP, 43, 182, 219, 379-82, 413
Goldberger, J., 216
Gorham, W., 23
Government, role of, 13-17, 37-38,
    44-47, 55-58, 398, 404, 406
Great Britain, 85, 118
Griliches, Z., 137
Grossman, M., 241, 258-59

Hadley, L.W., 262
Hambor, J.C., 259
Harrod-Domar model, 182-83
Harvard University School of Public
    Health, 52
Health care system, 1, 13-15, 315-18,
    333-37
Health expenditures, 37-40, 80, 267,
    316-25, 366, 376-77
  and biomedical research, 45-47,
    54-60, 316-18, 330-33, 345-47,
    353-56, 373-78
  effect of burden of illness on, 369
  by disease, 325-29, 337-41, 350-53,
    374-75
  and GNP, 379-81
  health services and, 333-37, 353-55
  and knowledge advances, 325-33
  model of, 345-53
Health hazard reduction, as objective,
    1, 28, 395, 397
Health Maintenance Organizations
    (HMOs), 316
Health programs, 117, 125-27, 421-29
Health research
  achievements of, 60-71
  and basic research, 46-47, 192-93,
    400-402, 406, 422
  effect on burden of illness, 35, 363,
    371, 375-76
  content of, 35-37
  and cost-benefit analysis, 13-15,
    21-25, 26-29
  cost of, 9-10, 411-13
  and cost of death, 23, 171-73,
    178-80, 200, 413-15
  effect on cost of health care,
    315-18, 325-26, 345
  and cost of sickness, 35-36, 53,
    253, 282-85
  and cost per death, 199-204
  definition of, 35-37
  effect on disease, 21-25, 243-44,
    315, 326, 337-41, 350-53,
    415-19, 422-23
  expenditures, 37-43, 197-204,
    398-400, 414-20
  funds for, 13-18, 36-37, 42, 44-47,
    56-58, 191-93, 195-204
  government support for, 15-17
  gains from, 183-84, 420
  and health expenditures, 345-53,
    353-56
  and health status, 257-63
  investment in, 398-400, 419-20
  military data and, 7, 402, 406
  and mortality, 80, 117-24, 124-27
  objectives, 1-2, 36, 395-97,
    398-402, 406-407
  and objective sickness, 250-53,
    263-64
  policy issues, 42-43
  quantity and quality of, 60-71

Health research, cont.
  rate of return on, 9, 19, 21-22, 25,
    403-405, 412-13
  vs. research and development
    policy, 44-54
  effect on sickness rates, 239-40,
    243
  in sickness rates model, 241
  size of, 37-42
  and willingness to pay, 435-38
Health services, 333-37, 345-46,
    354-55, 358
Health status of population
  and biomedical research, 48, 117,
    257-63, 409, 414
  and health expenditures, 318-19,
    358
  improvement in, 215-21
  indexes of, 206-208, 423-25
  influences on, 221-23
  as objective, 395-96, 406-407
  and research expenditures, 398
Heart disease, 111, 121-22, 192, 417,
    422
  and cost of sickness, 284, 289
  and debility, 302-304
  and mortality rates, 90-94, 99, 103,
    108, 111
Hemminki, E., 80, 118-19
Hirschleifer, J., 161
Hitch, C.J., 161
Hoover, E., 324
Hopkins, T.R., 259
Horton, M., 249
Housewives. See Women
Howard, L.O., 85
Hu, T., 259
Human capital valuation, 21, 23,
    26-28, 160-67, 180-83, 421-22,
    429-30

Iden, G., 259
Illich, I., 50, 80, 83
Illness. See Burden of illness; Sickness
Income, 3, 85, 90, 96-97, 162, 247
  in expenditures model, 346-50,
    356-58
  and health expenditures, 318-23,
    354-55
  in military data, 247
  in mortality rates model, 128-32,
    137-39, 142-46

  and sickness rates, 243, 259, 262
  in sickness rates model, 240-42,
    248, 252
  in work loss model, 255-57
Income maintenance, 222, 224,
    243-45, 247-48, 254-55
Index of Independence in Activities of
    Daily Living, 29, 206
Indexes, 16-17, 29, 43, 48, 206,
    369-75, 423-25, 428
Indirect costs, 2-3, 15, 18, 22-23,
    376-79
Industry, 37-38, 40-41, 44, 46-53,
    398, 402-405
Infant mortality rates, 5, 83-86, 111
Infectious disease, 1, 111, 178, 239,
    299
  and burden of illness, 370, 374-75
  and cost of death, 169-71, 365
  and cost of sickness, 280, 286-87,
    289
  and health expenditures, 325, 329,
    337-41, 351, 374
  and mortality rates, 85-86, 88, 90,
    94, 118-19
Inflation, 318, 323-25, 345-47,
    349-50, 356
Institutes, 16-17, 192-97, 436-41
Institutional population, 214, 227,
    244-45, 274, 287, 351, 378
International Classification of Diseases
    (ICDA), 100-101, 196, 337,
    363, 365
International health concerns, as ob-
    jective, 396-97, 401-402, 406
Investment, in biomedical research,
    398-407, 411-13, 416-20. See
    also Expenditures; Outlay; Re-
    search products

Jones, B., 328
Julius Rosenwald Fund, 56

Karnofsky, D.A., 29, 206
Kass, E.H., 80
Katz, S., 29, 206, 423
Kingston, J.L., 262
Klarman, H.E., 21-23, 162, 315,
    345-46, 429
Koos, E.L., 213
Kramer, M.J., 331

Labor force, 1, 165-67, 179-80, 227,
  255, 259, 411-13
  and cost of sickness, 269, 272-76,
  285-86
Laitin, H., 21
Landfeld, J.S., 309
Lando, M.E., 259, 262
Landsteiner, K., 61
Lave, J., and Lave, L., 331
Lave, L., and Seskin, E., 124, 145
Lee, R.I., 328
Legislation, 15, 17, 57
Lewinski-Cowin, E.H., 334
Life expectancy, 80-83, 94, 118, 125,
  148, 167, 169, 173, 179, 244-45
Lipscomb, J., 430
Lotka, A.J., 363
Luft, H.S., 259, 306-308

McCall, W., 326-29
McKean, R.N., 161
McKeown, T., 4, 118-19, 407
McKinlay, J.B., and McKinlay, S.M.,
  80, 118-19, 121
Mansfield, W.D., 404-405
Market behavioral models, 130-37,
  240-42, 248-49, 356-60. *See also*
  Econometric models
Market forces, 15, 28-30, 42-43
Market values, 431-35
"Maryland Disability Index," 29, 206,
  423
May, J.J., 331
Measles program, 23-24, 119-21,
  325-26
Medical procedures, 118-24, 125-27,
  148-49
Medicare/Medicaid, 43, 221-22, 259,
  262, 318-19, 325, 378
Mental illness, 214
  and burden of illness, 369-71,
  374-75, 378, 382, 385-86
  and cost of death, 18, 26, 171, 180,
  385-86
  and cost of sickness, 280-81,
  286-88, 382
  and debility, 306-308
  and health expenditures, 337,
  339-41, 351, 374-75
  and research expenditures, 417-18
Metropolitan Life Insurance Company,
  209-10, 212, 214-15

Milbank Memorial Fund, 56
Military data, 7, 215, 220-21, 233,
  246-48, 248-53, 279, 402, 406
Minority groups, 27, 422
Morbidity, 3, 239
Morbidity data, 191, 205, 208-13,
  215, 228, 377
  as criteria, 205, 423, 429
  and funds for research, 191-93,
  195-97
  research missions and, 193-96
  and willingness to pay, 432-33
Morbidity rates. *See* Sickness rates
Morbidity reduction
  and biomedical research, 5-9, 60,
  64, 251-53, 263-64, 407-13
  as objective, 1, 395-96, 400-401
Morgan, T.H., 61
Mortality rates, 103-10, 376-79, 384
  and age, 83, 86-87, 91, 94-96,
  99-100, 103-110, 121, 169,
  177-78
  age-adjusted, 79-80, 90, 94, 121,
  146-49
  effect of biomedical research on,
  3-5, 10-11, 14, 80, 127-28,
  137-44, 149, 245, 263-64, 422
  of children, 83, 86
  and cost of death, 11, 378
  vs. cost of sickness, 288-89
  and disease, 85-86, 87-94, 103-110,
  118-24, 148-49, 239, 353,
  364-65
  in econometric models, 5-6,
  130-37, 146-49
  environmental factors in, 80,
  128-31, 145-46, 414-15
  and firms for biomedical research,
  47-48, 50
  and funds for research, 191-92,
  193, 195-97, 200-201
  and health expenditures, 80,
  376-77
  and health status, 215
  of infants, 83-86
  and need, 205
  and policy evaluation, 205
  preventable deaths and, 110-13
  and research missions, 193-95
  and sex, 87, 94-96, 103-10, 377
  and sickness rates, 219, 228, 243
Mortality reduction, 376-79, 384

Mortality reduction, cont.
and age, 169, 171-73
effect of biomedical research on,
3-5, 7-9, 14, 29, 60, 63-64, 80,
133, 138-39, 263-64, 364-65,
407-413, 419
and cost of death, 169, 171-73,
176-80
economic values of, 8, 183-84
as objective, 1, 395-96, 400-401
and sickness rates, 244
and value of human life saved, 161,
167, 180-83
Mortality trends, 87, 79-96
and age, 79-87, 91, 94-96
determinants of, 124-25
and disease, 87-94, 239, 369-71
factors affecting, 127-30
future, 94-96, 103-110
methodology, 96-101
and sex, 87, 94-96
and sickness rates, 240, 244

Nagi, S.Z., 262
National Ambulatory Medical Care
Survey, 208
National Cancer Institute, 47, 192-93,
423
National Center for Health Statistics
(NCHS), 15, 173, 206, 242, 244,
296-303, 306, 321-22, 379
NCHS Health Interview Surveys,
208-210, 212, 258, 262, 296-97,
299, 306
National Conservation Commission
(1908), 36, 85, 110, 125, 148,
209, 213
National Disease and Therapeutic In-
dex (NDTI), 208
*National Drug and Therapeutic Index
and Pharmacological Facts and
Figures*, 148
National expenditures, 37-43, 80,
197-204
National health bill, 43
National Health Education Committee,
363
National Health Survey of 1935-36,
209
National Heart Institute, 192, 193
National Hygienic Laboratory, 57

National Institute of Arthritis, Meta-
bolic, and Digestive Diseases,
193-95
National Institute of Child Health and
Human Development, 193
National Institute of Dental Research,
195
National Institute of Environmental
Sciences, 192-95
National Institute of General Medical
Sciences, 192
National Institute of Health (NIH), 8,
36, 61, 364, 397, 400, 422, 428
cost of disease study, 2-3, 15
expenditures for research, 38, 55,
57
and funds for research, 47, 191-92,
197-99, 201, 403, 438
National Institute of Mental Health
(NIMH), 18, 306
National Institute on Aging, 192-93
National Office of Vital Statistics,
100-101
National Resources Committee report,
55
National Science Foundation, 45, 55
Need, for research
and disease, 191-93, 197-205
and funds for research, 42, 47-48
and mortality rates, 42, 47-48, 79,
191-92, 195-97, 205
Neoplasms, 193-95, 201, 280, 325,
337, 341, 370-71, 374-75,
417-18
Newhouse, J.P., 258
Niskanen, W.A., 395
Noneffective rates, 246, 250, *See also*
Military data
Nordhaus, W.D., 404
Nutrition, 117-18, 128-29, 241, 378,
407

Objectives
of biomedical research, 1-2, 36,
395-402, 406-407
common units for effectiveness of,
20, 28-30
of health programs, 30
Objective sickness rates, 6-8, 220, 224,
233. *See also* Noneffective rates
and biomedical research, 285,
409-413

and cost of sickness, 284, 285,
    289-90
definition of, 228-29
military data on, 7, 246-48
model of, 7, 248-49
Occupational Safety and Health Ad-
    ministration (OSHA), 160, 259,
    309-310
Opportunity costs, 9, 18, 27, 399-401,
    406-407, 419
Orcutt, G.H., 124, 136, 249
Orkand Corporation, 197, 201
Osler, W., 355-56
Outlay. *See also* Expenditures; Funds
    for health, 345, 371-77, 385-86
    for research, 54, 59-60, 398-401,
        403, 416-19

Paakkulainen, A., 80, 118-19
Parinja, L., 256, 259
Parsons, D.O., 259
Patents, 4-5, 62-64, 70-71, 132-37,
    142, 398
Patrick, D.L., 432
Peer group review, 17, 48-50, 315
Perception of illness, 209, 222-23,
    231, 242-43, 245, 247
Periodicals, 62-64, 70-71, 132-37, 360,
    398
Pharmaceutical firms, 53-54, 56, 58
Pharmaceutical Manufacturers Associa-
    tion, 54, 56, 58
Phd's, number of, 4, 60-63, 132-37,
    142-43, 249-50, 254, 360
Physician
    costs, 324, 331
    services, 333-35
    and sickness data, 208-210, 212
*Physician's Desk Reference and US
    Dispensatory*, 148
Pneumonia. *See also* Respiratory
        disease
    and cost of sickness, 288
    and debility, 299
    and mortality rates, 90, 108-109,
        118-19
Population growth, 276, 346-47, 350
Pregnancy, 85, 337, 339, 351
Premature death, 2-3, 8-9, 86, 110-13,
    159, 167-80, 407-13
    and burden of illness, 376-77, 379,
        381-82

Press, F., 44, 46
Preventable disease, 111-12, 125, 148,
    243-44
"Preventive Impairment Unit
    Decades," (PIUD), 29
Price, 159-67, 240, 429-30, 435
Private sector, 37, 40-41, 44-45, 47,
    54-58, 398, 403-405
Professional Review Organizations
    (PSROs), 316
Program evaluation, 205-208
Provider factors, 50-51, 245-46
    in expenditure model, 358
    in military data, 247-48
    and mortality rates, 122, 125-27,
        137-47
    in sickness rates model, 240, 243,
        252
    in work loss model, 254-55
    in mortality rate model, 128,
        130-32, 142, 144
Psychological cost, 267-68, 386-87,
    414
Publications. *See* Periodicals
Public Health Services Act of 1944, 57
Public policy, 1, 9-10, 13-15, 28
Public Services Laboratory (PSL),
    328-29

Quality-adjusted life years concept,
    24, 29, 206, 423, 428
Quality of biomedical research, 60-62
Quality of life
    effect of biomedical research on,
        60, 64
    and burden of illness, 384
    as criteria, 423, 428
    as objective, 1, 14, 395-96, 407
Quantity of biomedical research,
    60-70

Rao, P., 137
Rate of return, 9, 19, 21-22, 25,
    403-405, 412-13, 419
    internal, 9, 19, 21-22, 412-13
    social, 25, 403-406, 413
Record, R.G., 118
R&D, biomedical
    costs and benefits of, 9-10, 407-415
    by disease, 415-17
    and economic cost burdens, 417-20

R&D, biomedical cont.
  industry's involvement in, 25-26,
    402-405, 406
  and opportunity cost, 399-400,
    406-407
  rate of return on, 9, 19, 21-22, 25,
    403-406, 413, 419
  vs. R&D, 43, 44-54
Research expenditures, 37-42,
    197-204, 398-400, 402, 405,
    414-20
Research mission, 193-95, 422
Research product, 10-11, 398-400
Respiratory disease
  and burden of illness, 369-71
  cost of death and, 169-71, 178-79
  and cost of sickness, 280-81,
    286-88
  and debility, 299
  and funds for research, 438-41
  and health expenditures, 329, 351,
    374-75
  effect on mortality rate, 103,
    108-109
  prevalence of, 214-15
Restricted-activity days, 221-22, 242,
    244, 258, 262, 296-302
Rice, D., 15, 18, 22-23, 269, 315,
    363-64, 429
Rivlin, A.M., 23
Rockefeller Foundation, 47, 56
Rockefeller Institute for Medical Re-
    search, 47, 61
Rockefeller Sanitary Commission, 216
Rosen, S., 432
Russell Sage Foundation, 354
Rycroft, R.S., 330

Salkever, D., 331, 345
Savings, and biomedical research,
    167-80, 411-13, 415-16, 419
Scheffler, R.M., 259
Schonfeld, H.K., 328
Schulze, 430
Schwartzman, D., 25, 142
Science, and biomedical research, 37,
    407-409
Scientific advances. See Biomedical
    advances
Scitovsky, A.A., 326-29
Sex
  and cost of death, 167, 174, 179

  and cost of sickness, 275, 277-78,
    285
  effect on disability, 262
  and health expenditures, 319
  and mortality rates, 87, 94-96,
    103-110, 377
  in mortality rates model, 143
  and sickness rates, 232-33
  in value of human life, 162-67
Shepard, D., 24, 29, 206, 423
Shyrock, R.H., 55
Sick leave, 224, 241, 248, 255, 258
Sickness data, 208-13, 242-46. See
    also Disease; Morbidity data;
    Objective sickness rates
  and biomedical research, 5-9,
    257-64
  disease comparisons in, 214-15
  economic/social factors of, 221-23
  and improved health status, 215-21
  in military data, 248-49
  and objective sickness rate, 6,
    228-33
  and SES, 6-7, 228-31
  trends in, 223
Sickness Impact Profile (SIP), 206,
    296-97, 423
Sickness rates, 5-7, 232-33
  and biomedical research, 239-40,
    243-46, 250-53
  in market behavioral model,
    240-42, 248-49
  military data on, 215, 220-21,
    246-48
  in work loss model, 253-57
Sickness reduction. See Morbidity
    reduction
Silver, M., 221
Social costs, 14-15, 26, 28, 267-68,
    386-87, 414
Social rates of return, 25, 403-406,
    413
Societal factors
  and cost, 371
  in expenditures model, 356
  in mortality rates model, 128,
    130-31, 137-39, 146
  and sickness data, 221, 224, 228-33
  in sickness rate model, 240, 248
  and willingness to pay, 434-35
  in work loss model, 254
Socioeconomic status (SES), 6-7, 86

Social Security Act of 1935, 57, 85
Social Security Administration, 40,
    222, 256, 262
Steelman Report of 1947, 47-48
Stress, 36, 146
Strickland, S., 55
Summers, L., 161
Sweden, 85, 118
Sydenstricker, E., 212, 258
Syphilis control, 22-23, 409

Taylor, A., 331
Technology, new, 51-53, 315, 326,
    328-33, 345-47, 356, 398
Thaler, R., 432
Thedie, J., 159
Therapy, new, 4, 118-21, 125-27, 173
Third party payments, 13, 318-19,
    325, 346-50, 373-74
Time costs, 267-69
Time lags, 142-44, 412
    and investment in research, 398-99,
        419
    in mortality rates model, 133,
        138-41
    in sickness model, 249-51
    in work loss model, 257
Torrence, G.W., 29
Tuberculosis, 88, 90, 97, 111, 119,
    214, 239-40, 351, 355
Turner, R.D., 118

Unemployment, 222-23, 274
Urban Institute, 222

Vaccines, 2, 21-22, 86, 88, 121,
    325-26
Value-adjusted life expectancies, 206,
    423, 428
Value of human life, 159-67, 180-83,
    414, 431
Value of reduction of illness/prema-
    ture deaths, 8, 408-411
van Volkenburgh, V.A., 298, 300

Vascular disease, 103, 108
Vehorn, C.L., 330
Voluntary agencies, 436-37

Wages, *See* Earnings
Wales, 118
Weisbrod, B.A., 21-22, 162, 315, 429
White, B.K., 29, 206, 423
Williamson, J.W., 29
Willingness to pay criteria, 429-38
    and guide to resource allocation,
        438-41
Willner, S.G., 308
Women
    in cost-benefit analysis, 21-23,
        26-27
    and cost of premature death, 167
    and cost of sickness, 271-74
    in human capital valuation, 166,
        422
    and mortality rates, 94-96, 103-110
    in mortality rates model, 143
    and R&D, 414
Wooldridge Report of 1965, 204
Woolley, H.B., 14, 364
Work experience rates, 165-66
Work-loss days, 221-24, 278-79. *See
    also* Sickness reduction
    and biomedical research, 8-9,
        28-29, 253-57, 258-64, 284,
        407, 410-11
    and burden of illness, 376-77, 379
    and cost of debility, 294
    and economic cost of sickness,
        269-72, 275, 277-78, 285
    and sickness rates, 232-33
    in sickness rates model, 242
Worthington, N.L., 331
Wylie, C.M., 423

Yale Medical School, 52

Zeckhauser, R., 24, 29, 206, 423, 428

About the Author

Selma J. Mushkin is director of Georgetown University's Public Services Laboratory and a professor of Economics at the University. She is presently a Fellow of the Woodrow Wilson International Center for Scholars. Dr. Mushkin has published numerous works in the area of health economics as well as in public finance and management. She has served as a consultant to a number of state and federal agencies and to international organizations such as Pan American Health Organization, UNESCO, OECD and the International Institute of Educational Planning. She has served as a staff economist of the Office of Management and Budget and the Public Health Service and was Director of the Division of Financial Studies of the Social Security Administration.